Advances in Liposomal Therapeutics

Advances in Liposomal Therapeutics

Dr. S.P. Vyas

Ph.D. (Pharmaceutics)
Professor, Department of Pharmaceutical Sciences,
Dr. Harisingh Gour University,
Sagar - 470 003 (M.P.), India

Dr. V.K. Dixit

Ph.D. (Pharmacognosy)
Professor & Head, Department of Pharmaceutical Sciences,
Dr. Harisingh Gour University,
Sagar - 470 003 (M.P.), India

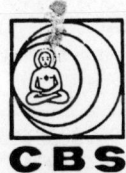

CBS

CBS Publishers & Distributors Pvt. Ltd.

New Delhi • Bengaluru • Chennai • Kochi • Kolkata • Mumbai
Hyderabad • Uttarakhand • Nagpur • Patna • Pune • Jharkhand

ISBN: 978-81-239-0713-0

First Edition: 2000
Reprint: 2012, 2018

Published by **Satish Kumar Jain** and produced by **Varun Jain** for

CBS Publishers & Distributors Pvt. Ltd.,
4819/XI Prahlad Street, 24 Ansari Road, Daryaganj, New Delhi - 110002
delhi@cbspd.com, cbspubs@airtelmail.in • www.cbspd.com
Ph.: 23289259, 23266861, 23266867 • Fax: 011-23243014

Corporate Office: 204 FIE, Industrial Area, Patparganj, Delhi - 110 092
Ph: 49344934 • Fax: 011-49344935
E-mail: publishing@cbspd.com • publicity@cbspd.com

Branches:
• *Bengaluru:* 2975, 17th Cross, K.R. Road, Bansankari 2nd Stage,
  Bengaluru - 70 • Ph: +91-80-26771678/79 • Fax: +91-80-26771680
  E-mail: cbsbng@gmail.com, bangalore@cbspd.com
• *Chennai:* No. 7, Subbaraya Street, Shenoy Nagar, Chennai - 600030
  Ph: +91-44-26681266, 26680620 • Fax: +91-44-42032115
  E-mail: chennai@cbspd.com
• *Kochi:* Ashana House, 39/1904, A.M. Thomas Road, Valanjambalam,
  Ernakulum, Kochi • Ph: +91-484-4059061-65
  Fax: +91-484-4059065 • E-mail: cochin@cbspd.com
• *Kolkata:* 6-B, Ground Floor, Rameshwar Shaw Road, Kolkata - 700014
  Ph: +91-33-22891126/7/8 • E-mail: kolkata@cbspd.com
• *Mumbai:* 83-C, Dr. E. Moses Road, Worli, Mumbai - 400018
  Ph: +91-9833017933, 022-24902340/41 • E-mail: mumbai@cbspd.com

Representatives:

• Hyderabad: 0-9885175004	• Nagpur: 0-9021734563
• Patna: 0-9334159340	• Pune: 0-9623451994
• Jharkhand: 0-9811541605	• Uttarakhand: 0-9716462459

Printed at:
J.S. Offset Printers, Delhi (India)

PREFACE

Liposomes and related developments and approaches have emerged as the most promising carrier stratagems for site specific optimized drug therapeutics. Targeted drug delivery which is a programmed kinetic behaviour, tissue distribution and pharmacodynamic activity of drug substances, seems to be an achievable goal with the advent of liposomes as a versatile, petite and bio-compatible drug carrier system. Furthermore, the products of biotechnological origin and bio-pharmaceuticals being complex, bio-susceptible potent molecules entail for bio-protected site specific delivery; which could be realized using liposomal system. At present not much is known about kinetic behaviour, tissue distribution and pharmacodynamic aspects of these complex bio-actives. Similarly, a little is known about site-specific behaviour of many bio-ligands. The need for site specific delivery of bio-actives and use of bio-ligands as sensing or homing modules for the purpose could be realized for optimized therapeutic effects.

Bangham bodies, the bio-molecular closed membrane system was initially developed as an artificial version to bio-membrane to study *in vitro* bio-membrane behavioural aspects. Nevertheless, later these closed systems were realized as effective and versatile drug carriers. These nano-constructs enticed G. Gregoriadis who appreciated their potential for site-specific and specialized drug and vaccine delivery. The ensuing era was obviously dominated by a great assortment of work on liposomes carried out at various levels in various laboratories in India and abroad. Many liposome-based therapeutics have already been approved by U.S. FDA and appeared in U.S. market. In order to discuss varied therapeutic aspects on which work is under progress and to take in account of general therapeutic perspective, *a National Symposium* on "Advances in Liposomal Research" was organized. This book records the proceedings of the same. It incorporates invited lectures, and research work presented during the symposium. Hope this effort shall interest many more to unravel the intriguing intricacies and future possibilities of targeted drug delivery using such versatile drug vectors and bio-cell mimics.

We are thankful to Dr. S.N. Sharma, Prof. Emeritus, New Delhi for delivering a key note and many distinguished scientists who participated in the symposium whose deliberations and works constitute the volume of this book. We are also indebted to U.G.C., New Delhi for financial support. The financial support from Panacea Biotec, New Delhi and their academic concern is gratefully acknowledged and appreciated. We remain thankful to our colleagues, on local advisory committees and to our publisher CBS, New Delhi.

We hope the book being very first of its own class would provide a useful review and perspective on liposomes and will stimulate research elements and collaborative ventures and investigations with a defined emphasis on optimized therapeutic benefits.

S.P. Vyas
V. K. Dixit

CONTENTS

LIPOSOMES : A HISTORICAL PERSPECTIVE AND PRESENT RELEVANCE

S.N. SHARMA
Professor Emeritus,
Block 5, H.No. 25 Eros Garden,
Surajkund Road, Harayana.

Drug therapeutics is now entering quite an exciting however, challenging era. The drug molecules, which are familiar to us, are relatively simple, and have been discovered by broad scale screening processes or conventional synthetic processes. These drugs generally demonstrate limited level of precision and specificity for pharmacodynamic activity and often accompanied by undesirable side effects. It is realized that drug should be precise, specific in action and they should be delivered to site that is in need of therapeutic effect. Obviously, these drug molecules by themselves are likely to be larger, more complex and more information rich structure than drugs we customarily deal with. Furthermore, for site specific target oriented delivery, they require a drug carrier system. The quest for the later generated continual scientific search and as a result of serendipity, liposomes were discovered and later introduced as a putative and effective drug carrier system.

It was early '60s, when A. D. Bangham and his colleagues made an observation that diffusion of univalent cations and anions out of spontaneously formed liquid crystals of lecithin is remarkably similar to the diffusion across the biological membrane. Bangham says that in Faraday's Society meetings, number of presentations were made on electromicrographic techniques to establish apparently ubiquitous bimolecular membrane to be bi-molecular leaflets. Later, it was the beginning of *ex vivo* preparations of credible membrane models as first suggested by Babraham based on black lipid membrane. Thus, Davson, Horne, Canni's Babraham, Bangham, Rodin, Wescott, and other were working on various aspects of artificial membane. In 1961, at Babraham, Bangham and his colleagues could observe these lipid mesophases following negative stains under electron microscope. They were used in expression of the integrity of bimolecular membrane of phospholipids that is dependent on the presence of water and it was found to be a structure vulnerable to the modification in such a way that water at large could be removed. Then, Horne who was the expert of negative staining of electron microscopy of that time could suggest that phospholipids in water form bag like uniform structure very closely resembled to what Bangham and colleagues envisioned. The subsequent study with incorporation of cholesterol, in phospholipids resulted into structural rearrangement that preciesely resemble biocell membrane in many regards. By that time it was well accepted that vigorous shearing of phospholipid in water, their solvation and associated entropic free energies altogether ensure spontaneous formation of unlimited closed membranes (smectic mesophases/Bangaham bodies). The ability of these mesophases (phospholipid based liquid crystals) was known latter to entrap solutes to which they were selectively permeable. These systems (mesophases) were presented as petite, putative and protean model for cell membrane and first time named as liposome (lipid-sphere) by Weissmann (1965) and thence forth heralded proliferation of studies on cell membrane biophysics, structure and functions. The versatility of the vesicular system was fully realized and expressed in a poetic way by Greogriadis as follows.

Little fatty vesicles of bilayer fame
Protean and elusive, fragile all the same,
aloof and enigmatic beneath your many skins,
unyielding to the vigour of the thousands of spins,
descended from the pastures of Babraham we are told,
you never ceased to wrinkle, expand and then fold
embracing sodium ions and such electrolytes.
Twinkling guide stars to throngs of acolytes
Desirous of your membranous semi-bilayers.
Precursors of bion, potential drug carriers.

The sequestration of aqueous phase what we more frequently refer to as entrapment/encapsulation, provided the basis to the liposomes drug-carrier concept which was realised, experimented, demonstrated and proposed in the early 70s, by Gregoriadis and Branda Ryman. They subsequently established that systems can be used with drugs, enzymes, anticancer chemotherapeutics, antimicrobial drugs, and as supplement adjuvants for potentiating the immune response. In the insuing years, the liposomes (lipid hollow spheres) were adopted by numerous researchers as the vehicle of choice for the drug as a class as well as for vaccine delivery and targeting. Need not to mention that confluence union of diverge applications has enriched the liposomal repertoire so much so that it has become a widely accepted scientific discipline in itself, with its applications covering biotechnology, biomedical, immunological, cosmetic, novel drug delivery systems and surrogative versions for various distinctive, well defined functionaries of the immune system. This is how it is pertinent to be realistic with the philosophy that an elusive voyage through daunting tides could eventually arrive at an optimistic ports as great leaps in liposome technology have culminated in the development of several liposomal formulations which are already knocking at for clinical applications while others are likely to be on the pharmacist's counter in the market.

It is behooved for the wisdom sake to know about liposomes. The phospholipids and other polar amphiphiles on confrontation with an excess water form closed concentric bilayers, which entrap water and dissolved solute in process. The formation of vesicular membrane involves aerodynamic, hydrodynamics and thermodynamic and the summing up effect provides them thermodynamically stable status and structure in turn.

Introduction of drug-containing carriers into the body is often accompanied by changes in their structure and function which may be brought about by elements in the biological milieu with which the carrier comes into contact or by carrier sequestration (uptake) by non-target tissues, or by other events (e.g., development of the immune responses against the carrier) which may be detrimental to effective carrier function. Such anatomical and physiological considerations have resulted over the years in systematic studies on carrier behaviour *in vivo* and, efforts have been made to design the construct with defined and specific biodisposition characteristics. Much of the relevant knowledge obtained so far concerns liposomes and other lipid-based vesicles.

Twenty five years of research into the use of liposomes in drug delivery have led to vastly improved technology in terms of drug capture, vesicle stability on storage, scaled-up production and the design of formulations for specialised tasks. In parallel, remarkable advances have been made in understanding and controlling liposomal behaviours *in vivo*. This has facilitated the application of a wide range of liposomal drugs in the treatment and prevention of diseases in experimental animals as well as clinically. Several liposomal preparations (one of them injectable) have already been licensed and a number of others are likely to follow soon. The future of liposomes in drug delivery systems appears to be elusive and secured. They will no doubt continue to contribute significantly to more efficient use of 'old' drugs providing them second life and will also find applications with agents now being produced by recombinant DNA technology.

The story of liposomes as drug-and vaccine-delivery systems hitherto appears to be a promising. It has come about as a result of the accumulated knowledge of their interaction with *in vivo* systems, which has allowed for the rational design of vesicle constructs, and through the sophisticated advances in liposome technology. Clearly this is only the beginning, and there are great challenges still to be met. The prolonged presence of liposomes in the circulatory system, which is essential for their applications involving targets other than the RES, has successfully been achieved, but only for small vesicles; this must be extended to include larger (micron size) vesicles if haemosomes are to have a future as a blood surrogate. Larger, long-circulating vesicles would also accommodate sufficient quantities of cytokines (for immunomodulation) and genetic material, (for gene therapy). Recent *in vivo* developments with liposome-mediated gene expression have demonstrated the potential use of the system in this respect. Liposomes have been appreciated and realised for their potential in immunomodulation applications, with the IRIV and oral vaccines, but there is still a lot to come before their use can become a clinical reality.

The symposium covered most of the application aspects of liposomes and intensive deliberations and content rich presentations offered opportunities to understand liposomes and related events from near. The proceedings include and integrate emerging biotrends with practical functional utility of liposomes as presented by different invited subject experts. Hope this volume will offer an effective venue of academic interactions for persons as diverse as basic pharmaceutical researchers, bioscientists and clinicians per se. I complement the authors for their academic concern and wish immense appreciation for their great efforts

TARGETING OF DRUGS TO LIPID BILAYER IN LIPOSOMES: AN APPROACH FOR THE SUCCESS OF LIPOSOMES AS DELIVERY SYSTEMS

SARANJIT SINGH* and MONICA GULATI[1]

National Institute of Pharmaceutical Education and Research (NIPER),
Sector 67, S.A.S. Nagar 160 062.
[1]University Institute of Pharmaceutical Sciences, Panjab University,
Chandigarh 160 014.

*Tel. +91 172 673848; Fax: +91 172 677185, e-mail: niper@chd.nic.in

INTRODUCTION

Liposomal formulations have proved to be very successful in improving the therapeutic efficacy of the drugs with very low therapeutic index where the difference between the effective and the toxic dose is very small. A number of successful liposomal formulations of such drugs have reached the market, e.g., AmBisome™ (amphotericin B), DaunoXome™ (daunorubicin citrate), and Doxil™ (doxorubicin). Lot many are presently under advanced stage of clinical trials [1].

Liposomal pharmaceuticals are, however, costly products. Doxil™ containing 20 mg doxorubicin costs about $ 485 & each single treatment for Kaposi's sarcoma costs around $ 1000, which is to be repeated every three weeks. The high cost of liposomal preparations is primarily due to the phospholipids that are high priced materials.

One good way of approaching the economic viability of liposomal formulations is to keep the drug:phospholipid ratio maximum in the favor of the drug. However, this is always not feasible as the extent of incorporation of a drug in the lipid vesicle strongly depends upon its solubility in aqueous mileau and/or the lipid bilayer. Based on whether the drug is hydrophilic, lipophilic, amphiphilic or biphasic insoluble, the degree of entrapment may range from nil to 100%. The partitioning characteristics, site of entrapment and examples of various categories of drugs are given in table 1.

Problems like poor entrapment efficiency and physical as well as chemical instability have been found to be associated with the liposomal entrapment of drug molecules, other than those that are highly lipophilic. Lipophilic drugs show very high degree of entrapment, which sometimes nears 100%. Over the last three decades, a large number of drugs that are not lipophilic by themselves have been structurally altered to render them to be more. Apart from using the appropriate hydrophobic anchors, approaches like complex-formation and pharmacosomes have also been utilised. The preparations of lipophilic drug derivatives are at different stages of development with several of them having already reached the stage of clinical trials. The topic has been recently reviewed [10].

Table 1. Types of drugs with the site of their incorporation and entrapment characteristics

Type of drug	Log P_{oct}	Site of entrapment	Entrapment characteristics	Drug Examples	Ref.
Lipophilic	>5	Lipid bilayer	High entrapment Low leakage Chemical stability	Cyclosporine	2, 3
Hydrophilic	<-0.3	Water mileu	Low entrapment Bilayer composition dependent leakage Hydrolytic degradation	CDP Choline	4
Amphiphilic	1.7<log P<4	Both aqueous and lipid phases	High Entrapment Rapid leakage	Mitomycin C Actinomycin D Vinblastin	5, 6
Biphasic Insoluble	–		Very poor entrapment	6-Mercaptopurine Azathioprine Allopurinol	7-9

DRUGS TRANSFORMED

The lists of drugs, category-wise, those have been transformed into lipophilic prodrugs are given in table 2.

Table 2. Examples of drugs for which lipophilic prodrugs and derivatives have been prepared

Anticancer Agents	Antiviral drugs	Steroids	Miscellaneous
Cisplatin Methotrexate Muramyl dipeptide 1-β-D-arabinofuranosyl cytosine 5-Fluorouracil Anthracyclin antibiotics Doxorubicin, Daunorubicn, Hydroxyrubicin Mitomycin C Boron Neutron-Capture Therapy Purine antimetabolites L-Asparginase	Phosphonoacids Nucleoside analogs, AZT, ddT, ddC, ddG Acyclovir	Cortisol Cortisone Dexamethasone Triamcinolone acetonide	Metronidazole Felbinac PABA Insulin

The drugs where complexes have been formed or the pharmacosome concept has been utilised for incorporation of drugs into the lipid phase of liposomes are listed in table 3.

Table 3. Dugs for which lipophilic prodrugs and derivatives have been prepared

Charge transfer complexes	Pharmacosomes
MRI Agents, Gd, Mn, and Fe	Pindolol
	AZT
^{51}Cr	Fenoprofen
Methantheline Br- Trichloroactetate	
Warfarin – Na (Ion pairs)	
Isopropamide iodide-	
Taurodeoxycholate (Ion-pairs)	

Table 4 gives a representative list of hydrophobic anchors attached to various drugs.

Table 4. Examples of the hydrophobic anchors attached to various drugs

Group attached	Structure	Examples
Hydrophobic attachments without spacers		
Alkyl-	(D)-R $R = -(CH_2)_nCH_3$,	N^4-hexadecyl-Ara-C Octadecydithiopurine
N- and O-acyl	(D-NH)-COR (N-acyl) (D-O)-COR (O-acyl) $R = -(CH_2)_nCH_3$; (alkyl) $= -CH_2)_7CH=CH(CH_2)_7CH_3$ (oleoyl)	N^4-oleoyl-Ara-C Acyclovir laurate Cortisol palmitate Cortisone hexadecanoate, etc.
Alkyloxycarbonyl	(D)-COOR $R = -(CH_2)_nCH_3$	Nonyloxycarbonyl-MMC
Cholesteryloxycarbonyl	$R = - C_{27}H_{45}$ (cholesteryl)	Cholesteryloxycarbonyl-MMC
Acyloxycarbamoyl	(D)-CONHR $R = -(CH_2)_nCH_3$	Octadecylcarbamoyl-5-FU
Phosphatidyl	(D)-R R = N = 12(myristoyl); 14(palmitoyl)	Dimyristoylphosphatidyl-ddT (Phosphatidyl-ddT) Dipalmitoylphosphatidylfluorouridine Dipalmitoylphosphatidyl-ddG
Hydrophobic attachments with spacers		
Phosphatidyl-Ethanolamine	(D)-R R =	MTX-α-dimyristoyl-phosphatidylethanolamine
Cholesteroyloxy-carbonylglycyl	(D)-R $R = COCH_2NHCOOC_{27}H_{45}$	N^4-(N-cholesteroyl-oxycarbonylglycyl-AraC N-Cholesteroyl-oxycarbonylglycyl-MMC

(D) = Drug   R = Substituent

molecules, other than those that are highly lipophilic. Lipophilic drugs show very high degree of entrapment, which sometimes nears 100%. Over the last three decades, a large number of drugs that are not lipophilic by themselves have been structurally altered to render them to be more. Apart from using the appropriate hydrophobic anchors, approaches like complex-formation and pharmacosomes have also been utilised. The preparations of lipophilic drug derivatives are at different stages of development with several of them having already reached the stage of clinical trials. The topic has been recently reviewed [10].

Table 1. Types of drugs with the site of their incorporation and entrapment characteristics

Type of drug	Log P_{oct}	Site of entrapment	Entrapment characteristics	Drug Examples	Ref.
Lipophilic	>5	Lipid bilayer	High entrapment Low leakage Chemical stability	Cyclosporine	2, 3
Hydrophilic	<-0.3	Water mileu	Low entrapment Bilayer composition dependent leakage Hydrolytic degradation	CDP Choline	4
Amphiphilic	1.7<log P<4	Both aqueous and lipid phases	High Entrapment Rapid leakage	Mitomycin C Actinomycin D Vinblastin	5, 6
Biphasic Insoluble	–		Very poor entrapment	6-Mercaptopurine Azathioprine Allopurinol	7-9

DRUGS TRANSFORMED

The lists of drugs, category-wise, those have been transformed into lipophilic prodrugs are given in table 2.

Table 2. Examples of drugs for which lipophilic prodrugs and derivatives have been prepared

Anticancer Agents	Antiviral drugs	Steroids	Miscellaneous
Cisplatin Methotrexate Muramyl dipeptide 1-β-D-arabinofuranosyl cytosine 5-Fluorouracil Anthracyclin antibiotics Doxorubicin, Daunorubicn, Hydroxyrubicin Mitomycin C Boron Neutron-Capture Therapy Purine antimetabolites L-Asparginase	Phosphonoacids Nucleoside analogs, AZT, ddT, ddC, ddG Acyclovir	Cortisol Cortisone Dexamethasone Triamcinolone acetonide	Metronidazole Felbinac PABA Insulin

The drugs where complexes have been formed or the pharmacosome concept has been utilised for incorporation of drugs into the lipid phase of liposomes are listed in table 3.

Table 3. Dugs for which lipophilic prodrugs and derivatives have been prepared

Charge transfer complexes	Pharmacosomes
MRI Agents, Gd, Mn, and Fe	Pindolol
	AZT
^{51}Cr	Fenoprofen
Methantheline Br- Trichloroactetate	
Warfarin – Na (Ion pairs)	
Isopropamide iodide-	
Taurodeoxycholate (Ion-pairs)	

Table 4 gives a representative list of hydrophobic anchors attached to various drugs.

Table 4. Examples of the hydrophobic anchors attached to various drugs

Group attached	Structure	Examples
Hydrophobic attachments without spacers		
Alkyl-	(D)-R	N^4-hexadecyl-Ara-C
	R = -(CH$_2$)$_n$CH$_3$,	Octadecydithiopurine
N- and O-acyl	(D-NH)-COR (N-acyl)	N^4-oleoyl-Ara-C
	(D-O)-COR (O-acyl)	Acyclovir laurate
	R = -(CH$_2$)$_n$CH$_3$; (alkyl)	Cortisol palmitate
	= -CH$_2$)$_7$CH=CH(CH$_2$)$_7$CH$_3$ (oleoyl)	Cortisone hexadecanoate, etc.
Alkyloxycarbonyl	(D)-COOR	Nonyloxycarbonyl-MMC
	R = -(CH$_2$)$_n$CH$_3$	
Cholesteryloxycarbonyl	R = - C$_{27}$H$_{45}$ (cholesteryl)	Cholesteryloxycarbonyl-MMC
Acyloxycarbamoyl	(D)-CONHR	Octadecylcarbamoyl-5-FU
	R = -(CH$_2$)$_n$CH$_3$	
Phosphatidyl	(D)-R	Dimyristoylphosphatidyl-ddT
	R = $\begin{array}{l} H_2C\text{-}O\text{-}\overset{O}{\overset{\|}{C}}\text{-}(CH_2)nCH_3 \\ HC\text{-}O\text{-}\overset{O}{\overset{\|}{C}}\text{-}(CH_2)nCH_3 \\ -\overset{O}{\overset{\|}{P}}\text{-}O\text{-}CH_2 \\ \quad\underset{OH}{} \end{array}$	(Phosphatidyl-ddT)
		Dipalmitoylphosphatidylfluorouri dine
		Dipalmitoylphosphatidyl-ddG
	N = 12(myristoyl); 14(palmitoyl)	
Hydrophobic attachments with spacers		
Phosphatidyl- Ethanolamine	(D)-R R = $\begin{array}{l} H_2C\text{-}O\text{-}\overset{O}{\overset{\|}{C}}\text{-}(CH_2)_{12}CH_3 \\ HC\text{-}O\text{-}C\text{-}(CH_2)_{12}CH_3 \\ -NH\text{-}CH_2CH_2O\text{-}\overset{O}{\overset{\|}{P}}\text{-}O\text{-}CH_2 \\ \quad\underset{OH}{} \end{array}$	MTX-α-dimyristoyl- phosphatidylethanolamine
Cholesteroyloxy- carbonylglycyl	(D)-R R = COCH$_2$NHCOOC$_{27}$H$_{45}$	N^4-(N-cholesteroyl- oxycarbonylglycyl-AraC N-Cholesteroyl- oxycarbonylglycyl-MMC

(D) = Drug   R = Substituent

THE SPECTRUM OF ADVANTAGES

A critical study of the literature reports on the use of lipophilic drug derivatives reveals that targeting of drugs to lipid bilayer offers several advantages, apart from simple enhancement of drug incorporation and reduction in leakage of drugs from liposomes. Table 5 gives a summary of the advantages.

Table 5. Advantages of lipophilic drugs/ derivatives

Improvement in Formulation Development and Processing	Modulation of Biological Response of the Drug

Enhancement of drug incorporation
Improvement of Stability
    Decreased leakage of entrapped drug
    Increase in stability of drugs against hydrolytic decomposition
Ease of Processing
    Removal of nonencapsulated drug
    Commercial Processing
    Sterilization
	Effect on Rate of Release
	Altered Biodistribution and Increase in Therapeutic Index
	Overcoming of Cross-Resistance

Improvement in formulation development and processing

For the development of commercially viable liposomal formulation for drugs, the major problems that have been identified include poor physical and chemical stability, drug leakage, difficulty in sterilization, etc. Fortunately, most of these problems are overcome by the use of the lipophilic derivatives.

Enhancement of drug incorporation

As discussed earlier, the way to reduce the cost of liposomal formulations is to increase the encapsulation efficiency of drugs to almost 100%. It reduces the amount of costly phospholipids, the basic raw materials required for preparation of liposomes. The lipophilic drugs carry an advantage in this regard as they are completely entrapped, being taken in the liposomal bilayer upto their "solubility". Accordingly, there is little chance of their being lost in the continuous aqueous phase. In comparison, water-soluble drugs show maximum encapsulation efficiency of about 70% which represents their theoretical maximum. This upper limit has been observed even at lipid concentrations as high as 600 mmol/ml. The reason is that at such lipid concentrations, the encapsulation of the aqueous volume is only about 70%, while the remaining 30% represents the unentrapped volume left in the void space due to the curvature of liposomes [11]. In literature some studies have been done in which direct comparison of relative encapsulation was made between hydrophilic and hydrophobic drugs. Stuhne-Sekalec and coworkers [12] investigated co-encapsulation of hydrophilic insulin and hydrophobic cyclosporin. It was observed that 2.3 nmol/mmol of insulin and 29.7 nmol/mmol of cyclosporin were entrapped in liposomes. It is thus a good example to show that lipophilic substances are preferentially uptaken by liposomes as compared to the hydrophilic compounds.

The extent of encapsulation of hydrophilic and amphiphilic drugs that either show rapid leakage and poor encapsulation can be improved by making them lipophilic through addition of hydrophobic side chains. A number of successful drug examples are there and a few of them are listed in table 6.

Table 6. Typical examples showing liposomal encapsulation achieved from drugs and their corresponding lipophilic derivatives

Drug	Encapsulation of drug, %	Maximum encapsulation from lipophilic drug derivative, %	Ref.
Asparaginase	12-50	72-100	13,14
Arabinosylcytosine	<0.1	99.8	15
5-Fluorouracil	0.03	99.96	16
Mitomycin	0.1	99.9	17
Triamcinolone acetonide	5	85	18

This approach seems to be applicable even in improving the encapsulation of biphasic insoluble drugs, like 6-mercaptopurine (6-MP). The water solubility of this drug is only 0.124 mg/mL and it is also poorly soluble in nonpolar solvents (log P=0.72±0.01) [19]. The liposomal entrapment of the drug is limited between 0.10 and 0.45% [7]. A dramatic improvement in the encapsulation efficiency was observed when 6-(octadecyldithio) purine (Fig.1), a lipophilic prodrug, was subjected to liposomal entrapment. This novel prodrug is reported to be taken up quantitatively by the liposomes [20].

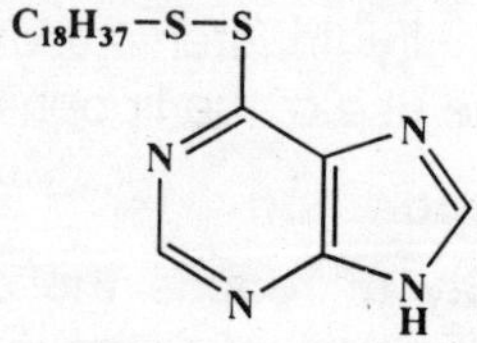

$$C_{18}H_{37}-S-S$$

Fig. 1 : 6-(Octadecylthio)purine (6-ODP)

Improvement of stability

To be of any clinical utility, the liposomal preparations must be stable for a period of 1.5-2 years. Several different stability problems are encountered with liposomes that include leakage of entrapped drug, change in liposome structure and the chemical instability of phospholipids as well as the entrapped drug. The stability problems are found to be more pronounced in liposomes containing low molecular weight and water-soluble drugs. On storage, hydrophilic drugs show marked loss from the liposomes, e.g., in case of 5-fluorouracil (5-FU), 15-35% of the encapsulated drug leached out within 6-7 h of storage [21]. In comparison to hydrophilic drugs, lipophilic drugs retain in the liposomes for longer periods. For example, the leakage of tacrolimus, a highly lipophilic drug, was negligible over a period of 40 h [22].

There are several instances in literature where polar drugs have been converted to their lipophilic derivatives to prevent drug leakage from liposomes. Some of the examples are listed in table 7.

Another example is that of cytosine arabinoside which is lost from liposomes to an extent between 40-70% within 24 h depending upon the concentration of cholesterol in the bilayer [2]. However, its lipophilic derivatives show no leakage from liposomes containing comparable amounts of cholesterol till a period of 30 days [15].

Table 7. Typical examples showing comparison of percent drug retained in liposomes containing drugs and their prodrugs

Drug	Prodrug	Time	% drug retained		Ref.
			Drug	Prodrug	
Cortisol	Cortisol palmitate	3 d	12	71	23
5-Fluorouracil	Octadecylcarbamoyl-5-fluorouracil	0.5 h	3	99.9	16, 21
Mitomycin C	Nonyloxycarbonyl mitomycin C	1h	12.8	99.9	5

Perez-Soler and Khokhar [24] have described the effect of lipophilicity of a prodrug on its in-vitro leakage from liposomal preparations. The drug leakage from liposomes containing cis-bis-neodecanoato-trans-R,R-1,2-diaminocyclohexane platinum compounds (Fig. 2), the lipophilic prodrugs of cisplatin, was found to be inversely related to the size of the leaving groups. The compounds with 5, 6, 7, 9 and 10 C-atoms showed drug leakage in a decreasing order of 25.9, 9.7, 11.9, 6.0 and 5.0%, respectively, in 6h.

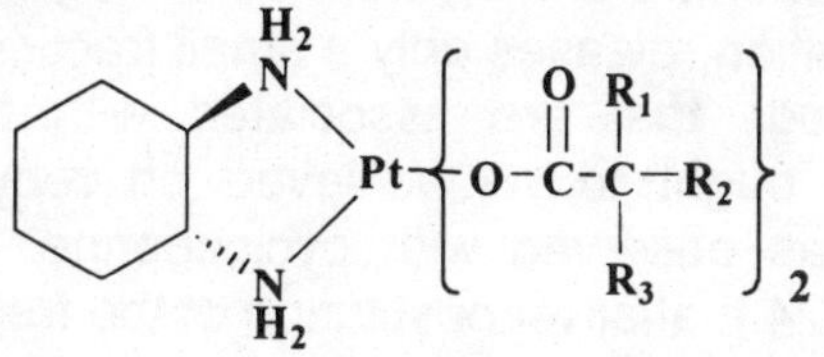

Fig. 2 : Structure of cis-bis-neodecanoato-trans-R,R-1,2-diaminocyclohexane platinum (NDDP) compounds. R_1, R_2, R_3 can be a group of 2-6 carbon atoms to yield a radical with $C_{10}H_{19}O_2$ as an emperical formula

The use of lipophilic drugs or derivatives has also been found fruitful in terms of reduced hydrolytic decomposition. While a water-soluble drug present in the aqueous compartment of liposomes is prone to hydrolytic attack, the lipophillic drugs/derivatives are located in the phospholipid bilayers and thereby show resistance to hydrolysis. Examples include cortisone [25], doxorubicin [26], and cisplatin [27]. An interesting case is that of campothecin, an antitumor drug. The drug is hydrophobic in nature and shows high binding affinity (97%) in liposomes. However, it contains a lactone ring that rapidly hydrolyzes to an inactive carboxylate form. This lactone functionality luckily partitions into the bilayer [28], by virtue of which no ring opening was observed till 72 h in liposomes composed of DMPC, a phospholipid with low transition temperature (Tc~24°C), that is in its unstable liquid crystal phase at 37°C. This was a significant improvement comparing the half-life of free campothecin which is just 16.6 min [29].

Ease of processing

The removal of non-encapsulated drug forms an essential step during the processing of liposomes. The entire purpose of liposomal incorporation of the drug is defeated if the unentrapped drug is present in the final product. When the drug itself is expensive, the recovery of unencapsulated drug becomes essential from the economics point of view. Furthermore, procedures such as dialysis and passage through exclusion columns that are employed for the removal of non-entrapped material are often time-consuming, tedious and expensive. Complete loading of the drugs in liposomes eliminates this step. In this respect the use of lipophilic drugs or derivatives is particularly beneficial as they are quantitatively incorporated into the liposomes.

The lipophilic drugs or lipophilic drug derivatives are also useful from the aspect of commercial processing of liposomal preparations. The first marketed liposomal preparation meant for parenteral use, i.e., AmBisome (amphotericin B), is marketed in the freeze-dried form [30]. In general, lyophilization assumes importance in development of liposomal formulations, as it is an excellent method to overcome most of the stability problems associated with liposomes, like chemical instability (of phospholipids as well as drugs), leaching, fusion, aggregation, etc. Freeze drying, however, can itself cause damage to the liposomes in different ways: crystallization of the internal water, formation of amorphous material, influence of osmotic forces and dehydration of the lipid bilayers. Hence it itself is not free from problems. The process can result in defects in the integrity of the bilayer causing leakage of the material present in the internal aqueous compartment of liposomes. As the association between liposomes and hydrophobic drug is more stable, the osmotic shock or brief ultrasonication releases only a small fraction of the encapsulated drug. Thus with lipophilic drugs that are associated with the lipid bilayer, excellent entrapment efficiencies ought to be achieved on rehydration of the lyophilized powder. This in fact was observed with cyclosporine, where 95% encapsulation efficiency was recorded 24 h after reconstitution of the freeze-dried powder [4].

Other than freeze drying, the formation of proliposomes is another approach to formulate liposomes in a dry powder form. The phospholipids as solid mixture with an inert water-soluble carrier like lactose and sodium chloride form proliposomes on rehydration immediately prior to use. With water-soluble drugs, one can expect usual problems like low entrapment and difficulty in the removal of non-encapsulated drug. The approach ideally suits hydrophobic drugs where the majority of the drug partitions into the lipid membrane and high encapsulation efficiencies can be achieved on hydration. Many lipophilic drugs have been successfully formulated into their proliposomal powders, e.g., amphotericin B [31] and ibuprofen [32]. The method has also been used to prepare liposomal delivery system of muramyl tripeptide phosphatidylethanolamine (MTP-PE), a lipophilic prodrug of muramyl dipeptide (MDP) (Fig. 3). The formulation has been put to clinical trials [33]. The details on the development of L-MTP-PE are discussed later in the chapter.

Sterilization

Streilization is must for liposomal preparations meant for parenteral administration. Almost all methods of sterilisation have been tried for liposomes but with varying success. This key issue in development of liposomal technology is not settled and is still live.

Gamma ray treatment has been found to disrupt the liposome membrane [34]. The sterilization of freeze dried liposomes by exposure to ethylene oxide has been carried out [35] but concern has been expressed on the toxicity likely to be caused by the residues of the incompletely removed sterilizing gas and/or contamination caused by it [11]. The sterilization by filtration although useful for SUVs of size <0.22 mm in diameter, however, cannot be used for larger liposomes [11].

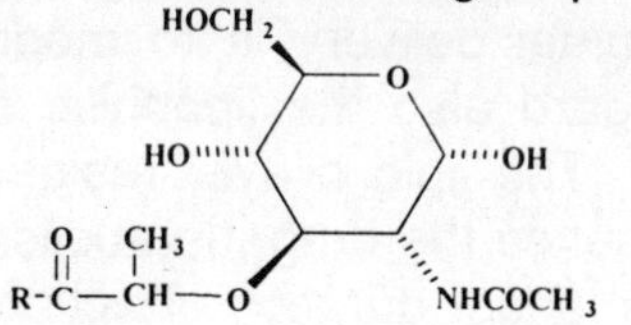

Compound	R
N-acetylmuramyl-L-alanyl-D-isoglutamine (N-acetylmuramyl dipeptide, MDP)	L-Ala-D-isoGln
N-acetylmuramyl-L-alanyl-D-isoglutaminyl-L-alanine (Muramyl tripeptide, MTP)	L-Ala-D-isoGln-L-Ala
N-acetylmuramyl-L-alanyl-D-isoglutaminyl- L-alanyl-phosphatidylethanolamine (MTP-phosphatidylethanolamine, MTP-PE)	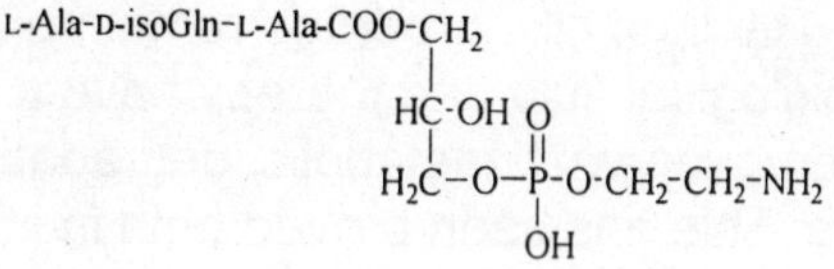

Fig. 3 : Structures of MDP, MTP and MTP-PE

Heat sterilization has been used as a convenient alternative for certain types of MLVs and extruded liposomes without much damage to their integrity [36]. However, the major issue in sterilisation of liposomes by autoclaving is the drug leakage. Zuidam et al. [37] investigated the extent of leakage of various types of drugs on heat treatment and observed a pronounced outflow of a water-soluble compound, calcein. The same behaviour was seen with doxorubicin, an amphipathic compound. The lipophilic bilayer associated prodrug of the latter, N-trifluoroacetyl doxorubicin-14-valerate (AD-32), however, was retained in the liposomes after autoclaving and the liposomes were stable with no aggregation. The values are given in table 8. Similarly, in another study, lipophilic perfluoroalkylated bipyridine platinum and palladium complexes in egg phospholipid liposomes showed complete retention after autoclaving [27].

Table 8. The % leakage and % degradation on sterilisation of various drugs

Lipid composition	pH	Drug	% Leakage	% Degradation
DPPC/DPPG/CHOL 10/1/4	4.0	Doxorubicin	20 ± 5	26 ± 8
EPC/EPG 10/1	4.0	AD-32	--	39 ± 4
DPPC/DPPG/CHOL 10/1/4	7.4	Calcein	44 ± 4	--
DPPC/DPPG/CHOL 10/1/4	7.4	a-Tocopherol	--	--

Although it is yet to be extensively investigated and further confirmed, it seems from the studies of Zuidam et al. [37] and Garelli and Vierling [27], that hydrophobic drugs or the lipophilic drug derivatives carry an advantage over water-soluble or amphiphilc compounds even with respect to sterilization of liposomal preparations.

Modulation of biological response of the drug

One of the goals of liposomal delivery is to modulate the response of drugs in biological mileu. In this regard also the lipophilic drugs or derivatives have been found to be advantageous. The lipid bilayer resident drug is slowly released from liposomes and as a conseuence the drug metabolism to inactive metabolites is also slowed down, resulting in a longer duration of action. The biodistribution of the drug is altered and generally the activity is enhanced resulting in better therapeutic index. Even the toxic effects normally associated with the therapeutic doses of the drug are reduced or even removed in some cases. Reports also exist which show that the use of liposomal formulations containing lipophilic drug derivatives has succeeded in overcoming the cross-resistance, particularly of antitumor drugs.

Rate of release

The release of hydrophilic materials from disrupted liposomes is immediate, while it is delayed for the lipophilic material because of its association with the lipid bilayers [38]. The lipophilic prodrugs remain entrapped when liposomes come in contact with the biological fluid and thereby have a potentially longer life in-vivo. The protection of the drug against metabolic degradation results in longer lasting therapeutic drug levels. This has been proved both in in-vitro and in-vivo studies.

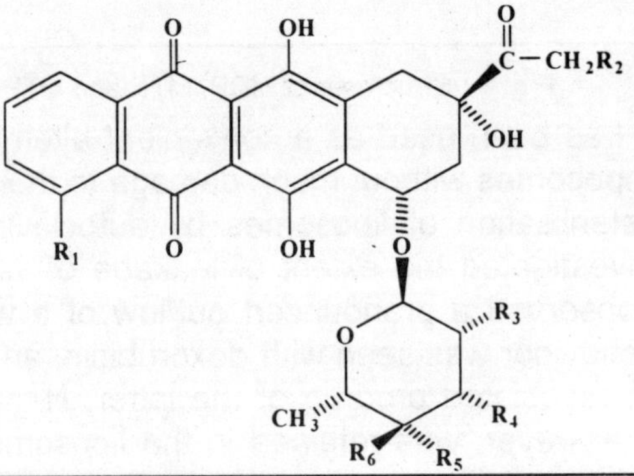

Compound	R_1	R_2	R_3	R_4	R_5	R_6
Doxorubicin	Ome	OH	H	NH_2	OH	H
Annamycin	H	OH	I	OH	H	OH
Daunorubicin	Ome	H	H	NH_2	OH	H
N-palmitoyl daunorubicin	Ome	H	H	$NHCO(CH_2)_{14}CH_3$	OH	H

Fig. 4 : Structures of doxorubicin, annamycin, duanorubicin and its lipophilic derivative

Bard et al. [39] showed that there was no leakage of *N*-palmitoyl daunorubicin (Fig.4) from liposomes in 10% new-born calf serum for as long as 5 days. In comparison a more than 10% of the unconverted drug was leaked out from liposomes within 2 h in buffer medium. Similarly, the stability of cortisone hexadecanoate (Fig. 5) from liposomes in the aspirated cell-free human rheumatoid synovial fluid is reported to be very high [25]. It is hypothesised that even after the liposome integrity is lost in the biological medium, the drug remains adhered to the liposomal fragments, thus resulting in prolonged stability.

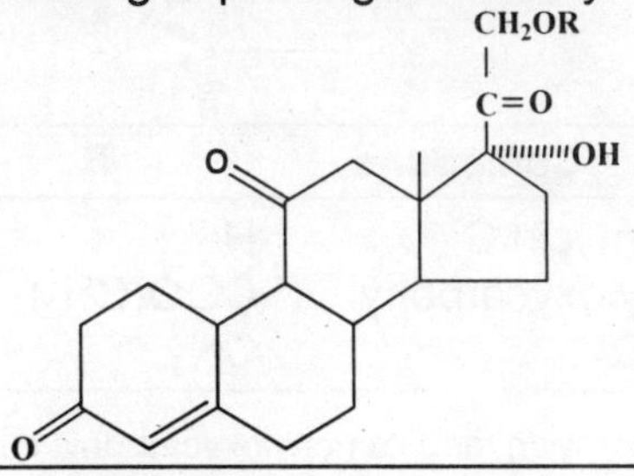

CH_2OR

$C=O$

OH

Compound	R
Cortisone	H
Cortisone	$CO(CH_2)_{15}$
hexadecanoate	CH_3

Fig. 5 : Structure of cortisone hexadecanoate

The liposomal formulation of octadecylcarbamoyl-5-FU (C18FU) (Fig. 6), a lipophilic prodrug of 5-FU, on i/m injection was retained at the injection site and in the regional lymph nodes for a considerably longer periods of time as compared to similar formulation of 5-FU [16]. In a parallel in-vivo study, on intramuscular injection of liposomal formulation into the thigh muscle of rats, nonyloxycarbonyl derivative of mitomycin-C (MMC) (Fig. 7) was retained much longer at the site of injection and more than70% of the dose remained as the prodrug in muscle even 120 min post injection. In comparison, the plain drug was rapidly absorbed from the injection site and little drug was found after 30 min [40]. The lymphotropic retention of the liposomal formulation of the lipophilic prodrug was also found to be much more as compared to that of the original water-soluble drug.

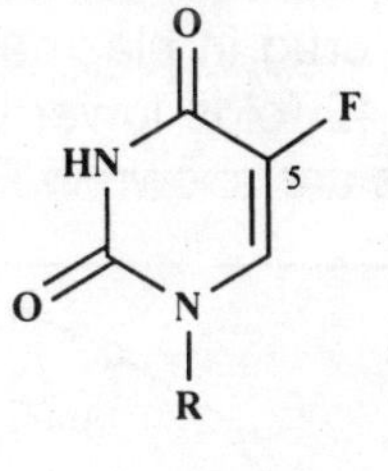

O

F

HN

5

O

N

R

Compound	R
5-Fluorouracil (5-FU)	H
Octadecylcarbamoyl-5-FU (C18FU)	$CONH(CH2)_{17}CH_3$
Cholesteryl-5-(5-FU-carbamoyl)capronate (ChFU)	$CONH(CH_2)_5COO\text{-}C_{27}H_{45}$

Fig. 6 : Structures of FU and the lipophilic deivatives C18FU and ChFU

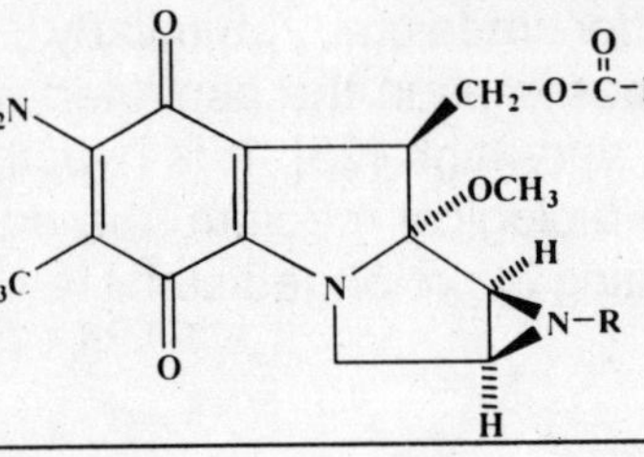

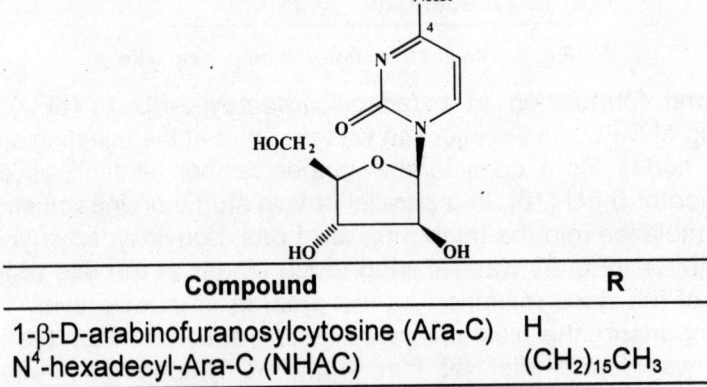

Compound	R
Mitomycin C	H
Nonyloxycarbonyl-	COO(CH$_2$)$_8$
MMC	CH$_3$

Fig. 7 : Mitomycin and its nonyloxycarbonyl derivative

The increase in stability to metabolic conversion of drug is reported for N^4-Hexadecyl-1-β-D-arabinofuranosyl cytosine (NHAC) (Fig. 8), a prodrug of 1-β-D-arabinofuranosyl cytosine (Ara-C).

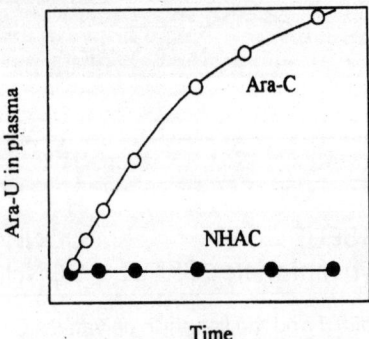

Compound	R
1-β-D-arabinofuranosylcytosine (Ara-C)	H
N^4-hexadecyl-Ara-C (NHAC)	(CH$_2$)$_{15}$CH$_3$

Fig. 8 : Structures of Ara-C and NHAC

On delivery of NHAC as liposomal formulation, there was almost complete resistance to deamination of the drug in plasma. The formation of Ara-U, the major metabolite of Ara-C, was about 42 folds lower with NHAC as compared to the free drug [41]. Representative profiles are shown in Fig. 9.

Fig. 9 : Profiles showing formation of Ara-U from Ara-C and NHAC

Altered biodistribution and increase in therapeutic index

The altered biodistribution on encapsulation of drugs in liposomes as lipophilic derivatives perhaps is also the key factor responsible for increase in the efficacy and a decrease in the toxic effect of drugs. For example, liposomal NDDP is more active than cisplatin in murine models of experimental liver metastasis and melanoma [42]. It is also associated with markedly less in-vitro toxicity as compared to cisplatin. While the most prominent side effect of cisplatin is severe renal dysfunction, L-NDDP is devoid of any nephrotoxicity, the dose limiting side effect being myelosuppression alone.

The phospholipid conjugates of methotrexate (MTX, Fig. 10) in their liposomal formulation (MTX-LIPO) strongly inhibit the release of both IL-1-beta and TNF in human blood monocytes, whereas free MTX or empty liposomes fail to show any such effect [43].

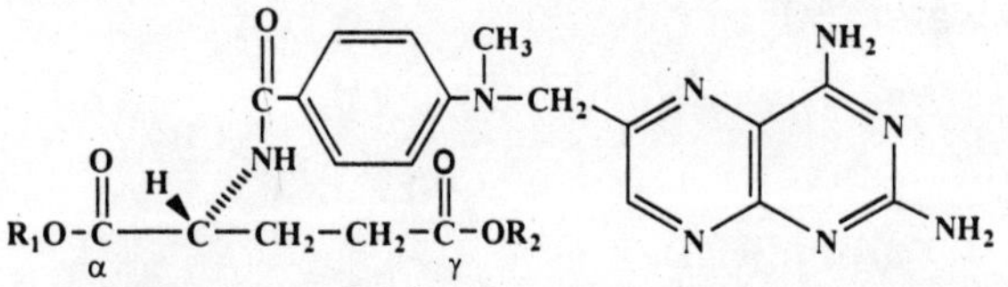

Compound	R_1	R_2
Methotrexate (MTX)	OH	OH
MTX--dimyristoylphosphatidyl-ethanolamine (MTX-α-DMPE)	DMPE*	OH
MTX-γ-DMPE	OH	DMPE
MTX-α,γ-diDMPE	DMPE	DMPE

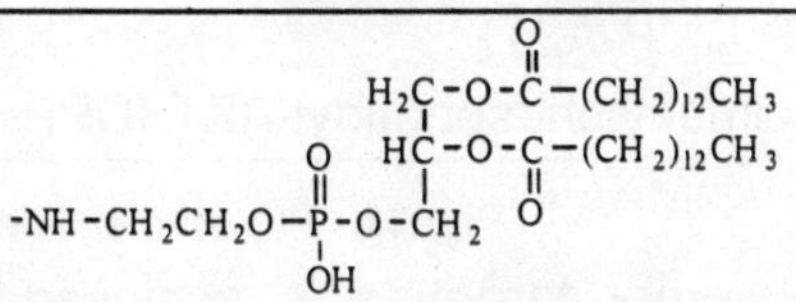

Fig. 10 : Structure of methotrexate and some of its lipophilic derivatives

During the studies, difference was also observed in the course of action. The free drug showed anti-inflammatory activity if treatment was started on the day of arthritis induction, however, it was ineffective in established arthritis. MTX-LIPO, on the other hand, was ineffective if dosing was started on day 0 but exerted a significant effect in established arthritis. The incorporation of lipophilic derivatives of MTX in liposomes results in reduction in hemotoxic effect [44].

When doxorubicin (Fig. 4), a water soluble compound, is delivered dissolved in aqueous mileau of liposomes, its plasma clearance and heart drug levels are reduced while distribution into RES is enhanced [45]. On encapsulation in stealth liposomes composed of phospholipids with high transition temperatures, the magnitude of changes in biodistribution and tumor targeting of doxorubicin is increased [46]. The stealth liposomes containing annamycin (Fig. 4), the lipophilic derivative of doxorubicin, however, fails to exhibit any tumor targeting advantage as compared to the regular liposomes [47]. The stealth bilayer is relatively impermeable to water soluble doxorubicin leading to longer retention and higher tumor selectivity of the drug. In case of annamycin, due to its high affinity for lipid membranes, the tendency of the drug to partition into plasma constituents, blood cells and endothelial cells, etc., is not effected and, therefore, its pharmacokinetics is not altered much. The plasma distribution of annamycin is influenced when the plasma HDL lipid compositions and HDL structure are altered [48].

Phospholipid analogs of AZT (Fig. 11), an antiviral drug, on incorporation in liposomes exhibit an altered biodistribution showing increased drug levels in liver, spleen and lymph nodes as compared to the free drug [49]. These organs being important sites of viral replication, the liposomal formulations containing lipophilic analogs showed an increase in the antiviral effect. In a comparative study, a single intraperitoneal injection of liposomal formulation was sufficient to prevent increased spleen weight and reverse transcriptase levels in serum, comparable to that of AZT given continuously in water [50].

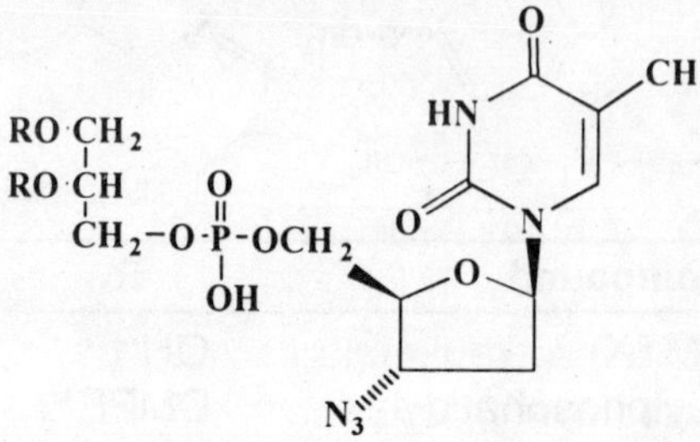

Compound	R
Dimyristoylphosphatidyl-AZT (Phosphatidyl-AZT, DMP-AZT)	$CO(CH_2)_{12}CH_3$
Dipalmitoylphosphatidyl-AZT (DPP-AZT)	$CO(CH_2)_{14}CH_3$

Fig. 11 : Phospholipid derivatives of AZT

Successful tumor targeting is achieved on incorporation of boron salts into liposomes [51]. However, the salts show very low entrapment efficiency. As a solution to the problem, Feakes et al. [52] synthesized lipophilic boron compounds and liposomes containing both water soluble salts and the lipophilic derivatives. The combined formulation was successful in delivering the highest tumor boron concentrations.

The liposomal incorporation of palimitoyl-L-asparaginase results in a marked increase in the circulation time (MRT, 32.1h) as compared to the free prodrug (MRT, 4.1h) or the unmodified drug (MRT, 2.9h) [14]. The pharmacosomes of pindolol, prepared from the lipophilic diglyceride derivative of the drug (Fig. 12), enhances the plasma concentrations of the drug 3-5 folds higher as compared to its free form [53]. The administration of pharmacosomes further results in a lower renal clearance.

Overcoming of cross-resistance

One of the remarkable advantages of delivering lipophilic prodrugs in liposomes is with respect toovercoming of resistance to the original drug. This has been observed in several cases, e.g. Cisplatin, MTX, Ara-C, etc. The liposomal delivery system containing NDDP (Fig. 2) displayed in-vitro a significant antitumor effect on human colon carcinoma LoVo cells resistant to cisplatin [54]. A similar effect was also seen in-vivo against L1210/PDD leukemia resistant to cisplatin [55].

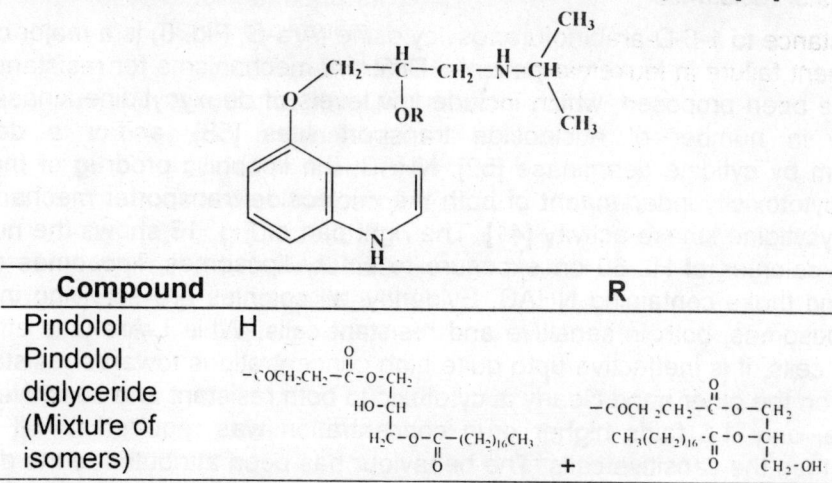

Compound	R
Pindolol	H
Pindolol diglyceride (Mixture of isomers)	

Fig. 12 : Pindolol and its diglycerides

Liposomes containing MTX in their aqueous compartments partially inhibit the growth of MTX resistant human leukemia cells (CEM/MTX), but only if the cells are exposed to fresh liposomes every day. The liposomes containing MTX-γ-DMPE (Fig. 10) instead completely by-pass the resistance [56]. The behaviour is depicted in left part of Figure 13. It is shown that to show equal cytotoxic effect, the resistant CEM/MTX cells require exposure of 2.5 μM drug than 0.025 μM needed for noresistant CEM/0. In case of MTX-γ-DMPE, the liposomal formulation yields a similar profile at a dose of 0.3 μM both for CEM/0 and the resistant CEM/MTX cells. The mechanism by which MTX-γ-DMPE contained in liposomes It is hypothesised that CEM cells become resistant to MTX due to defective transport and/or elevated levels of dihydrofolate reductase.

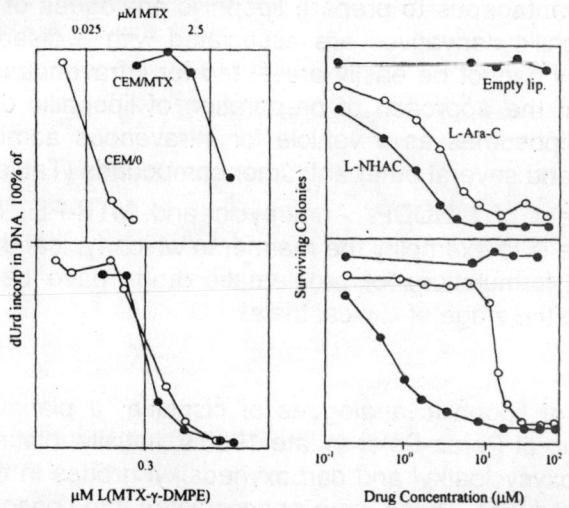

Fig. 13 : Profiles showing the overcoming of cross resistance upon exposure of resistant cells to lipophilic derivatives of methotrexate (left and Ara-C (right)

The liposomes apparently enter the target cells as a consequence of phagocytosis and not via the MTX transport system and are thus able to overcome both types of resistance.

Resistance to 1-β-D-arabinofuranosylcytosine (Ara-C, Fig. 8) is a major cause for its treatment failure in leukemia patients. Different mechanisms for resistance to the drug have been proposed, which include low levels of deoxycytidine kinase G [57], decrease in number of nucleoside transport sites [58], and/or a decreased catabolism by cytidine deaminase [59]. NHAC, the lipophilic prodrug of the Ara-C, exhibits cytotoxicity independent of both the nucleoside transporter mechanism and the deoxycytidine kinase activity [41]. The right part of Fig. 13 shows the number of surviving colonies of HL-60 on exposure to empty liposomes, liposomes containin Ara-C, and those containing NHAC. Evidently, all colonies are surviving in case of empty liposomes, both in sensitive and resistant cells. Whie L-Ara-C is effective in sensitive cells, it is ineffective upto quite high concentrations towards resistant cells. L-NHAC on the other hand clearly is cytotoxic to both resistant and sensitive cells. In this case, only 1.6 folds higher drug concentration was required to kill resistant colonies than the sensitive cells. The behaviour has been attributed to the difference in mechanism of cytotoxic action of NHAC and Ara-C. The cytotoxicity of Ara-C is known to be S-phase specific [60] whereas NHAC exhibits no phase specific toxicity at therapeutic concentrations [41].

DEVELOPMENT OF FORMULATIONS OF LIPOPHILIC DERIVATIVES CURRENTLY UNDER CLINICAL TRIALS

The lipophilic prodrugs currently under clinical studies include liposomal neodecanoato-trans-R,R-1,2-diaminocyclohexane-platinum II (L-NDDP) [61,62], liposomal annamycin [63] and liposomal muramyl tripeptide phosphatidyl ethanolamine (MTP-PE) [64]. Evidently, all these three are anticancer agents. Especially for antitumour drugs, the organ distribution, cellular distribution, cellular uptake and hence the spectrum of activity is largely determined by their lipophilicity. Therefore, it is advantageous to prepare lipophilic analogues of this class of drugs. However, the lipophilic derivatives are associated with a disadvantage that being water insoluble they cannot be easily presented for intravenous administration. It is for this reason that the approach of preparation of lipophilic derivatives and their incorporation into liposomes as a vehicle for intravenous administration has been explored for these and several other antitumor compounds (Table 2).

The development of L-NDDP, Annamycin and MTP-PE, is briefly discussed below. The purpose is to exemplify the manner in which typical difficulties associated with the liposomal formulations of problematic drugs have been tackled and the products brought to the stage of clinical trials.

L-NDDP

The development of lipophilic analogues of cisplatin, a platinum compound, was taken up by a group of Perez-Soler in late 1980's. Initially, platinum complexes with carboxyalkyl, carboxycycloalkyl and carboxyneoalkyl groups in the range of 5-15 C-atoms were prepared [65]. These were encapsulated into liposomes prepared using DMPC and DMPC:DMPG mixed in the ratios of 7:3 and 3: 7. For all the derivatives, liposomal entrapment efficiency of >80% was observed in all type of liposomes. The entrapment was correlated directly to the number of C-atoms in the hydrophobic side chain. Compounds containing more than nine C-atoms showed encapsulation of >95% [66]. Unexpectedly in in-vivo studies, no antitumour activity was seen for the prodrugs, either when in free form or when encapsulated in liposomes prepared from dimyristoylphosphatidylcholine (DMPC). However, an interesting observation was that the activity in-vivo was directly related to the amount of dimyristoyl phosphatidylglycerol (DMPG) in the bilayer. The critical role of DMPG was attributed to the formation of complex between the drug and DMPG.

The antitumor activity of NDDP (Fig. 2), one of the platinum derivatives, was subsequently looked for on entrapment in liposomes composed of varying ratios of DMPC and DMPG. Based on this study, an active drug-DMPG complex containing one or two DMPG molecules as side chains was proposed [24]. L-NDDP, the liposomal prodrug-phospholipid complex, was found to be significantly more cytotoxic than free NDDP and cisplatin against tumor cell lines sensitive and resistant to cisplatin [54]. In in-vivo studies, it was as active as cisplatin against L-1210 leukemia and more active against M-5076 reticulosarcoma [67]. In toxicology studies in mice and dogs, L-NDDP proved to be less toxic than cisplatin. The main side effect of L-NDDP was myelosuppression unlike cisplatin that shows severe renal dysfunction.

Studies are also reported on the effectiveness of NDDP formulation in conventional liposomes. The preparation proved to be effective in murine models of experimental liver metastases, attributed to the avid uptake by liver. For treatment of solid tumors outside the liver, NDDP was also formulated in long-circulating liposomes composed of phosphatidylcholine (PC), cholesterol, and polyethylene glycol (PEG) conjugated to phosphatidylethanolamine (PE) [42,68]. These were found to localise preferentially in melanomas in mice. The in-vivo toxicities were significantly less than those for cisplatin. On treatment of the tumor with local hyperthermia, after the injection of long-circulating liposomes, the tumor uptake of NDDP was increased by 60% and its tumor inhibitory effect was also found to improve significantly.

Annamycin

The development of liposomal preparations of anthracyclin antibiotics, especially doxorubicin, has been the subject matter of several studies [45,69]. Doxorubicin is very effective for the treatment of acute leukemia, lymphoma, breast carcinoma, osteosarcoma and soft tissue sarcomas [70] but its use is severely limited due to its serious side effects, including acute myelosupression and chronic cumulative cardiotoxicity [71,72]. On delivery of the drug in liposomes, reduced cardiotoxicity and increased activity against tumors were observed. The drug, however, presented formulation problems, as being amphiphilic in nature, it tended to partition between lipid bilayers and aqueous compartments of liposomes resulting in suboptimal entrapment and significant leakage with time. The entrapment was limited to 45-55% in liposomes composed of cardiolipin/PC/cholesterol/ stearylamine [45,73]. Similarly, encapsulation efficiency between 60-80% was obtained in liposomes composed of egg PC/egg derived PG/cholesterol/ d□□□tocopherol succinate [69].

The pH driven active drug loading technique was successful in yielding 100% liposomal incorporation. However, doubts have been expressed on the wide and daily use of the procedure requiring reconstitution of the lyophilized powder with isotonic saline and addition of sodium carbonate solution of pH 10.8-12.0, followed by subsequent heating of the preparation in-situ at 60°C [74].

As an alternate solution to the formulation problem of anthracyclines, Perez-Soler et al. [66] worked upon the approach of synthesizing different lipophilic analogues of doxorubicin. The compounds were incorporated into MLVs and based on the structure-liposome entrapment relationship studies, 2-iodo-3'-hydroxy-4'-epi-4-demethoxy-doxorubicin (Annamycin, Fig. 4) was selected for biological testing. Liposomal annamycin proved to be more active than doxorubicin in L-1210 leukemia and M 5076 reticulosarcoma in mice [75]. Also, it was found to be non-cross-resistant in-vitro [76,77] and in-vivo [78] in a number of non-resistant and multi-drug-resistant cancer cells. The therapeutic index of annamycin was shown to be dependent on the liposomal size, with SUVs showing better anticancer activity than the large liposomes [47]. Unlike doxorubicin, annamycin did not show any enhancement in therapeutic effect when encapsulated in long circulating non-leaky liposomes [47]. Plasma distribution of liposomal annamycin is currently being studied [63,79].

MTP-PE

The activation of the macrophages to make them tumoricidal through the use of an immunostimulant agent is one amongst the numerous approaches being employed in cancer research [80]. The in-vivo activation of macrophages with muramyl dipeptide (MDP, Fig. 3) was not very successful in the initial studies as the activator was rapidly cleared from the system, within 60 min after injection [81]. The liposomal delivery was subsequently tried to decrease the clearance rate. It proved useful and the macrophage activation and tumoricidal activity was seen both in-vitro and in-vivo [82]. Studies were done to further prolong the intracellular residence time of the drug for which lipophilic derivatives of MDP were prepared and incorporated into liposomes [83,84]. The other purpose of making lipophilic drug derivatives and their incorporation into liposomes was to decrease leakage of the water-soluble peptide from liposomes.

Out of the various derivatives, MTP-PE (Fig. 3) worked out to be promising analogue as it could be incorporated into multilamellar liposomes with a high degree of efficiency [80,85]. This synthetic acyl derivative of MDP in liposomes showed 100-folds enhancement of activity of murine macrophages [80,86] and human monocytes [87]. It was also found to give good response in eradication of malignant and highly spontaneous tumors in a variety of animal models [86-91]. The effect of L-MTP-PE in humans was first studied by Murray et al. [92] who conducted phase I trial in 28 metastatic cancer patients employing a stable reproducible preparation developed by CIBA-GEIGY Ltd., Basel, Switzerland [33]. Although the preparation expectedly did not give significant antitumor activity, because systemic macrophage activation is effective when the disease is in a minimal state [93], a clear evidence was provided on in-situ activation of tumoricidal properties [92,94,95]. Other salient findings were that liposomal preparation of MTP-PE was safe at the dosage schedule used and that the optimal biological dose of MTP-PE was below that recorded for the maximum tolerated dose. A similar finding of the absence of objective antitumoral effect and macrophage activation was made by Sculier et al. [94] in a pilot study on eleven lung cancer patients.

OPTIMISATION OF LIPOSOMAL FORMULATIONS CONTAINING LIPOPHILIC DERIVATIVES

There are some interesting findings on development and evaluation of liposomal formulations containing lipophilic derivatives.

The lipophilicity cannot be taken as the only criterion for the solubility of a lipophilic drug or a lipophilic derivative into the phospholipid bilayers. Geometrical constraints of the lipophilic molecules also govern their distribution into the liposomes. For example, triacylglycerols and cholesterol esters are poorly incorporated into the phospholipid bilayers [96].

Some very hydrophobic compounds tend to phase-separate and form microscopic and macroscopic subphases. Sampedro et al. [97] studied the liposomal entrapment of eight lipophilic anticancer drugs. While good entrapment was obtained with hexamethylmelamine, penclomedine, mitindomide and fazarabine, presence of either free drug crystals or microaggregates of lipid/drug complex were seen in liposomes containing taxol, batracylin, trimelamol and diaziquone.

It is not necessary that the drugs that are completely incorporated within a series of compounds would give similar release behaviour. Two lipophilic prodrugs of 5-FU, C18FU and Cholesteryl-5-(5-FU-carbamoyl)capronate (ChFU) (Fig. 6) were prepared by Hashida et al. [98] and both showed complete incorporation into liposomes. However, on studying the release characteristics, the release half-life of FU from ChFU was found to be only about 1 hr, while it was more than 24 h for C18FU. Interestingly, the partition coefficient of the first was much higher than second.

Even an increase in the lipophilicity of the drug and its successful incorporation into liposomes does not guarantee that the final liposomal preparation will give the desired effect in-vivo. Several formulation factors like the nature and composition of the phospholipid, the type of liposomes, etc., and pharmacodynamic/ pharmacological factors like mechanisms of action, toxicity, uptake, etc., tend to play a significant role. To quote the examples, lipophilic derivatives of cisplatin showed encapsulation efficiencies of 80-95%, but no antitumour activity was seen from the liposomes composed of DMPC [55]. Instead, a good in-vivo activity was observed when DMPC was replaced with DMPG. Similarly, in L-asparginase, a strong effect of the charge on liposomes was observed. While the negatively charged liposomes showed elimination of toxicity, the positive charged were rather more toxic [14]. In the same manner, the effect of the type of liposomes was observed with methotrexate (MTX). The lipophilic complex of the drug with γ-dimyristoyl-phosphatidylethanolamine (γ-DMPE) (Fig. 10) was found to be more effective in suppressing the knee joint inflammation when delivered in MLVs than in SUVs [99]. When the MTX-γ-DMPE (Fig. 10) complex and its glycerol-PE analogs were tested for cytotoxic activity, they were found to be less active in comparison to the free drug.

The difference in mechanisms of uptake of the drug and liposomes is reported to be the governing factor in this case [100].

The findings as above suggest that detailed studies that identify the influence of side chain and linkage/spacer structures and the effect of formulation and other in-vivo factors need to be carried out to optimise the liposomal delivery systems containing lipophilic drug derivatives.

CONCLUSION: THE KEY TO SUCCESS

Knight in 1981 [101] strongly advocated the design of lipophilic prodrugs for the ultimate success of liposomes as drug delivery systems. Over the years, apart from preparing prodrug and non-prodrug lipophilic derivatives, approaches like complex-formation and pharmacosomes have also been utilised for increasing the lipophilicity of the drugs with the purpose of enhancing their liposomal encapsulation. The concept has been applied to hydrophilic, amphiphilic and biphasic insoluble drugs. The major achievement is that several liposomal preparations containing lipophilic derivatives have reached the clinical trial stage. A number of others are in different stages of development. Table 9 gives a comprehensive list of the derivatives prepared for various drugs and the benefits achieved for each of them.

Table 9. Lipophilic drug derivatives and the stage of their development

In clinical and preclinical stage

Drug	Lipophilic modification	Objectives achieved	Stage of development	Ref.
Arabinosyl-cytosine	N^4- & 5'-oleyl- and N^4-palmitoyl derivatives	↑ Encapsulation efficiency ↑ Antitumor effect	Clinical trials	102,103
Cisplatin	Neodecanoato-trans-R,R-1,2-diamino cyclohexane platinum II)	↑ Encapsulation efficiency ↑ Antitumor effect ↓ Toxicity	Clinical trials	24,54,55, 61,62,65, 67
Cortisol	Alkyl esters	↑ Encapsulation efficiency ↑ Physical stability ↑ Anti-inflammatory activity	Clinical trials	23,104,1 05
Doxorubicin	2-Iodo-3'-hydroxy-4'-epi-4-demethoxy-doxorubicin (annamycin)	↑ Encapsulation efficiency ↑ Antitumor effect Non-cross-resistant	Clinical trials	47,63,75-79

(Contd.)

Muramyl dipeptide (MDP)	Muramyl tripeptide ethanolamine (MTP-PE)	↑ Encapsulation efficiency ↑ Physical stability ↑ Immunomodulating effect	Clinical trials	87,88,92, 94
Arabinosyl-cytosine	N^4-hexadecyl derivative (NHAC)	↑ Encapsulation efficiency ↑ Antitumor effect Non-cross-resistant	Preclinical studies	41,106-108,109

At the stage of animal studies

Drug	Lipophilic modification	Objectives achieved	References
Arabinosyl cytosine	N^4-[N-(cholesteryloxy carbonyl)glycyl] derivative	↑ Encapsulation efficiency ↑ Antitumor effect	15
	Phospholipid-N^4-palmitoyl conjugates	↑ Encapsulation efficiency	110
	Phospholipid-N^4-hexadecyl conjugates	↑ Encapsulation efficiency	111
L-Asparaginase	Palmitoyl derivative	↑ Encapsulation efficiency ↑ Antitumor activity ↓ Toxicity	14,112,113
Azidothymidine	Phospholipid derivatives	↑ Encapsulation efficiency ↓ Toxicity	49,50,114
Boron	K[nido-7-$CH_3(CH_2)_{15}$-7,8-$C_2B_9H_{11}$]	↑ Encapsulation efficiency ↑ Antitumor effect	52
Cortisone	Alkyl esters	↑ Encapsulation efficiency ↑ Physical stability Alteration in biodistribution	25,115-117
5-Fluorouracil	Alkylcarbamoyl derivatives	↑ Encapsulation efficiency ↑ Antitumor effect	16
	Palmitoyl and dipalmitoyl derivatives of 5-fluoro-2'-deoxyuridine	↑ Encapsulation efficiency ↑ Antitumor effect	118-120
	Dipalmitoylphosphatidyl	↑ Encapsulation	121

(Contd.)

	fluorouridine	efficiency ↑ Antitumor effect	
	5'-Palmitoyl –and 5'-succinyl derivatives of 5-fluorouridine	↑ Encapsulation efficiency ↑ Antitumor effect	122
Gadolinium	DTPA-stearate complex	↑ Encapsulation efficiency ↑ Physical stability Signal enhancement of MRI	123
Hydroxyrubicin	14-O-palmitoyl derivative	↑ Encapsulation efficiency ↑ Physical stability ↑ Antitumor effect	124
Indium	DTPA-stearate complex	↑ Encapsulation efficiency	125
Manganese	Mn-EDTA-DDP	↑ Encapsulation efficiency	126
Methotrexate	α- & γ- DMPE and α,γ-di DMPE derivatives	↑ Antiarthiritic activity	43,44,99,127,128
Mitomycin C	Benzyl, benzoyl, benzyl-carbonyl, benzyloxycarbonyl & benzyloxymethyl derivatives	↑ Encapsulation efficiency	40,129,130
Mitomycin C	Alkoxycarbonyl derivatives	↑ Encapsulation efficiency Altered biodistribution	5,131,132
Mitomycin C	Stearoyl MMC and cholesterol derivatives with different spacers	↑ Encapsulation efficiency ↑ Stability Sustained release	17,133,134
Mitoxantrone	Lipophilic complex	↑ Encapsulation efficiency	135,136
Pindolol	Pharmacosomes	↑ Encapsulation efficiency Altered biodistribution	53

At the stage of cell-culture studies

Drug	Lipophilic modification	Objectives achieved	Reference
Methantheline Br	Ion pairs with trichloroacetic acid	↑ Encapsulation efficiency	137

(Contd.)

Azidothymidine	N⁴-palmitoyl and N⁴-hexadecyl-2'-deoxycytidinyl- (3,5')-3'-azido-2',3'-dideoxythymidine	↑ Encapsulation efficiency	138
Acyclovir	Laurate and palmitate esters	↑ Encapsulation efficiency ↑ Antiviral effect	139
	Diphosphate dimyristoyl glycerol derivatives	↑ Encapsulation efficiency ↑ Antiviral effect	140
Daunorubicin	N-acyl derivatives	↑ Encapsulation efficiency ↑ Physical stability ↑ Antitumor effect	39
Foscarnet Sodium	Sphingolipid-, glycerolipid-, phospholipid- and fatty acid analogs	↑ Encapsulation efficiency Prolonged antiviral activity	141,142
	1-O-octadecyl-sn-glycero-3-phosphonoformate	↑ Encapsulation efficiency ↑ Antiviral activity	143
Fosfonet Sodium	Sphingolipid-, glycerolipid-, phospholipid- and fatty acid analogs	↑ Encapsulation efficiency Prolonged antiviral activity	141,142
Methotrexate	α- & γ- DMPE and α,γ-di DMPE derivatives	↑ Encapsulation efficiency Non-resistant anticancer effect	56,100,144-146
Metronidazole	Myristic and lauric esters	↑ Encapsulation efficiency ↑ Antiprotozoal activity	147,148
Muramyl dipeptide (MDP)	MDP-L-alanyl-cholesterol (MDP-CHOL) Glycerol dipalmitate derivatives of MDP, MDP-n-butyl ester and N-acetyl-muramyl-D-alanyl-D-isoglutamine	↑ Encapsulation efficiency ↑ Immunomodulating effect	84,149
Triamcinolone acetonide	Myristic and lauric esters	↑ Encapsulation efficiency	18

(Contd.)

At the stage of in-vitro studies

Drug	Lipophilic modification	Objectives achieved	Reference
[51]Cr	Complex with 3-cholesteryl-6-[N'-iminobis(ethylenenitrilo)-tetraacetic acid] hexyl ether	↑ Encapsulation efficiency Better biodistribution	150
Insulin	Phosphatidyl ethanolamine derivative	↑ Encapsulation efficiency	151
Isopropamide Iodide	Ion pairs with taurodeoxy cholate	↑ Encapsulation efficiency	152
6-Mercaptopurine	(6-Octadecyldithio)purine	↑ Encapsulation efficiency	153

At the stage of physicochemical studies

Drug	Lipophilic modification	Objectives achieved	Reference
Acyclovir	Nucleolipid with 17-C side chain	↑ Encapsulation efficiency	154
Dexamethasone	Palmitate ester	↑ Encapsulation efficiency	155
Diatrizoic acid	Long chain esters	↑ Encapsulation efficiency Better contrast medium	156
Enkephalin	DPPE-enkephalin conjugate	↑ Encapsulation efficiency	157
Felbinac	α-β-Poly(N-hydroxyethyl)-DL-aspartamide conjugate	↑ Encapsulation efficiency	158
Fenoprofen	Pharmacosomes	↑ Encapsulation efficiency	159,160
5-Fluorouracil	Pentyl- & hexyl- 5-fluorouracil-1-acetate	↑ Encapsulation efficiency	160
PABA	Ester derivatives	↑ Encapsulation efficiency	161
Warfarin	Ion pairs with sodium ions	↑ Encapsulation efficiency	162

The approach of incorporating drugs as lipophilic derivatives in liposomes provides solutions to most of the problems encountered with liposomal formulations. Looking into the potential, it is hoped that the drug derivatisation would continue to be applied in future on problematic drugs, both old and new.

REFERENCES

1. Sharma, A. and Sharma, U.S. (1997). **Int. J. Pharm.** 154, 123-140.

2. Mayhew, E.G., Rustum, Y.M., Szoka, F. and Papahadjopoulos, D. (1979). **Cancer Treat. Rep.** 63, 1923-1928.

3. Fresta, M., Puglisi, G., Panico, A.M., Di Marco, S. and Mazzone, G. (1993). **Drug Dev. Ind. Pharm.** 19, 559-585.

4. Vadiei, K., Lopez-Berestein, G., Perez-Soler, R. and Luke, D.R. (1989). **Int. J. Pharm.** 57, 133-138.

5. Sasaki, H., Takakura. Y., Hashida, M., Kimura, T. and Sezaki, H. (1984). **J. Pharm. Dyn.** 7, 120-130.

6. Defrise-Quertain, F., Chatelain, P., Delmelle, M. and Ruysschaert, J. (1984). Model studies for drug entrapment and liposome stability. In : Liposome Technology: Incorporation of drugs, proteins and genetic material (Gregoriadis, G. Ed.), CRC Press, Boca Raton, pp. 183-204.

7. Tsujii, K., Sunamoto, J. and Fendler, J.H. (1976). **Life Sci.** 19, 1743-1750.

8. Gulati, M., Grover, M., Singh, M. and Singh, S. (1998). **J. Microencapsul.** (In Press).

9. Philippot, J.R. and Liautard,J.P. (1993). A mild method for the preparation of very large unilamellar liposomes. In : Liposome Technology: Liposome preparation and related techniques (Gregoriadis, G. Ed.), CRC Press, Boca Raton, pp. 81-98.

10. Gulati, M., Grover, M., Singh, S. and Singh, M. (1998). **Int. J. Pharm.** 165, 129-168.

11. Betageri, G.V., Jenkins, S.A. and Parsons, D.L. (1993). Industrial applications of liposomes. In : Liposome Drug Delivery Systems, Technomic Publishing Co., Pennsylvania, pp. 109-125.

12. Stuhne-Sekalec, L., Chudzik, J. and Stanacev, N.Z. (1986). **J. Biochem. Biophys. Methods** 13, 23-27.

13. Fishman, Y. and Citri, N. (1975). **FEBS Lett.** 60, 17-20.

14. Jorge, J.C.S., Perez-Soler, R., Morais, J.G. and Cruz, M.E.M. (1994). **Cancer Chemother. Pharmacol.** 34, 230-234.

15. Tokunaga, Y., Iwasa, T., Fujisaki, J., Sawai, S. and Kagayama, A. (1988). **Chem. Pharm. Bull.** 36, 3574-3583.

16. Sasaki, H., Matsukawa, Y., Hashida, M. and Sezaki, H. (1987). **Int. J. Pharm.** 36, 147-156.

17. Tokunaga, Y., Iwasa, T., Fujisaki, J., Sawai, S. and Kagayama, A. (1988). **Chem. Pharm. Bull.** 36, 3060-3069.

18. Goundalkar, A. and Mezei, M. (1984). **J. Pharm. Sci.** 73, 834-835.

19. Newton, D.W., Suphalerk, R. and Murray, W.J. (1982). **Int. J. Pharm.** 11, 209-213.

20. Daniel, P.T., Holzschuh, J., Müller, C.E., Roth, H.J. and Berg, P.A. (1989). **Arch. Toxicol.** (Suppl.) 13, 179-182.

21. Fresta, M., Villari, A., Puglisi, G. and Cavallaro, G. (1993). **Int. J. Pharm.** 99, 145-156.

22. Lee, M.J., Straubinger, R.M. and Jusko, W.J. (1995). **Pharm. Res.** 12, 1055-1059.

23. Shaw, I.H., Knight, C.G. and Dingle, J.T. (1976). **Biochem. J.** 158, 473-476.

24. Shaw, I.H., Knight, C.G. and Dingle, J.T. (1976). **Biochem. J.** 158, 473-476.

25. Arrowsmith, M., Hadgraft, J. and Kellaway, I.W. (1983). **Int. J. Pharm.** 17, 91-98.

26. Bekers, O., Beijnen, J.H., Storm, G., Bult, A. and Underberg, W.J. (1989). **Int. J. Pharm.** 56, 103-109.

27. Garelli, N. and Vierling, P. (1992). **Biochim. Biophys. Acta** 1127, 41-48.

28. Burke, T.G., Staubus, A.E., Mishra, A.K. and Malek, H. (1992). **J. Am. Chem. Soc.** 114, 8218-8219.

29. Burke, T.G., Mishra, A.K., Wani, M.C. and Wall, M.E. (1993). **Biochemistry** 32, 5352-5364.

30. Gulati, M., Bajad, S., Singh, S., Ferdous, A. and Singh, M. (1998). **J. Microencapsul.** 15, 137-151.

31. Payne, N.I., Timmins, P., Ambrose, C.V., Ward, M.D. and Ridgway, F. (1986). **J. Pharm. Sci.** 75, 325-329.

32. Katare, O.P., Vyas, S.P. and Dixit, V.K. (1990). **J. Microencapsul.** 7, 455-462.

33. van Hoogevest, P. and Frankhauser, A. (1989). An industrial liposomal dosage form for muramyl-tripeptide-phosphatidyl ethanolamine (MTP-PE). In: Liposomes in the Therapy of Infectious Diseases and Cancer (Lopez-Berestein, G. and Fidler, I.J. Eds.), Liss, New York, pp. 117-125.

34. Lanzini, F., Guidoni, L., Viti, V., Errivi, G., Onnis, S. and Randaccio, P. (1984). **Rad. Res.** 98, 154-166.

35. Ratz, H., Freise, J., Magerstedt, P., Schaper, A., Preugschat, W. and Keyser, D. (1989). **J. Microencapsul.** 6, 485-492.

36. Kikuchi, H., Carlsson, A., Yachi, K. and Hirota, S. (1991). **Chem. Pharm. Bull.** 1018-1022.

37. Zuidam, N.J., Lee, S.S. and Crommelin, D.J.A. (1993). **Pharm. Res.** 10, 1591-1596.

38. Juliano, R.L., Stamp, D. and McCullogh, N. (1978). **Annals N.Y. Acad. Sci.** 308, 411-423.

39. Bard, D.R., Knight, C.G. and Page-Thomas, D.P. (1982). **Br. J. Cancer** 45, 783-785.

40. Sasaki, H., Fukumoto, M., Hashida, M., Kimura, T. and Sezaki, H. (1983). **Chem. Pharm. Bull.** 31, 4083-4090.

41. Horber, D.H., Schott, H. and Schwendener, R.A. (1995). **Br. J. Cancer** 71, 957-962.

42. Li, S., Khokhar, A.R., Perez-Soler, R. and Huang, L. (1995). **Oncol. Res.** 7, 611-617.

43. Williams, A.S., Camilleri, J.P., Topley, N. and Williams, B.D. (1994). **J. Pharmacol. Toxicol. Methods** 32, 53-58.

44. Williams, A.S., Camilleri, J.P., Amos, N. and Williams, B.D. (1995). **Clin. Exp. Immunol.** 102, 560-565.

45. Rahman, A., Treat, J., Roh, J.K., Potkul, L.A., Alvord, W.G., Forst, D. and Woolley, P.V. (1990). **J.Clin. Oncol.** 8, 1093-1100.

46. Gabizon, A.A. (1992). **Cancer Res.** 52, 891-896.

47. Zou, Y., Ling, Y.H., Reddy, S., Priebe, W. and Perez-Soler, R. (1995). **Int. J. Cancer** 61, 666-671.

48. Wasan, K.M., Ng, S. and Cassidy, S.M. (1997). **J. Pharm. Sci.** 86, 872-875.

49. Hostetler, K.Y., Korba, B.E., Sridhar, C.N. and Gardner, M.F. (1994). **Antiviral Res.** 24, 59-67.

50. Hostetler, K.Y., Richman, D.D., Sridhar, C.N., Felgner, P.L., Felgner, J., Ricci, J., Gardner, M.F., Selleseth, D.W. and Ellis, M.N. (1994). **Antimicrob. Agents Chemother.** 38, 2792-2797.

51. Feakes, D.A., Shelly, K., Knobler, C.B. and Hawthorne, M.F. (1994). **Proc. Natl. Acad. Sci. USA**, 91, 3029-3033.

52. Feakes, D.A., Shelly, K. and Hawthorne, M.F. (1995). **Proc. Natl. Acad. Sci.** USA, 92, 1367-1370.

53. Vaizoglu, M.O. and Speiser, P.P. (1986). **Acta Pharm. Suec.** 23, 163-172.

54. Perez-Soler, R., Yang, L.Y., Drewinko, B., Lautersztain, J. and Khokhar, A.R. (1988). **Cancer Res.** 48, 4509-4512.

55. Perez-Soler, R., Lautersztain, J., Clifton, S.L., Wright, K. and Khokhar, A.R. (1989). **Cancer Chemother. Pharmacol.** 24, 1-8.

56. Perez-Soler, R., Lautersztain, J., Clifton, S.L., Wright, K. and Khokhar, A.R. (1989). **Cancer Chemother. Pharmacol.** 24, 1-8.

57. Chu, M.Y. and Fisher, G.A. (1965). 14, 333-341.

58. Wiley, J.S., Jones, S.P., Sawyer, W.H. and Paterson, A.R. (1982). **J. Clin. Invest.** 69, 479-489.

59. Steuart, C.D. and Burke, P.J. (1971). **Nature New Biol.** 233, 109-110.

60. Gorczyca, W., Gong, J., Ardelt, B., Traganos, F. and Darzynkiewicz, Z. (1993). **Cancer Res.** 53, 3186-3192.

61. Perez-Soler, R., Lopez-Berestein, G., Lautersztain, J., Al-Baker, S., Francis, K., Macias-Kiger, D., Raber, M.N. and Khokhar, A.R. (1990). **Cancer Res.** 50, 4254-4259.

62. Chase, J., Wood, J., Pazdur, R., Khokhar, A.R., Perez-Soler, R., Siddik, Z.H. and Roh, M. (1991). **Proc. AACR** pp. 420.

63. Wasan, K.M. and Morton, R.E. (1996). **Pharm. Res.** 13, 462-468.

64. Gano, J.B. and Kleinerman, E.S. (1995). **Oncol. Nurs. Forum** 22, 809-816.

65. Khokhar, A.R., Al-Baker, S., Krakoff, I.H. and Perez-Soler, R. (1989). **Cancer Chemother. Pharmacol.** 23, 219-224.

66. Perez-Soler, R., Khokhar, A.R., Preibe, W. and Krakoff, I.H. (1993). Use of liposomes as carriers of lipophilic antitumor agents. In : Liposomes in Drug Delivery, (Gregoriadis, G., Florence, A.T. and Patel, H.M. Eds.), Harwood Academic Publishers, Switzerland, pp. 1-11.

67. Perez-Soler, R., Khokhar, A.R. and Lopez-Berestein, G. (1987). **Cancer Res.** 47, 6462-6466.

68. Morl, A., Wu, S.P., Han, I., Khokhar, A.R., Perez-Soler, R. and Huang, L. (1996). **Cancer Chemother. Pharmacol.** 37, 435-444.

69. Gabizon, A.A., Peretz, T., Sulkes, A., Amselem, S., Ben-Yosef, R., Ben Baruch, N., Catane, R., Biran, S. and Barenholz, Y. (1989). **Eur. J. Cancer Clin. Oncol.** 25, 1795-1803.

70. Tan, C., Etcubanas, E., Wollner, N., Rosen, G., Gilladoga, A., Showel, J., Murphy, M.L. and Krakoff, I.H. (1973). **Cancer** 32, 9-17.

71. Benjamin, R.S., Wiernik, P.H. and Bachur, N.R. (1974). **Cancer** 33, 19-27.

72. Rinehart, J.J., Lewis, R.P. and Balcerzak, S.P. (1974). **Ann. Internal Med.** 81, 475-478.

73. Treat, J., Greenspan, A.R. and Rahman, A. (1989). Liposome encapsulated doxorubicin: preliminary results of phase I and phase II trials. In: Liposomes in the Therapy of Infectious Diseases and Cancer (Lopez-Berestein, G. and Fidler, I.J. Eds.), Alan R. Liss. Inc., New York, pp. 353-365.

74. Creaven, P.J., Cowens, J.W., Ginsberg, R., Ostro, M. and Browman, G. (1990). **J. Liposome Res.** 1, 481-490.

75. Perez-Soler, R. and Priębe, W. (1990). **Cancer Res.** 50, 4260-4266.

76. Ling, Y.H., Priebe, W. and Perez-Soler, R. (1993). **Cancer Res.** 53, 1845-1852.

77. Ling, Y.H., Priebe, W., Yang, L.Y., Burke, T.G., Pommier, Y. and Perez-Soler, R. (1993). **Cancer Res.** 53, 1583-1589.

78. Zou, Y., Ling, Y.H., Van, N.T., Priebe, W. and Perez-Soler, R. (1994). 54, 1479-1484.

79. Wasan, K.M. and Perez-Soler, R. (1995). **J. Pharm. Sci.** 84, 1094-1100.

80. Fidler, I.J. (1986). Immunomodulation of macrophages for cancer and antiviral therapy. In : Site Specific Drug Delivery (Tomlinson, E. and Davis, S.Eds.), Wiley, New York, pp. 111-134.

81. Parant, M., Parant, F., Chedid, L., Yapo, A., Petit, J.F. and Lederer, E. (1979). 1, 35-41.

82. Fidler, I.J., Sone, S., Fogler, W.E. and Barnes, Z.L. (1981). **Proc. Natl. Acad. Sci.** USA , 78, 1680-1684.

83. Lopez-Berestein, G., Mehta, K., Mehta, R., Juliano, R.L. and Hersh, E.M. (1983). **J. Immunol.** 130, 1500-1502.

84. Phillips, N.C., Chedid, L., Bernard, J.M., Level, M. and Lefrancier, P. (1987). **J. Biol. Response Modif.** 6, 678-691.

85. Schroit, A.J. and Fidler, I.J. (1982). **Cancer Res.** 42, 161-167.

86. Fidler, I.J., Sone, S., Fogler, W.E., Smith, D., Braun, D.G., Tarcsay, L., Gisler, R.H. and Schroit, A.J. (1982). **J. Biol. Response Modif.** 1, 43-55.

87. Kleinerman, E.S., Erickson, K.L., Schroit, A.J., Fogler, W.E. and Fidler, I.J. (1983). **Cancer Res.** 43, 2010-2014.

88. Kleinerman, E.S., Gano, J.B., Johnston, D.A., Benjamin, R.S. and Jaffe, N. (1995). **Am. J. Clin. Oncol.** 18, 93-99.

89. Talmadge, J.E., Lenz, B.F., Klabansky, R., Simon, R., Riggs, C., Guo, S., Oldham, R.K. and Fidler, I.J. (1986). **Cancer Res.** 46, 1160-1163.

90. Mac Ewen, E.G., Kurzman, I.D., Helfand, S., Vail, D., London, C., Kisseberth, W., Rosenthal, R.C., Fox, L.E. and Keller, E.T. (1994). **J. Drug Target.** 2, 391-396.

91. Goldbach, P., Dumont, S., Kessler, R., Poindron, P. and Stamm, A. (1996). **Am. J. Physiol.** 270, L429-L434.

92. Murray, J.L., Kleinerman, E.S., Cunningham, J.E., Tatom, J.R., Andrejcio, K., Lepe-Zuniga, J., Lamki, L.M., Rosenblum, M.G., Frost, H., Gutterman, J.U., Fidler, I.J. and Krakoff, I.H. (1989). **J. Clin. Oncol.** 7, 1915-1925.

93. Fidler, I.J. (1988). **Adv. Drug Deliv. Rev.** 1, 69-106.

94. Sculier, J.P., Gerain, J., Body, J.J., Markiewicz, E., Klastersky, J., Frost, H., Gutterman, J.U., Fidler, I.J. and Krakoff, I.H. (1993). **Drug Invest.** 6, 276-284.

95. Favaro, D., Santarosa, M., Quaia, M., Spada, A., Freschi, A., Talmini, R. and Galligioni, E. (1995). **Eur. J. Cancer** 31A, 1027.

96. Barenholz, Y. and Crommelin, D.J.A. (1988). Liposomes as pharmaceutical dosage forms. In : Encyclopedia of Pharmaceutical Technology (Swarbrick, J. and Boylan, J.C. Eds.), Marcel Dekker Inc., New York, pp. 1-39.

97. Sampedro, F., Partika, J., Santalo, P., Molins, P., Bonal, J. and Perez, S.R. (1994). **J. Microencapsul.** 11, 309-318.

98. Hashida, M., Sato, K., Takakura, Y. and Sezaki, H. (1988). **Chem. Pharm. Bull.** 36, 3186-3189.

99. Williams, A.S., Camilleri, J.P., Goodfellow, R.M. and Williams, B.D. (1996). **Br. J. Rheumatol.** 35, 719-724.

100. Kinsky, S.C., Loader, J.E. and Hashimoto, K. (1987). **Biochim. Biophys. Acta** 917, 211-218.

101. Knight, C.G. (1981). Hydrophobic pro-drugs in liposomes. In : Liposomes : From physical structure to therapeutic applications, (Knight, C.G. Ed.),Elsevier / North Holland Biomedical Press, Netherlands, pp. 381-390.

102. Rubas, W., Supersaxo, A., Weder, H.G., Hartmann, H.R., Hengartner, H., Schott, H. and Schwendener, R. (1986). **Int. J. Cancer** 37, 149-154.

103. Schwendener, R.A., Pestalozzi, B., Berger, S., Schott, H., Hengartner, H. and Sauter, C. (1989). Treatment of acute myelogenous leukemia with liposomes containing N⁴-oleyl-cytosine arabinoside. In : Liposomes in the Therapy of Infectious Diseases and Cancer (Lopez-Berestein, G. and Fidler, I.J. Eds.), Alan R Liss, Inc., New York, pp. 95-103.

104. Fildes, F.J.T. and Oliver, J.E. (1978). **J. Pharm. Pharmacol.** 30, 337-342.

105. de-Silva, M., Hazleman, B.L., Page-Thomas, D.P. and Wraight, P. (1979). **Lancet** 1, 1320-1322.

106. Schwendener, R.A. and Schott, H. (1992). **Int. J. Cancer** 51, 466-469.

107. Schwendener, R.A. and Schott, H. (1992). **Int. J. Cancer** 51, 466-469.

108. Horber, D.H., von Ballmoos, P., Schott, H. and Schwendener, R.A. (1995). **Br. J. Cancer** 72, 1067-1073.

109. Schwendener, R.A., Horber, D.H., Ottiger, C. and Schott, H. (1995). **J. Liposome Res.** 5, 27-47.

110. Schott, H. and Schwendener, R.A. (1996). **Liebigs Ann.** 3, 365-369.

111. Schott, H. and Schwendener, R.A. (1996). **Anticancer Drug Del.** 11, 451-162.

112. Martins, M.B.F., Jorge, J.C.S. and Cruz, M.E.M. (1990). **Biochimie** 72, 671-675.

113. Cruz, M.E.M., Martins, M.B., Carvo, M.L., Jorge, J.C.S. and Gaspar, M.M. (1994). **Proc. Int. Symp. Controlled Release Bioact. Mater.** pp. 346-347.

114. Cruz, M.E.M., Martins, M.B., Carvo, M.L., Jorge, J.C.S. and Gaspar, M.M. (1994). **Proc. Int. Symp. Controlled Release Bioact. Mater.** pp. 346-347.

115. Arrowsmith, M., Hadgraft, J. and Kellaway, I.W. (1983). **Int. J. Pharm.** 16, 305-318.

116. Arrowsmith, M., Hadgraft, J. and Kellaway, I.W. (1983). **Int. J. Pharm.** 14, 191-208.

117. Arrowsmith, M., Hadgraft, J. and Kellawy, I.W. (1984). **Int. J. Pharm.** 20, 347-362.

118. Schwendener, R.A., Supersaxo, A., Rubas, W. and Weder, H.G. (1984). Proc. Liposomes as Drug Carriers, Symposium, Stuttgart, FRG, pp. 170-181.

119. van Borssum, W.M., Fichtner, I., Dontje, B., Lenn, N.M., Becker, M., Arndt, D. and Scherphof, G.L. (1992). **J. Microencapsul.** 9, 335-346.

120. Mori, A., Kennel, S.J. and Huang, L. (1993). **Pharm. Res.** 10, 507-514.

121. Doi, K., Oku, N., Toyota, T., Shuto, S., Sakai, A., Itoh, H. and Okada, S. (1994). **Biol. Pharm. Bull.** 17, 1414-1416.

122. Crosasso, P., Brusa, P., Dosio, F., Arpicco, S., Pacchioni, D., Schuber, F. and Cattel, L. (1997). **J. Pharm. Sci.** 86, 832-839.

123. Schwendener, R.A., Wuethrich, R., Duewell, S., Wehrli, E. and Von Schulthess, G.K. (1990). **Invest. Radiol.** 25, 922-932.

124. Perez-Soler, R. and Priebe, W. (1992). **Cancer Chemother. Pharmacol.** 30, 267-271.

125. Grant, C.W.M., Karlik, S. and Florio, E. (1989). **Magn. Reson. Med.** 11, 236-243.

126. Unger, E.C. and Shen, D. (1991). **US Patent** 704, 542, 23.

127. Williams, A.S., Love, W.G. and Williams, B.D. (1992). **Int. J. Pharm.** 85, 189-197.

128. Williams, A.S., Punn, Y.L., Amos, N., Cooper, A.M. and Williams, B.D. (1995). **Br. J. Rheumatol.** 34, 241-245.

129. Sasaki, H., Mukai, E., Hashida, M., Kimura, T. and Sezaki, H. (1983). **Int. J. Pharm.** 15, 49-59.

130. Sasaki, H., Mukai, E., Hashida, M., Kimura, T. and Sezaki, H. (1983). **Int. J. Pharm.** 15, 61-71.

131. Sasaki, H., Kakutani, T., Hashida, M., Kimura, T. and Sezaki, H. (1985). **Chem. Pharm. Bull.** 33, 2968-2973.

132. Sasaki, H., Kakutani, T., Hashida, M. and Sezaki, H. (1985). **J. Pharm. Pharmacol.** 37, 461-465.

133. Tokunaga, Y., Iwasa, T., Fujisaki, J., Sawai, S. and Kagayama, A. (1988). **Chem. Pharm. Bull.** 36, 3557-3564.

134. Tokunaga, Y., Iwasa, T., Fujisaki, J., Sawai, S. and Kagayama, A. (1988). **Chem. Pharm. Bull.** 36, 3565-3573.

135. Schwendener, R.A. (1990). **German Patent** 3,825,374,

136. Schwendener, R.A., Fiebig, H.H., Berger, M.R. and Berger, D.P. (1991). **Cancer Chemother. Pharmacol.** 27, 429-439.

137. Jay, M. and Digenis, G.A. (1982). **J. Pharm. Sci.** 71, 958-960.

138. Schott, H., Haussler, M.P., Gowland, P., Horber, D.H. and Schwendener, R.A. (1994). **Antiviral Chem. Chemother.** 5, 387-394.

139. Tong, P., Hou, X.P., Shao, S., Zhang, Y.M. and Zhang, C.H. (1992). **Acta Pharm. Sinica** 27, 15-21.

140. Shakiba, S., Freeman, W.R., Flores-Aguilar, M., Munguia, D. and Hostetler, K.Y. (1995). **Antimicrob. Agents Chemother.** 39, 1383-1385.

141. Hostetler, K.Y. and Kumar, R. (1993). **US Patent** 5,194,654.

142. Hostetler, K.Y. and Kumar, R. (1995). **US Patent** 5,463,092.

143. Hostetler, K.Y., Kini, G.D., Beadle, J.R., Aldern, K.A., Gardner, M.F., Border, R., Kumar, R., Darshak, L. and Sridhar, C.N. (1996). **Antiviral Res.** 31, 59-67.

144. Hashimoto, K., Loader, J.E. and Kinsky, S.C. (1985). **Biochim. Biophys. Acta** 816, 163-168.

145. Hashimoto, K., Loader, J.E. and Kinsky, S.C. (1985). **Biochim. Biophys. Acta** 816, 163-168.

146. Noe, C., Hernandez-Borrell, J., Kinsky, S.C., Matsuura, E. and Leserman, L. (1988). **Biochim. Biophys. Acta** 946, 253-260.

147. Hou, X.P., Cui, D.H., Yi, Y.y., Li, X.Y. and Yang, L.P. (1990). **Yaxue Xuebao** 25, 854-858.

148. Hou, X.P., Ning, B., Li, X. and Tan, A. (1994). **Beijing Yike Daxue Xuebao** 26, 481-483.

149. Phillips, N.C., Moras, M.L., Chedid, L., Petit, J.F., Tenu, J.F., Lederer, E., Bernard, J.M. and Lefrancier, P.L. (1985). **J. Biol. Response Modif.** 4, 464-474.

150. Tilcock, C., Ahkong, Q.F., Koenig, S.H., Brown, R.D., Davis, M. and Kabalka, G. (1992). **Magn. Reson. Med.** 27, 44-51.

151. Wu, H.L. (1980). Ph.D. Thesis, Ohio State Univ., Columbus, OH, USA.

152. Lee, J.H., Shim, C.K., Lee, M.H. and Kim, S.K. (1988). **Drug Dev. Ind. Pharm.** 14, 451-463.

153. Müller, C.E. (1988). Synthese und eigenschaften chiraler amphiphile und liposomaler prodrugs mit unsymmetrischer substituierter disulfid brucke. Ph.D. Thesis, University of Tubingen, FRG.

154. Rosenmeyer, H., Ahlers, M., Schmidt, B. and Seela, F. (1985). **Angew Chem.** 97, 500-502.

155. Benameur, H., De-Gand, G., Brasseur, R., Van-Vooren, J.P. and Legros, F.J. (1993). **Int. J. Pharm.** 89, 157-167.

156. Charles, I. and Robinson, M. (1986). **US Patent** 4,567,034.

157. Tetsui, S., Kimura, S. and Imanishi, Y. (1992). **Proc. Jpn. Symp.** Leiden, The Netherlands, pp. 381-383.

158. Castelli, F., Giammoma, G., Puglisi, G., Carlisi, B. and Gurrieri, S. (1990). **Int. J. Pharm.** 59, 19-25.

159. Müller-Goymann, C.C. and Hamann, H.J. (1991). **Eur. J. Pharm. Biopharm.** 37, 113-117.

160. Jee, U.K., Park, M.S., Lee, G.W. and Lyu, Y.G. (1995). **Yakche Hakhoechi** 25, 249-264.

161. Ma, L., Ramachandran, C. and Weiner, N.D. (1991). **Int. J. Pharm.** 70, 209-218.

162. Cools, A.A. and Janssen, L.H.M. (1984). **Int. J. Pharm.** 20, 335-346.

3

LDL AS A CARRIER IN SITE SPECIFIC DRUG DELIVERY

R. S. R. MURTHY

Pharmacy Department, Faculty of Technology and Engineering,
M.S. University of Baroda, Vadodara 390 001.

INTRODUCTION

One of the major drawbacks in systemic drug therapy is the existence of side effect, which entails for a site specific drug delivery especially in pathological conditions such as cancer and severe viral infections. In some cases the chemical modification of drug can some how enhance the targetability however, most of the time a specific carrier is required that is designed for transport and delivery of the drug to its target tissue.

Recently, the possibility of using lipoproteins as drug carriers has attracted much attention due to their endogenous nature and capability to target onto the tissues rich in the lipoprotein receptor. Physiologically lipoproteins have been recognized as the cholesterol/fatty carriers through the vascular and extracellular fluid compartments of body. They are composed of a lipid component and a proteinaceous coat as their structural components. Structurally, the lipoproteins are consisted of a hydrophobic core comprised of triglycerides and esterified cholesterol solubilized by mono-molecular film of amphipathic phospholipid intervened with the free cholesterol and apolipoproteins with hydrophilic domains projected into aqueous phase [1] (Fig. 1). Being endogenous in origin they are almost non-immunogenic vis-à-vis comply the major requirements of the drug carrier.

CLASSIFICATION

Natural lipoproteins could be classified based on density (density gradient centrifugation), size (gel filtration), net surface charge (electrophoresis) and other surface properties (precipitation methods or affinity columns). However, commonly accepted classifications of lipoproteins is based on density wherein they could be categorized as very low density lipoproteins (VLDL), low density lipoproteins (LDL), intermediate density lipoproteins (IDL), high density lipoproteins (HDL). HDL particles are often separated into two subclasses i.e., HDL_2 and HDL_3. Chylomicrons are formed after fatty diet and have a density lower than 1.006 g/ml [2]. The characteristics of lipoproteins are listed in table I. and their biological fate is schematically presented in fig.1.

Table1. Physical characteristics of plasma lipoproteins

Class	Density in g/l	Electrophoretic mobility	Diameter (A°)
Chylomicron	0.95	--	800-10,000
VLDL	0.95-1.006	Per-β	300-800
IDL	1.006-1.020	Slow Per-β	250-350
LDL	1.020-1.063	β	180-220
HDL2	1.063-1.125	α	95-120
HDL3	1.125-1.210	α	55-95

* taken from Patsch & Gotto, 1987 [3]

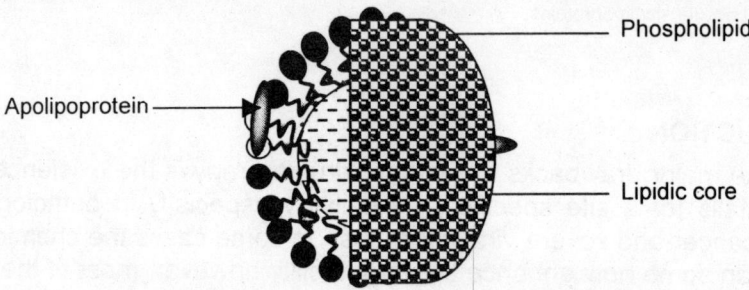

Fig. 1 : Schematic representation of the structure of Lipoprotein

CHYLOMICRONS

Chylomicrons are the originative lipoproteins, which are formed after ingestion of fatty diet/fat. Triglyceride lipids are first digested within the intestinal lumen via enterocytes and secreted into the intestinal lymphatics for the transport of fats [4,5]. Normally they are within the size range of 80-100 nm and have density less than 0.950 g/ml. The chylomicrons transverse through lymph and subsequently enter blood circulation via thoracic duct. During circulation, the triglyceride component of the particles is rapidly hydrolyzed by lipoproteins lipase, an enzyme present on surface of epithelial cells cells [6,7] which leads to the formation of chylomicron remnants a different class of lipoprotein enriched in cholesterol and apoprotein E [8,9]. The remnants are subsequently cleared from the systemic pool by liver involving receptor-mediated mechanism however, specific receptor proteins for their binding are yet to be identified.

VERY LOW DENSITY LIPOPROTEINS (VLDL)

VLDLs are colloidal particulates with size ranging from 30-90 nm. These are commonly synthesized by liver for translocation of fats to diverse sites in body. After secretion from liver, VLDLs are metabolized in the circulation via the hepatic remnant receptor uptake [10,11] and further catabolized via intermediate density lipoproteins (IDL) to low density lipoproteins.

LOW DENSITY LIPOPROTEINS (LDL)

Low-density lipoproteins (LDLs) have a density of 1.019-1.063 g/ml and consist of homogenous population of particles with 20-25 nm size that results from the catabolism of VLDL remnants. They consist of 1500 molecules of cholesteryl ester in the core whereas 800 molecules of phospholipid and 500 molecules of unesterified cholesterol. Each LDL particle consists of a single copy of apoprotein B-100 (5,14,000 Da). LDLs are slowly cleared from circulation (half-life in rats more than 4 h) [12] via specific LDL receptor that interacts through apoprotein apoprotein [13].

HIGH DENSITY LIPOPROTEINS (HDL)

HDL fraction of the serum consists of relatively small particulate of 8-12 nm diameter and relatively high density of 1.063-1.210 g/ml. The HDL particles are rich in cholesterol, protein and phospholipids content as compared to their relative counterparts. The metabolic fate of the HDL depends upon the apoprotein composition [14,15].

LOW DENSITY LIPOPROTEINS (LDL)

Low-density lipoproteins have attracted a major attention in drug delivery because of ease of their availability and better stability.

Formation of LDL

Very low-density lipoprotein remnants or intermediary density lipoproteins are largely removed from the plasma by LDL receptor of the liver where part of it is converted directly to LDL by an unknown mechanism. The crucial loss of VLDL is that of apo E, a process that has been ascribed to the action of hepatic LDL; thus the resulting LDL retains only the apo B-100.

The liver represents the major site of LDL removal from plasma by a predominantly receptor-mediated pathway [16,17]. The hepatic LDL receptor has a higher affinity for IDL than for LDL, which is due to high IDL content in apo E. The hepatocytes have additional recognition sites for LDL other than LDL receptor; they perform a less efficient endocytosis.

Low-density lipoprotein is also taken up by extrahepatic tissues, as a function of the rate of transcapillary transport and the LDL receptor activity on the surface of those cells. In addition, both in liver and extrahepatic tissues, receptor-independent endocytosis of LDL takes place at rates that vary with the organ. The receptor-independent pathway is especially prominent in the receptor-negative FH homozygotes and the WHHR, in which virtually all plasma LDL is degraded (in the liver and extrahepatic tissues) by a receptor-independent process. However, in normal conditions, in most species, including humans, the receptor-mediated clearance of plasma LDL in vivo amounts to 70-80% of the whole uptake [18-20] (Fig. 2).

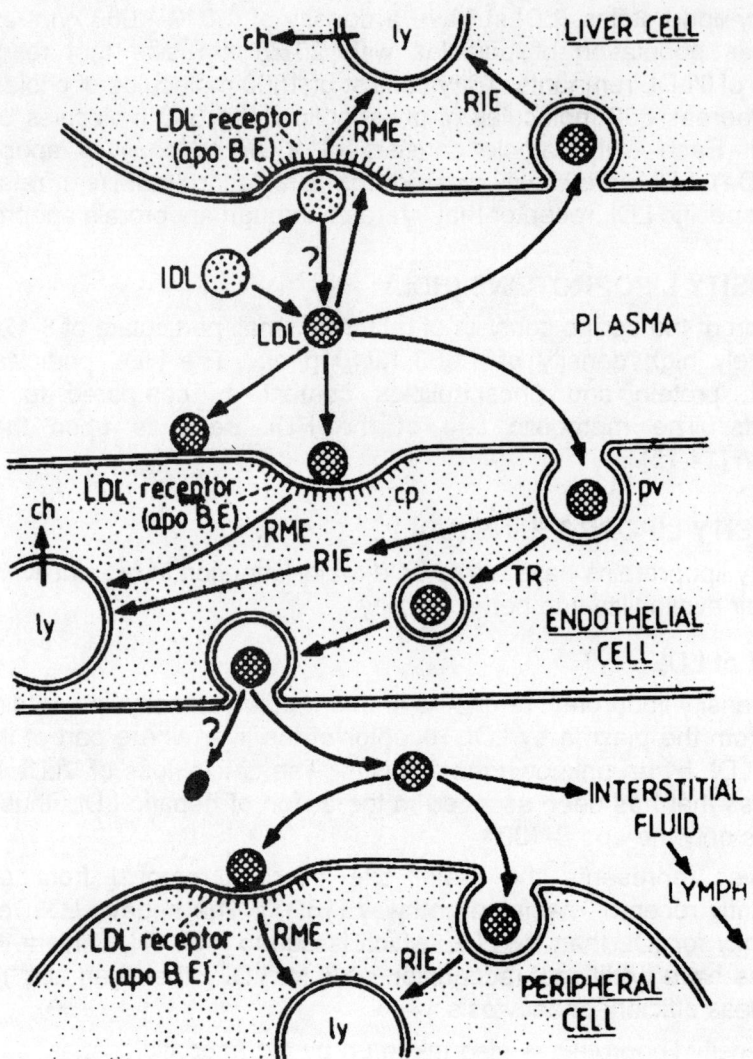

Fig. 2 : General metabolic pathways of LDL and their interaction with endothelium

Mechanism of LDL Transport

LDL are cleared from plasma by two basic pathways, i.e. receptor-mediated process and receptor independent process. Uptake of LDL by tissues may be mediated by LDL receptor (receptor-dependent transport) or by a less well understood process that is independent of the LDL receptor pathway (receptor-independent transport).

Receptor mediated uptake

Specific receptors that bind LDL were first described on the surface of cultured human fibroblasts and have subsequently been found on a variety of cell types. These receptors mediate the binding and internalization of lipoproteins containing apoB-100 or apoE. Following binding of LDL to its receptor, the LDL -receptor complex is incorporated into coated pits and internalized into endosomes [21]. Apparently, due to a drop in the pH of the endosome the LDL dissociates from its receptor.   The LDL is then delivered to the lysosomal compartment where it is completely degraded while LDL receptor is returned to the cell surface (Fig. 3). The entire cycle takes 10 to 20 minutes and continues whether or not ligand is present in the media.   The endosome containing LDL fuses with lysosome to form large secondary lysosome. ApoB protein is degraded to amino acids and cholesterol ester to fatty acid and cholesterol, liberated into cytosol [22].

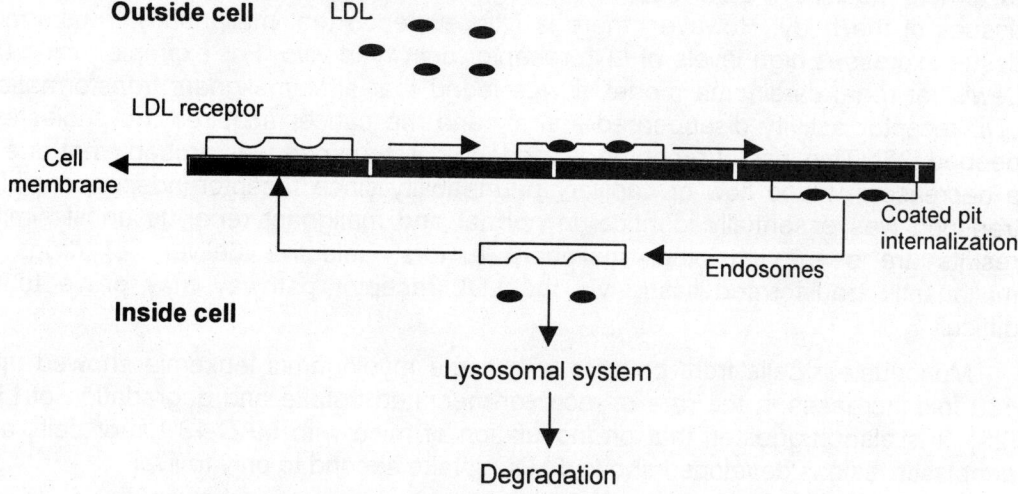

Fig. 3 : Fate of LDL particles and LDL receptor after endocytosis

Distribution of LDL receptor

Many tissues in the human body have a fewer LDL receptors probably due to high LDL blood level in humans compared to the other animal species except hamsters. For example tissues like CNS, heart, skeletal muscle and skin do not show significant receptor mediated LDL uptake. It has been found that in almost all the species highest level of LDL was detected in endocrine organs, liver, small intestine and spleen followed by some lower concentrations as detected in kidney, lungs, colon, heart and stomach. Absolutely no levels are detected in skeletal muscles, adipose tissue, skin and brain. After taking the weight consideration of the organ it was concluded that liver at large could be accounted for 60-80% of total clearance where a major part of accumulation is contributed by the receptor mediated uptake.

Tissues showing substantial LDL uptake include liver, endocrine glands, spleen and small intestine. Liver predominantly expresses and houses 75% of total body LDL receptor.

Moreover, the number of LDL receptors on many cells is not constant and can be up or down regulated. For instance with HepG2 cells pre incubation with HDL or lipoprotein depleted serum will increase the number of LDL receptor on the other hand pre incubation with LDL (high concentration) will down regulate LDL receptors [23].

Regulation of LDL receptor during malignancy

All cells of the body require at least some new cholesterol to support membrane synthesis and turnover. After malignant transformation, requirements for cholesterol may increase, especially during periods of rapid proliferation and growth of the tumor. In vivo, tumors derive cholesterol via two tightly regulated pathways, de novo synthesis and receptor-dependent LDL uptake [24].

Many cell lines derived from malignant tissue express LDL receptor activity in vitro [25]. Thus the possibility exists that chemotherapeutic agents could be delivered to tumors via LDL if LDL receptor activity in the tumor was high relative to other tissues of the body. However, there is little evidence that malignantly transformed tissue expresses high levels of LDL receptor activity in vivo. For example, using the Lewis rat renal carcinoma model, it was found that after malignant transformation, LDL receptor activity disappeared entirely and the cancer acquired the cholesterol needed [26]. This loss of receptor-dependent LDL transport was probably not due to a decrease in blood flow or capillary permeability since receptor-independent LDL transport was essentially identical in normal and malignant renal tissue. If similar results are seen with other malignant tumors, selective delivery of drugs to malignantly transformed tissue via the LDL receptor pathway may prove to be difficult.

Mononuclear cells from patients with acute myelogemic leukemia showed upto 100 fold increases in the rate of receptor-mediated uptake and degradation of LDL [25]. It is also suggested that on inoculation of mice with MAC-13 tumor cells and neoplastic lesions developed showed LDL uptake second to only to liver.

Receptor-independent process

More than two third of the LDL turnover is mediated by receptor dependent process, however, one third is accounted for by the involvement of receptor independent process [27]. The contribution of receptor-dependent and receptor independent process to total LDL turnover can be determined in normal individuals by comparing the turnover rates of native LDL and modified LDL to prevent recognition by LDL receptor [28]. This approach is rationalized on the basis that arginine and lysine residues of apoB are essential for binding of LDL to its receptor.

The techniques such as selective glucosylation, reductive methylation and treatment with cyclohexanedione, could most effective in eliminating receptor binding of LDL. Further these modified LDL particles are cleared from circulation. 20-35% portion is cleared more rapidly than the native LDL indicating that 65-80% of total LDL turnover is mediated by LDL receptors [29-31]. Utilizing the primed continuous infusion of methylated LDL, receptor independent LDL transport could be measured in several tissues. As is apparent, the high rates of LDL transport is mediated largely by LDL receptor (>90%). In contrast low rates of uptake in the larger tissue compartments such as skin, heart, skeletal muscles and fats could be accounted for the receptor independent process. Thus 80-90% of whole LDL is localized within the liver. Hence it could be appreciated that LDL could serve as an effective drug(s) carriers for targeting to and within the liver compartment.

LDL AS DRUG CARRIER

Being endogenous in nature the LDL could serve as efficient drug carrying modules for delivery of drugs to the selective sites expressing lipoprotein receptors in abundance. The major sites for targeting could be liver or tumor cells, which express high amount of lipoprotein receptors. The lipoproteins being endogenous in nature could serve as better carriers as compared to the others as they are non-immunogenic, biodegradable and occur as natural entities. The apolar pool of the lipoproteins comprising of triglycerides/cholesterol could serve for a reserve of the (pro)drug molecules as per the requisites for the site specific delivery. The lipoproteins are processed biologically by receptor mediated endocytosis hence it is expected that the drug molecule associated with the lipoproteins will figure a similar behavior, will get presented to the lysosomal enzymal system of the target cells. The advantages of LDL as the drug carriers include:

1. Being endogenous components it can avoid such typical carrier problem as immunological reaction and rapid plasma clearence due to uptake by reticuloendothelial cells.
2. Receptor-mediated endocytosis enables interacellular uptalke of the drug.
3. They are biodegardable in nature.
4. The small particle size avoids size related problems like lungs embodi and promotes diffusion to extravascular compartments
5. It provides a biocompatable vehicle for lipophilic drugs, which is of special importance if the drug is sensitive to decomposition.

On the other hand, lipoprotein have disadvantages as drug carrier:

1. Their complex and unstable nature.
2. Potential drug cytotoxicity to normal cells through defective targeting.

Choice of drug

Lipophilic drugs offer best potential for incorporation into the oily pool of the lipoproteins. Moreover, a pre-requisite for the entrapment of drug is that it should not disturb the normal recognition pattern of the lipoproteins. The amphipathic molecules on the other hand could be incorporated as they get arranged concomitantly in a polar pool as well as a polar phospholipid pool with the polar portion projected outside.

Many lipophilic drug molecules like porphyrin containing compounds, diphenyl-hydantoin, reserpine and estradiol have been successfully incorporated within the lipoproteins [32,33]. However, most of the drugs ought to be lipophilic, could be derivitized into their respective prodrugs by anchoring some lipophilic moieties. Oleyl, retinyl palmitoyl and cholesterol residues are most suitable for this purpose [34]. Furthermore, the conversion of the prodrug may lead to a loss in the activity of the drug molecules, hence, it is desirable to use the linkages which can be broken within the lysosomal compartment releasing active moiety. Ester and peptidic linkages are the most suitable for the purpose. If the original drug is desired to act pharmacodynamically at a diverse site(s) other than the lysosomes, then it is desirable that the drug should permeates across the membranes to reach the site of action. Moreover, the ionization, hydrophobicity and steric configuration may affect the penetration. Hence as a rule of thumb the molecules for entrapment into lipoproteins should be:

(a) Fairly hydrophobic
(b) Remain associated with the carrier throughout the shipment
(c) Derivatives should be easily degraded by the lysosomal compartment
(d) Incorporated drug should be sufficiently stable within the lysosomal compartment.

Model drug for LDL mediated tumor targeting is Cholesteryl oleate with the Nitrogen mustard attached to its D ring side chain.

$(CH_2)_3OCON(CH_2CH_2Cl)$

Oleoyl —— O

Structure of Cholesteryl oleate

Incorporation methods

Lipoprotein isolation: The initial step in the use of lipoproteins as drug carriers is to find a suitable method for preparation of lipoproteins. There is no problem for basic research, since there are many good routine methods available. When it comes to large-scale separation of lipoproteins for clinical use as drug carriers, however, more emphasis must be placed on simple and cheap, but still reproducible and pharmaceutically acceptable methods. One alternative is centrifugation, preferably single spin gradient or zonal ultra centrifugation. The precipitation methods in common clinical use could be another possibility. The methods based on use of polyethylene glycol 6000 or heparin should be gentle ones. A simple method, which, however, yields the lipoproteins in a diluted form, is gel filtration on agarose or corresponding gels. The use of plasmaphoaresis for the isolation of LDL and the preparation of drug-lipoprotein complex from the patients own LDL has also been proposed. Such a procedure might have the advantage of reducing the endogenous LDL level and hence the competition between LDL-drug complex and native LDL.

Solvent extraction: The first method for the reconstitution of biologically active LDL was presented by Krieger et al. (35). This so-called Krieger method used potato starch to stabilize an apo B-phospholipid complex. While the neutral lipid core was extracted with heptane and replaced with an exogenous cholesteryl ester. The reconstituted LDL retained its β mobility on agarose gel electrophoresis and its ability to be precipitated by an antibody to native LDL and by heparin-manganese. The Krieger method (Fig. 4) has been used to incorporate a variety of hydrophobic compounds into the core of LDL, including dioleyl methotrexate, 25-hydroxycholesteryl oleate, cholesteryl nitrogen mustard (phenesterine) and pyrene coupled to a derivative of cholesteryl oleate.

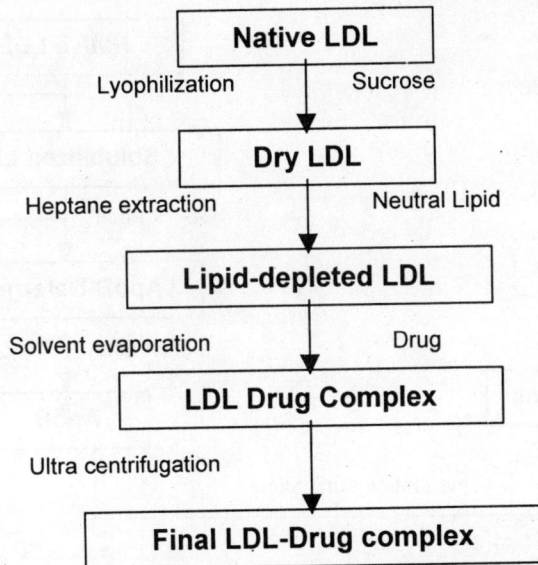

Fig. 4 :   Schematic representation of modified Krieger method for reconstitution of LDL

Detergent solubilization : Detergents can be used for the delipidation and solubilization or the water-insoluble apo B. The isolated apoprotein can then be used for reassembly of LDL with lipid (-drug) microemulsions. Such a method has been applied to the incorporation of cholesteryl oleate and a cytotoxic steroid mustard carbamate into the core of the reconstituted LDL particle. The procedures, schematically shown in figure 5, included solubilization of apo B from LDL with sodium deoxycholeate (SDOC), separation of apo B-SDOC complexes by gel filtration and then completion of the LDL reconstitution by association of the solubilized apo B with a neutral lipid (or drug)-EYPC microemulstion prepared by the injection-sonication method. By these procedures an optically clear preparation of reassembled LDL was obtained, which was stable as determined by density gradient ultracentrifugation and gel filtration. The LDL particles had a mean diameter of 21 nm and exhibited β migration at agarose electrophoresis. The in vivo cellular uptake and metabolization were found to be similar to that of native LDL.

Enzymatic digestion : Delipidation methods involving organic solvents or detergents involve a risk for changes in the protein structure. A presumably more gentle method uses enzymatic delipidemic of LDL. The cholesteryl ester core was hydrolyzed with sterol ester hydrolase in the presence of EYPC vesicles and albumin in order to bind the reaction products; free cholesterol and free fatty acids. The resulting apo B-polar lipid complexes were associated with a suspension of the lipophilic drug in buffer. After purification by centrifugation and filtration the cytotoxic activity of the LDL-drug complex was tested on cells in culture. It was demonstrated that the preparation was able to kill all the cells by uptake via the LDL receptor pathway. *In vivo* studies have not been performed.

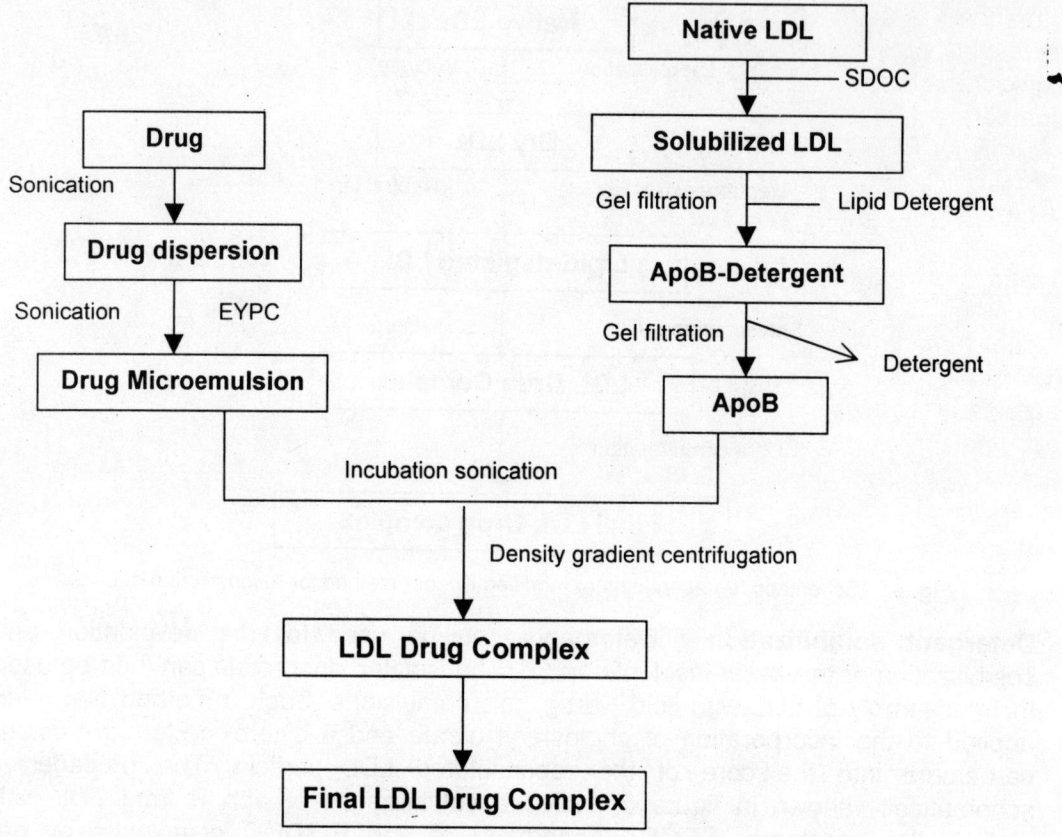

Fig. 5 : Schematic representation of detergent method for reconstitution of LDL

MODIFIED LDL

LDLs are extensively internalized by the LDL specific receptors up to 80-85%. The apoprotein fragments serve as the pilot molecules for determining their specific uptake. The uptake of LDL could be changed in turn directing the LDL to non-lipoprotein receptors by providing the surface with new recognition markers.

Lactosylated LDL

The asialoglucoprotein receptor located on parenchymal liver cells has been extensively studied [36]. Low-density lipoproteins could be easily derivatised with 200-250 lactose using lactose (D-galactosyl-D-glucose) in presence of sodium cyanoborohydride [37]. The latter reduces the Schiff's base between the glucose moiety of lactose and the amino group of lysine residues of the apoproteins and facilitates their covalent linkage [38]. The involvement of the galactose receptor in the uptake of lactosylated LDL has been evidenced by delivering an initial dose of N-acetyl galactosamine leading to decreased uptake of lipoprotein [39]. This receptor pathway has a high capacity transport system located almost exclusively on parenchymal cells of the liver, which mediates the binding, internalization and lysosomal catabolism of asialofetuin. The mechanism of uptake is however size dependent suggested by the higher uptake of lactosylated HDL as compared to lactosylated LDL [40]. Thus, LDL whose apo B has been extensively lactosylated could serve as vehicle for rapid and quantitative delivery of drugs to the lysosomal compartment of hepatocytes.

Acetylated low-density lipoproteins

When the apo B function is annihilated it will be possible to store drugs in LDL core while taking other routes than the conventional LDL pathway. LDL when placed with acetic anhydride leads to the modification of lysine residue of apoprotein, which results into more negatively charged particles, which are cleared by the scavenger receptors on hepatocytes [41]. The scavenger receptor is expressed on blood monocytes and macrophages derived from a variety of tissues as well as liver parenchymal cells. Moreover, the macrophages incubated with modified LDL may accumulate large amounts of cholesteryl ester and eventually assume the appearance of foam cells. In fact, when chemically modified LDL was administered to animals *in vivo* the vast majority was found to be cleared by endothelial cells of liver [42].

Tris-Gal-Chol anchored lipoproteins

Tris-gal-chol (tri antennary galactose terminated cholesterol derivative could be anchored onto the lipoproteins. This leads to their increased uptake by the parenchymal liver cells.

Structure of Tris Gal-chol

Tris-gal-cholesterol addition to LDL leads to immediate incorporation. The incorporation of Tris-gla-chol into LDL markedly increases serum clearance with a parallel quantitative recovery of the LDL in liver. The decay and clearance could however be blocked by a preinjection of N-acetylgalactosamine. Similar effects have been recorded with preinjection of asialofetuin suggesting asialoglycoprotein receptors on parenchymal cells are responsible for this uptake. Alternatively this system could serve as a strategem for selective delivery to the parenchymal cells of liver.

The ability to introduce chylomicron and derivatized VLDL into parenchymal cells, acetyl LDL into endothelial cells, Tris-gal-chol LDL into Kupffer cells and Tris-gal-chol into parenchymal cells suggest that in case of complex tissue based organs like liver targeting to target cell type could be possible. The quantitative levels of uptake may be enhanced or modulated via individual lipoprotein or through surface characteristic modification.

REFERENCES

1. Edelstein, C., Kezdy, F.J., Scanu, A.M. and Shen, B.W. (1979). **J. Lipid Res.** 20, 143-153

2. Havel, R.J., Goldstein, J.L. and Brown, M.S. (1980). Lipoprotein and lipid transport, In: Metabolic control of diseases (Bondy, P.K. and Rosenberg, L.E. Eds.), W.B. Saunders, Philadelphia, pp. 393-494

3. Patsch, J.R. and Gotto, A.M. (Jr) (1987). Metabolism of high density lipoproteins, In: Plasma lipoproteins (Gotto, A.M. (Jr) Ed.), Amsterdam, Elsevier, pp. 299-333.

4. Tso, P. (1985). **Adv. Lipid Res.** 21, 143.

5. Tso, P. and Balin, J.A. (1986). **Am. J. Physiol.** 250, G715.

6. Fielding, C.J. and Havel, R.J. (1977). **Arch. Pathol. Lab. Med.** 101, 225.

7. Bengtson, G. and Olivercrona T. (1980). **Eur. J. Biochem.** 106, 549.

8. Lakshman, M.R., Muesing, R.A. and LaRose J.C. (1981). **J. Biol. Chem.** 265, 3037.

9. Borenztan, J., Getz, G.S. and Kotlar, T.J. (1988). **J. Lipid Res.** 29, 1087.

10. Van Barkel, T.J.C., Kruijt, V.G. and VanTol, A. (1981). **Biochim. Biophys. Acta.** 665, 22.

11. VanTol, A. and Van Barkel, T.J.C. (1980). **Biochim. Biophy. Acta.** 619, 156.

12. Pittman, R.C, Attie, A.D., Carew, T.W. and Sterhberg, D. (1982). **Biochim. Biophys. Acta.** 710, 7.

13. Brown, M.S. and Goldstein, J.L. (1986). **Science** 232, 34.

14. Hamilton, R.L., Williams, M.C., Fielding, C.J. and Harvel, R.J. (1976) **J. Clin. Invest.** 58, 667.

15. Marsh, J. (1974). **J. Lipid Res.** 15, 544.

16. Brown, M.S. and Goldstein, J.L. (1984). **Science American** 251, 58.

17. Brown, M.S. and Goldstein J.L. (1985). **Ann NY Acad. Sci.** 454, 178.

18. Alderson, L.M., Endemann, G., Lindsey, S., Pronzcuk, A., Hoover, R.L. and Hayes, K.C. (1986). **Am J. Pathol.** 123, 334-342.

19. Spady, D.K., Bilheimer, D.W. and Dietschy, J.M. (1983). **Proc. Natl. Acad. Sci.** USA, 80, 3499-3503.

20. Spady, D.K., Turley, S.D. and Dietschy, J.M. (1985). **J. Clin. Invest.** 76, 1113-1122.

21. Brown, M. S. and Goldstein, J.L. (1974). **Proc. Natl. Acad. Sci.** USA, 71, 788.

22. Goldstein, J.L., Brown, M.S., Anderson, R.G.W., Russell, D.W. and Schneider, W.J. (1985). **Ann. Rev. Cell Biol.** 1, 1.

23. Harekes et. al., (1986). **Biochem. Biophys Acta** 875, 236.

24. Faust, J., Goldstein, J. L. and Brown, M.S. (1977). **J. Biol. Chem.** 252, 4861.

25. Ho, Y.K., Smith, G.S., Brown M.S. and Goldstein, J.L. (1978). **Blood**, 52, 1099.

26. Vitols, S., Gahrton, G., Ost, A. and Peterson, C.O. (1984). **Blood** 63, 1186.

27. Bilheimer, D.W., Stone, N.J. and Grundy, S.M. (1979). **J. Clin Invest.** 64, 524.

28. Shepherd, J., Bicker, S., Lorimer, A.R. and Packard, L.J. (1979). **J. Lipid Res.** 20, 999.

29. Spady, D.K., Bilheimer, D.W. and Dietschy, J.M. (1983). **Proc. Natl. Acad. Sci.** USA, 80, 3499.

30. Kesaniemi, Y.A., Witatum, J.L. and Steinbrecher, U.P. (1983). **J. Clin. Invest.** 71, 950.

31. Steinbrecher, U.P., Witztum, J.L., Kesaniemi, Y.A. and Elam, R.L. (1983). **J. Clin. Invest.** 71, 960.

32. Reyftmann, J.P., Morliere, P., Goldstein, S., Santus, R., Dubertret, L. and Lagrange, D. (1984). **Photochem. and Photobiol.** 6, 721.

33. Counsell, R.E. and Pohland, R.C. (1982). **J. Med. Chem.** 25, 1115.

34. Firestone, R.A., Pisano, J.M., Fakk, J.R., McPhaul, M.M. and Kreiger, M. (1984). **J. Med. Chem.** 27, 1037.

35. Krieger, M., Brown, M.S., Faust, J.R. and Goldstein, J.L. (1978). **J. Biol. Chem.** 253, 4093-4101.

36. Ashwell, G. and Morell, A.G. (1974). **Enzymol.** 41, 99.

37. Attie, A.D., Pittman, R.C. and Steinberg, D. (1980). **Proc. Natl. Acad. Sci.** USA, 77, 5923.

38. Gray, G.R. (1974). **Arch. Biochim. Biophys.** 163, 426.

39. Bijsterbosch, M.K., Ziere, G.J. and Van Barkel, T.J.C. (1989). **Mol. Pharmacol.** 36, 484.

40. Schipper-Schafter, J., Hulsmann, D., Dj Meyer, H.E., Herbertz, L., Kolb, H. and Kolb-Bachofen, V. (1986). **Exp. Cell Res.** 165, 494.

41. Pitas, R.E., Boyles, J., Mahley, R.W. and Montgomery, B.D. (1985). **J. Cell Biol.** 100, 103.

42. Blomhoff, R., Drevon, C.A., Eskild, W., Hilgerud, P., Norum, K.K. and Berg, T. (1984). **J. Biol. Chem.** 254, 1658.

4

FORMULATION ASPECTS OF LIPOSOMES

SANJAY K. JAIN

Department of Pharmaceutical Sciences,
Doctor Harisingh Gour Vishwavidyalaya,
Sagar (M.P.) 470 003 India.

- • Introduction
- • Basic components of liposomes
- • Physical structure of liposomes
- • Preparation of liposomes
- • Physical dispersion methods
- • Solvent dispersion methods

- • Detergent solubilization methods
- • Purification of liposomes
- • Characterization of liposomes
- • Stability of liposomes
- • Conclusion
- • References

INTRODUCTION

Liposomes have been widely considered as a potential drug delivery system since being first reported in 1965 by Bangham [1]. The accumulated evidence has confirmed their usefulness in avoiding some practical problems raised by the administration of different drugs. Thus, it has been reported that the toxicity of many therapeutic drugs can be significantly reduced when administered in conveniently designed liposomes [2,3]. In addition, adsorption [4,5], biodistribution and pharmaco-kinetics [6] of many drugs may be altered or improved by liposome encapsulation. Liposomes can be defined as simple microscopic vesicles in which an aqueous volume is entirely enclosed by a bilayered membrane composed of lipid molecule [1]. The drug molecules can either be encapsulated in aqueous space or intercalated into the lipid bilayers. The exact location of drug depends upon its physico-chemical characteristics and the composition of lipids [7,8].

BASIC COMPONENTS OF LIPOSOMES

There are number of structural and non-structural components of liposomes. Phospholipids and cholesterol are the major structural components amongst the various components of liposomes. Phospholipids vary in their purity, depending upon the manufacturer and the batch. Hence, it is essential to ascertain their purity before use either by TLC or HPLC. It is also reported that phospholipids are degraded if not stored properly. These phospholipids should be stored at -20° C in dark, under an inert gas e.g., N_2 or argon. The most common phospholipid used in the formulation of liposomes is phosphatidylcholine (PC) molecule. PC is an amphipathic molecule in which a glycerol bridge links a pair of hydrophobic acyl hydrocarbon chains, with a hydrophilic polar headgroup, phosphocholine [9]. Phosphatidylcholine is also known as "lecithin". It can be derived from natural and synthetic sources. PC is not soluble in water and in aqueous media. They align themselves closely in planar bilayer sheets in order to minimize the unfavorable action between the bulk aqueous phase and the long hydrocarbon fatty chain. Such interactions are completely eliminated when the sheet fold on themselves to form closed sealed vesicles. The lecithin membranes can exist in different phases. At elevated temperature lipid membrane passes from tightly ordered gel to a liquid crystal phase where freedom of movement of individual molecule is higher. As the temperature increases, the fatty acid chains tend to adopt conformation other than the all trans-straight chain configuration, such as Gauche conformation state (Fig. 1). This tends to expand the area occupied by the chains, and hence the membranes, at the same time as it reduces the overall length of hydrocarbon chains, giving rise to a decrease in bilayer thickness upon transition from gel to liquid crystalline phase. The transition from gel to liquid crystal does not occur in a single step for lecithin, but involves two transitions- the main transition and the pretransition, about 5° below the main transition, at which a change in head group orientation may occur. The heat of pretransition is very slow as compared with main transition. In the temperature range between the two transitions, the membrane adopts ruffled appearance in which it is transformed from a planar to an underlining surface with a fairly long regular periodicity.

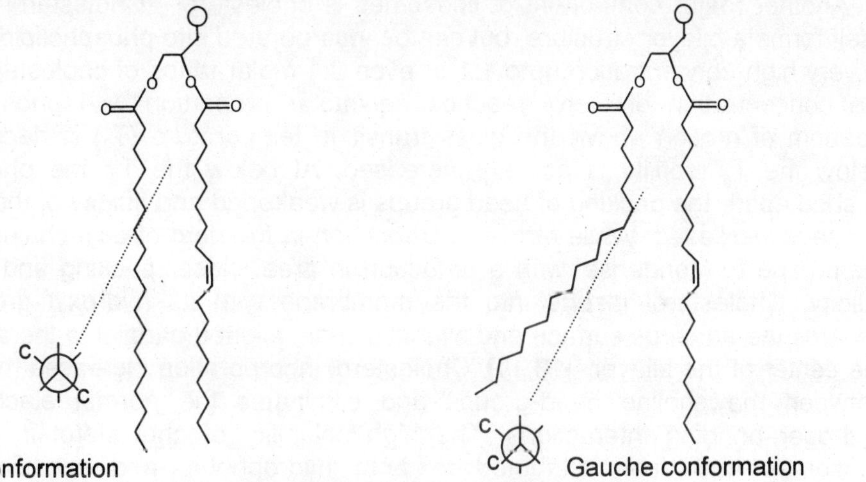

Trans conformation   Gauche conformation

Fig. 1: Disposition of phospholipid diacyl chains

Liposome membranes are semipermeable, in that the diffusion of molecules and ions across the membrane varies considerably for molecules with a high solubility in both organic and aqueous media. A phospholipid membrane clearly constitutes a very dense barrier; on the other hand, polar solutes such as glucose, and higher molecular weight compounds pass across membrane only very slowly. Smaller molecules with neutral charge (e.g. water and urea) can diffuse across quite rapidly, while charged ions differ greatly in their behavior. Proton and hydrogen ions cross the membrane fairly quickly, probably as a result of transfer of hydrogen bonds between the water molecules (water molecules are found as deep in the bilayer interior as the lower carbonyl group, so the distance to be bridged is considerably reduced). Sodium and potassium ions, on the other hand, traverse the membrane very slowly, not only with respect to protons, but also to anions such as chloride and nitrite.

Moreover, the diffusion of proteins and metal ions depends on phase transition temperature (Tc). The protein's permeabilities increase at Tc, and remain high as the temperature is increased whereas sodium ions (of other solutes) showed lower permeation at lower temperature and below the Tc. Thus, protons of water molecules whose transport is considerably faster than sodium ions have extra routes across the membrane which are qualitatively different, possibly in the form of water channels. This discussion refers to liposomes in which inner and the other outer aqueous compartments are in equilibrium with each other. Because, phospholipid membranes are semipermeable, however, a concentration gradient of solute between one side and side of the membrane can generate an osmotic pressure which will lead to accumulation of water molecules (being the faster diffusion species) on one side. In case of high concentration of solute entrapped inside liposomes, bathed in low concentration of buffer outside, the liposomes will swell up as the internal volume of water increases. This results in an accelerated leakage through the membrane for solutes of molecular size equivalent to or smaller than glucose. In some cases, pressure generated may be sufficient to rupture the membrane completely.

Another major component of liposomes is cholesterol. Cholesterol does not by itself forms a bilayer structure, but can be incorporated into phospholipid membranes in very high concentration upto 1:1 or even 2:1 molar ratios of cholesterol to PC. As the concentration of sterol reaches equimolar proportion with phospholipid, the freedom of motion above the glass transition temperature (T_g) is decreased while below the T_g motility is actually increased. At below the T_g, the phospholipid is pushed apart, the packing of head groups is weakened and fluidity of the ordered gel phase is increased. While above T_g, reduction in freedom of acyl chains causes the membrane to 'condense' with a reduction in area, closer packing and decrease in fluidity. Cholesterol inserts into the membrane with its hydroxyl group oriented towards the aqueous surface and aliphatic chain aligned parallel to the acyl chains in the center of the bilayer [10,11]. Cholesterol incorporation increases the separation between the choline head-groups and eliminates the normal electrostatic and hydrogen-bonding interactions. The high solubility of cholesterol in phospholipid liposomes has been attributed to both hydrophobic and specific headgroup interaction [12,13], but there is no unequivocal evidence for the arrangement of cholesterol in the bilayer. Cholesterol has relatively little effect on the position of the phase transition but can abolish completely the heat of transitions.

Non-structural components (lipophilic/hydrophilic/amphiphilic) can be accommo-dated at a concentration range of 1-10% w/w without serious disruption of basic bilayer structure. On incorporating these non-structural components, the membrane integrity (fluidity or permeability) may well be altered. These components are easily incorporated by physical means.

PHYSICAL STRUCTURE OF LIPOSOMES

Generally, the chemical constituents incorporated into liposomes will affect the membrane fluidity, charge, density and permeability of liposomes. The liposomes are characterized by size and shape. Liposomes are composed of simple bilayer membrane lamellae. Liposomes of different sizes require completely different method of preparation. The different applications of liposomes demand the use of liposomes within a particular size range. On the basis of size and shape, the liposomes are classified as:

- Multilamellar vesicle (MLVs): They have a size range of 100-1000 nm and consist of five or more concentric lamellae. Vesicles, which are composed of just few concentric lamellae are called oligo-lamellar vesicles.
- Small uni-lamellar vesicles (SUVs): They are lower sized liposomes. The size limit depends on ionic strength of aqueous media and lipid composition. Pure lecithin in normal saline produces unilamellar liposomes of 15-nm size.
- Large unilamellar vesicles (LUVs): These vesicles are approximately 1000 nm in size with single lamellae.
- Intermediate size unilamellar vesicles (ULVs): They are having 100-nm size.
  - ➢ REVs- Reverse phase evaporation vesicles
  - ➢ DRVs- Dried reconstituted vesicles

PREPARATION OF LIPOSOMES

Before discussing the different methods of preparation, it is necessary to understand the handling of liposomes.

Handling of liposomes

Generally, liposomes have a standard composition egg lecithin:cholesterol: phosphatidyl glycerol in molar ratio of 0.9:1.0:0.1. These lipids are oxidized if not stored or handled properly. Therefore, it is advised to store these lipids either as solids, or in organic solution at -20°C or at -70°C. All lipid solutions should be stored in dark, in glass vessels with a securely fastened ground glass stopper. Polypropylene containers may also be used, although it is difficult to find caps, which fasten tightly enough to prevent evaporation of the solvents, which can take place even under refrigeration. Inert rubber (e.g. neoprene) can be used as a seal, but it does not tend to swell in chloroform. In order to reduce the possibility of oxidation of lipids, nitrogen is most commonly used. Since nitrogen is lighter than air, yet, a strong flow of gas is needed to ensure complete exchange with air. The use of argon gas is preferable since this is heavier than air and forms an effective blanket with just a very gentle stream of gas. These lipids are easily soluble in a mixture of chloroform and methanol in a volume ratio of 2:1. Compounds, which are sparingly soluble in either chloroform or methanol alone, will often dissolve readily in 2:1 solvent mixture. Solvents used to dissolve these lipids should be of high purity because some contamination may be chemically reactive and cause the lipids to deteriorate. Ether degrades over time to form peroxides, while chloroform gives rise to phosgene on standing. Formation of the latter can be prevented by addition of 1% ethanol to stabilize the chloroform and most commercial sources of chloroform are sold in this form.

Methods of preparations

Generally, all the methods of liposome preparation involve three or four basic stages

(Fig. 2). These include (i) Drying down lipids from organic solvent, (ii) Dispersion of lipids in aqueous media, (iii) Purification of resultant liposomes, and (iv) Analysis of the final product.

Large volume of organic solution of lipids is most easily dried in a rotary evaporator fitted with a cooling coil and a thermostatically controlled water bath. Rapid evaporation of solvent is carried out by gentle warming (20-40°C) under reduced pressure (400 -700 mm Hg). Rapid rotation of the solvent-containing flask increases the surface area for evaporation.

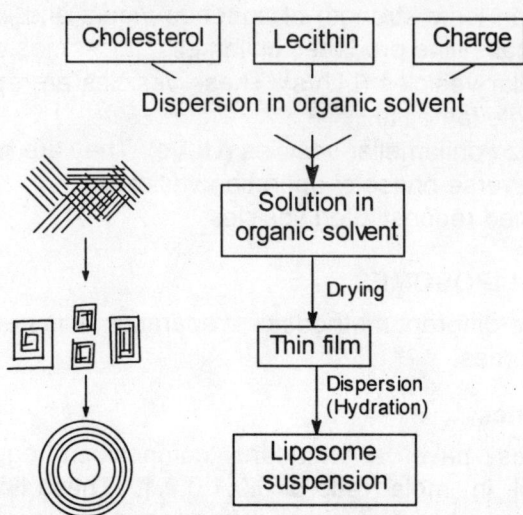

Fig. 2 : Common stages involved in various methods of liposome preparation

In cases where sufficient vacuum is not attainable or if the concentration of lipids is particularly high, it may be difficult to remove the last traces of chloroform from the lipid film. Therefore, it is recommended as a matter of routine that after rotary evaporation some further means be employed to bring the residue to complete dryness. Attachment of the flask to the manifold of lyophilizer, and overnight exposure to high vacuum is a good method.

The methods of liposome preparations have been classified according to the three basic modes of dispersion (Fig. 3).

- Physical dispersion methods
- Solvent dispersion methods
- Detergent solubilization methods

PHYSICAL DISPERSION METHODS

In this method the aqueous volume enclosed within the lipid membrane is usually 5-10%, which is a very small proportion of the total volume used for swelling. Therefore, large amounts of water-soluble compounds are wasted during swelling. On the other hand, lipid soluble compounds can be encapsulated to 100% efficiency, provided they are not present in quantities, which overwhelm the structural component of the membrane.

There are four basic methods of physical dispersion, i.e. hand shaking, non-shaking, freeze dry and proliposomes.

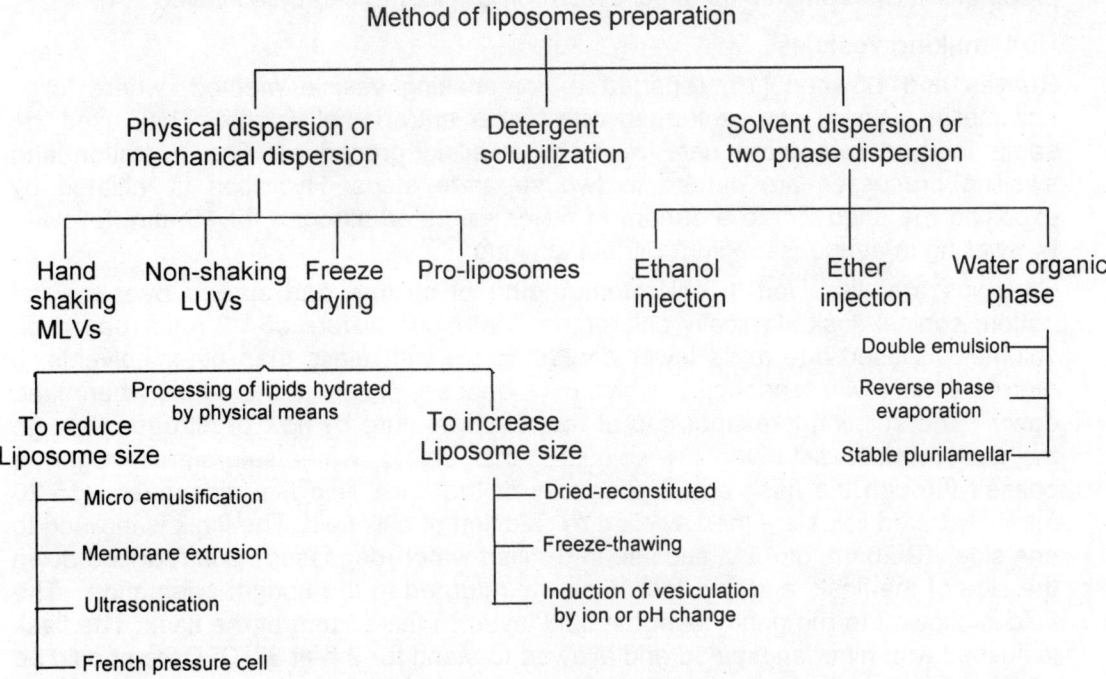

Fig. 3 : Classification of methods of liposome preparation

Hand-shaken multilamellar vesicles (MLVs)

This is a simplest and most widely used method of physical dispersion were the lipid mixture of different phospholipids and charge components are dissolved first in chloroform: methanol solvent mixture (2:1 v/v) in a 250mL round bottom flask. Then, the solvent was evaporated using a rotary evaporator, at about 30°C or above the transition temperature of the used lipids. The rotation is continued for 15 minutes after the dry residue first appears. Subsequently, the nitrogen is introduced into the evaporator and the pressure at the cylinder head is gradually raised until there is no pressure difference between inside and outside of the flask. The flask is removed from the evaporator and fixed on to the manifold of lyophilizer to remove residual solvents. After releasing the vacuum and removal from the lyophilizer, the flask is flushed with nitrogen and then 5 mL of saline phosphate buffer (containing solute to be entrapped) is added. The flask is rotated again at room temperature and pressure at the same speed or below 60rpm. The flask is left rotating for 30 minutes or until all lipids have been removed from the wall of the flask and have turned into a homogeneous milky-white dispersion free of visible particles. The dispersion is allowed to stand for another 2 h at room temperature or at a temperature above t_g of the lipid in order to complete swelling.

The MLVs of entirely neutral lipids tend to pack tightly in the form of, multilayer assemblies with very little aqueous space between them. The presence of negatively charged lipids in the membrane repels the bilayers apart from each other, and increases the volume of aqueous domain significantly. The same effect can be achieved with neutral lipid by freezing and thawing repeatedly the final liposome preparation. Entrapments up to 30% (at 100mg lipid/mL) can be achieved [14].

Non-shaking vesicles

Reeves and Dowben [15] reported a non-shaking vesicle method, where large unilamellar vesicles can be formed with higher entrapment volume. They used the same method with more care over the swelling procedure. The hydration and swelling processes are carried in two separate steps. Hydration is initiated by exposing the dried film to a stream of water saturated nitrogen for 15 min, followed by swelling in aqueous medium without shaking.

Lipids are dissolved in chloroform:methanol mixture and spread over the flat bottom conical flask. Typically chloroform: methanol mixture of 1:2 ratio (based on volumes) is used due to its lower contact angle with glass than other solvents. It therefore has fewer tendencies to give thick deposits of lipid at the edges when dried down. The solution is evaporated at room temperature by flow of nitrogen through the flask without disturbing the solution. After drying, water saturated nitrogen is passed through the flask until the opacity of the dried lipid film disappears (15-20 min). Hydrated lipids are then swelled by addition of bulk fluid. The flask is inclined to one side, 10-20 mL of 0.2M sucrose in distilled water (degassed) is introduced down the side of the flask, and the flask is slowly returned to the upright orientation. The fluid is allowed to run gently over the lipid layer on the bottom of the flask. The flask is flushed with nitrogen, sealed and allowed to stand for 2 h at 37°C. Care should be taken not to knock the flask or agitate the medium in any way during this period. After swelling, the vesicles are harvested by swirling the contents of the flask gently, to yield a milky-dispersion. The dispersion is centrifuged at 12,000g for 10 min at room temperature. The layer of multilamellar vesicles floating on the surface is removed. To the remaining fluid, an equal volume of iso-osmomolar glucose is added and centrifuged again at 12,000g. Large unilamellar vesicles form a soft pellet, which can be resuspended in any required medium of an appropriate osmolarity.

Further, this method was modified by Lasic et al. [16], where thin film of lipid is casted on a finely-etched silicon wafer because the total area of wafers is much greater than an ordinary flat surface. In addition, irregular surfaces with many different angles and planes encourage the lipid to break up into small sheets upon hydration, which may help to define the size of the final liposome.

Pro-liposomes

Pro-liposome method, increase the surface area of dried lipid film by drying the lipid over a finely divided particulate support, such as powdered sodium chloride, or sorbitol or other polysaccharide [17]. These dried lipid coated particulates are called pro-liposomes. Pro-liposomes form dispersion of MLVs on adding water into it, where support is rapidly dissolved and lipid film forms MLVs. The size of the carrier influences the size and heterogeneity of the liposomes. This method also overcomes the stability problems of liposomes encountered during their storage in liquid, dry or frozen form. It is ideally suited for preparations where the material to be entrapped incorporates into lipid membrane. In cases where 100% entrapment of aqueous components is not essential, this method is also of value.

A Buchi rotary evaporator 'R' with water-cooled condenser coil and a stainless steel covered thermocouple connected to a digital thermometer is used to prepare pro-liposomes. The end of the glass solvent inlet tube is modified to a fine point, so that the solvent is introduced into the flask as a fine spray.

The sorbitol powder is introduced into 100mL flask and flask is fitted into the evaporator. The flask is rotated slowly so that the powder tumbles gently off the walls to ensure good mixing. The flask is lowered into a water bath at 50-55°C when a good vacuum has developed (around 100 KPa). An aliquot of 5 mL of lipid solution (60mg/ml in chloroform) is introduced into the flask via the solvent inlet tube. The solvent is absorbed completely by the powder and the temperature of the bed is monitored. As evaporation proceeds, the temperature decreases. A second aliquot is then introduced slowly, when the temperature begins to rise again. The temperature is allowed to rise to 30°C, the vacuum is released and the drying process is completed by connecting the flask containing the powder to lyophilizer, and leaving it evacuated overnight at room temperature. The powder is transferred into a 10mL glass vial containing 600mg solid (100mg lipid and 500mg sorbitol) flushed with nitrogen, sealed well and stored.

For use, introduce 10mL of distilled water into one vial and mix on a whirl mixer for 30 sec or in a shaking water bath above the lipid phase transition temperature. This will give a 5% w/v solution of sorbitol (isotonic with normal saline) and a lipid concentration of 10mg/mL. Care must be taken not to allow temperature rise too high if working with low melting temperature lipids (e.g. egg PC) otherwise agglomeration of powder particles may result.

Freeze-drying

Freeze drying is another method of dispersing the lipid in a finely divided form where lipids dissolved in suitable solvent is freeze dried prior to addition of aqueous media [18]. The solvent choice depends on the freeze point which needs to be above the temperature of the condenser of the freeze dryer, and its inertness with regard to rubber seals which form a part of most commercial lyophilizers. From this point of view tertiary-butanol is considered to be the most suitable solvent. After obtaining the dry lipid, which is expanded foam like structure, water or saline can be added with rapid mixing above the phase transition temperature to give MLVs.

Processing of lipids hydrated by physical means

MLVs prepared by hydration of dried lipids are further processed in order to modify the size and other characteristics of liposomes. There are two sets of methods used to modify the size of MLVs. In general, MLVs are too large or too heterogeneous hence a number of methods have been devised to reduce their size. These include techniques such as microencapsulation, extrusion, ultrasonication and use of French pressure cell. Another set of methods involve MLVs size enlargement by increasing the entrapment volume of hydrated lipids, or breaking the lamellarity of the vesicles employing procedures such as freeze drying, freeze thawing, or induction of vesiculation by ions or pH change.

Micro emulsification liposomes (MEL)

"Micro fluidizer" is used to prepare small MLVs from concentrated lipid dispersion [19]. Microfluidizer pumps the fluid at very high pressure (10,000psi, 600-700bar) through a 5 um orifice. Then, it is forced along defined micro channels, which direct two streams of fluid to collide together at right angles at a very high velocity, thereby effecting a very efficient transfer of energy. The lipids can be introduced into the fluidizer, either as a dispersion of large MLVs, or as slurry of unhydrated lipid in an organic medium. The fluid collected can be recycled through the pump and interaction chamber until vesicles of the spherical dimension are obtained.

After a single pass, the size of vesicles is reduced to a size 0.1 and 0.2 mm in diameter. The exact size distribution depends on the nature of the components of the membrane and hydration medium. The presence of negative lipids tend to decrease their size, while increasing cholesterol concentration gives larger liposomes.

In addition to the high rate of production, this method has the advantages of being able to process samples with a very high proportion of lipid (20% or more by weight). This process is very efficient for encapsulation of water-soluble materials. Percentage capture values up to 70% have been reported, starting with lipid concentration of approximately 200mg/mL.

Sonicated unilamellar vesicles (SUVs)

This method reduces the vesicles size utilizes energy at a high level. This was first achieved by exposure of MLVs to ultrasonic irradiation [20-22] and is still remains the method most widely used for producing small vesicles. There are two methods of sonication, which essentially use either a probe or a bath ultrasonic disintegrator. The probe is employed for dispersions which require high energy in a small volume (e.g. high concentration of lipids, or a viscous aqueous phase) while the bath is more suitable for large volumes of diluted lipids, where it may not be necessary to reach the vesicle size limit [22,23]. Probe sonication has the disadvantage of contaminating the preparation with metal from the tip of the probe and if one is not careful, it can lead to degradation of lipid [23].

SUVs are purified by centrifugation method devised by Barenholtz et al., [24]. Liposome dispersion after sonication is placed in a clear plastic walled ultracentrifuge tube. The dispersion is centrifuged at 100,000g for 30 min at 20°C to sediment titanium particles and large MLVs followed by higher speed centrifugation at 1,59,000g for 3-4 h. After spinning, the tube is carefully removed from the rotor and with the help of a Pasteur pipette, the liquid with top clear layer is decanted leaving the central opalescent layer (containing small multilamellar vesicles) and the pellet behind. The top layer constitutes pure dispersion of SUVs having radius 105Å.

French Pressure Cell Liposomes

The ultrasonic radiation degrades not only the lipids but also macromolecules and other sensitive compounds to be entrapped inside the liposomes. One of the first and still very useful method developed is extrusion of preformed large liposomes in a french press under very high pressure [25,26]. This technique yields rather uni- or oligo- lamellar liposomes of intermediate size (30-80nm in diameter depending on the applied pressure). These liposomes are more stable as compared to sonicated liposomes. One of the few drawbacks of this technique is the high initial cost of purchase an entire new system, which consists of an electric hydraulic press and pressure cell.

The heart of french press is pressure cell, manufactured in stainless steel and designed to resist up to 20,000 or even 40,000psi. Two pressure cells of different size are available. The large one holds up to 40mL (the operational minimum is approximately 40mL) while the smaller one is the cell of choice and may hold <4mL volume. The pressure cell is comprised of the body, containing a precision bored cylindrical cavity (the pressure chamber) with small outlet orifice (valve), a bottom seal, a piston, valve closure and outlet tubing. The bottom seal and piston are fitted each with the different 'O' rings, to ensure a tight seal even at very high pressures. The valve closure will close the outlet orifice with the aid of a plastic ball placed in a groove at its tip (Fig. 4).

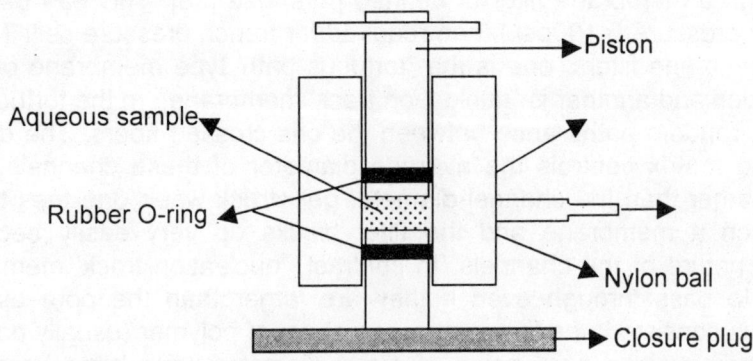

Fig. 4 : French pressure cell

Liposome (or cell) dispersion is filled into the pressure chamber, the piston is inserted a short distance into the body and the cell is turned upside down. The liquid sample is introduced into the cavity. The height of the piston is adjusted by pressing down on the outer wall of the cell, so that the chamber is completely filled with liquid. It should be ensured that the chamber is filled right up to the outlet hole. It is important to fill the chamber up to the hole in order to prevent compression of trapped air, which will result in uncontrollable splashing during extrusion. Upon filling the chamber, the bottom seal is inserted, and with the pressure cell still held upside down, it is closed gently but firmly, and turned to an upright position. Following insertion of the pressure cell into the hydraulic press, proper gear is selected and power is switched on. The pressure inside the chamber is adjusted by manually selecting the appropriate setting of the hydraulic press. Once this pressure is reached inside the cell, the valve closure is released very gently, so as to create a pressure gradient across the outer orifice. The outflow is collected in a suitable container. The flow rate will be about 0.5-1.0 mL/min

It applies a tremendous shear force at the orifice, which is sufficient to disrupt multilamellar liposomes mechanically. At higher force, the smaller liposomal fragments are formed and these fragments form liposomes spontaneously due to hydrophobic interactions. The homogeneity of the resulting liposome dispersion is inversely proportional to the flow rate through the orifice. The chances of disruption of liposomes passing though the orifice are better at the slower flow rate. Therefore, it is imperative to open the valve very carefully and let the contents bleed out very slowly drop by drop.

The size of the resulting french-pressed liposomes (FPL) is variable, depending on the lipid composition, the temperature and most important, on the pressure [27]. The liposomes prepared by this technique are less likely to suffer from the structural defects and instabilities known to arise in sonicated vesicles. Leakage of vesicle contents from liposomes prepared using french press has been found to be slower than from sonicated liposome. French press has also been used to reduce the heterogeneity of populations of proteo-liposomes obtained by detergent dialysis technique.

Membrane extrusion liposomes

In membrane extrusion method, the size of liposomes is reduced by gently passing them through a membrane filter of defined pore size [28]. This can be achieved at much lower pressure (<100psi.) than required for french pressure cell. There are two types of membrane filters, one is the `tortuous path' type membrane often used for sterile filtration and another is `nucleation track' membrane. In the tortuous path type membrane, random paths arise between the cris crossed fibers. The density of the fibers in the matrix controls the average diameter of these channels. Liposomes, which are larger than the channel diameter get struck when one tries to pass them through such a membrane and the filter blocks up very easily because of the convoluted nature of the channels. In contrast, 'nucleation track' membrane allows liposomes to pass through even if they are larger than the pore diameter. This membrane is consisted of a thin continuous sheet of polymer (usually polycarbonate) in which straight-sided pore holes of exact diameter have been bored through a combination of laser and chemical etching. As the pores go straight through one side to the other, they offer much less resistance to material that is passing through than does tortuous path membrane. The inherent flexibility of phospholipid lamellae enables liposome to change their conformation so that they can squeeze through the pores. However, liposomes, which are much larger than the pore size are broken up in the process, and emerge from the membrane pore smaller than before. After several passes through the membrane population of liposomes will be reduced in size to an average diameter somewhat smaller than the membrane pore diameter, but with a small proportion still slightly larger than the pores having managed to squeeze through without breaking up. The apparatus used for extrusion is the same as that employed for other membrane filtration applications [29].

The integrity testing of assembled unit with regards to defective membrane or leaking in the cell is carried out by a `bubble point test'. After testing the integrity of the membrane, the liposome dispersion is filled into the cell and pressure taken quickly upto 100 psi in order to trace the liposomes through the membrane. The membrane extrusion technique can be used to process LUVs as well as MLVs. In this process, the vesicle contents are exchanged with the dispersion medium during breaking and resealing of phospholipid bilayers as they pass through the polycarbonate membrane. In order to achieve high entrapment, the water-soluble compounds should be present in suspending medium during the extrusion process. The material, which is not entrapped can be removed subsequently. The liposomes produced by this technique have been termed LUVETs by their originator [30]. The 30% capture volume can be obtained using high lipid concentration (300mM PC). The trapped volume in this process is 1-2 L/mol. of lipids.

A new continuous high-pressure extrusion apparatus for generation of liposomes was designed by Schneider and co-workers [31]. The extruder basically consisted of an open supply vessel and a high-pressure filter holder mounted on a gas-driven pump, which exhibited superior performance compared to currently available, discontinuous extrusion devices. Due to continuous flow upto 500 mL/min (filter diameter 47 mm), large batches on a liter scale could be extruded in one step. The maximum pressure employed is 10.5 Mpa, which enables the rapid passage of liposomal preparations with various lipid composition at lipid concentration as high as 400 mg/g, through polycarbonate membrane without any clogging of the system. Further, it is suggested that large volume of stable, contrast-carrying liposomes with increased encapsulation efficiencies may be obtained by this method [32].

Dried-reconstituted vesicles (DRVs)

The solid lipids are dispersed in finely divided form using freeze drying technique before contact with the aqueous fluid, which will form medium for the final dispersion. Freeze-drying has again been used but this time, a dispersion of empty SUVs is frozen and lyophilized instead of drying the lipids from an organic solution [33]. Thus, in contrast to the preparation dried from solvent, SUVs dried lipid is already very highly organized into membrane structure, which on addition of water can rehydrate, fuse and reseal to form vesicles with a high capture efficiency. The water-soluble materials to be entrapped are added to the dispersion of empty SUVs and they are dried together, so the material for inclusion is present in the dried precursor lipid before the final step of addition of aqueous medium.

Liposomes obtained by this method are usually uni- or oligo- lamellar of the order of one micron or less in diameter. Entrapment yield can vary, but 40% is fairly standard compared with 2-10% for MLVs prepared by hand-shaking method.

Freeze thaw sonication (FTS)

The DRV method is a variant of an earlier one developed by Pick [34] after Kasahara & Hinckle [35] in which the entrapped material is again introduced into liposomes after they have been formed. A freezing and thawing process is used to rupture and re-fuse SUVs during which the solute equilibrates between inside and outside, and the liposomes themselves fuse and increase markedly in size. The entrapment volume can rise to 30% of the total volume of the dispersion (10μL/mg phospho-lipids). The starting preparation of empty liposomes is made by sonication and after thawing, the liposomes are subjected to brief sonication again. The second step sonication considerably reduces the permeability of the liposome membrane, perhaps by accelerating the rate at which packing defects are eliminated.

The FTS method has several disadvantages compared to DRVs in terms of encapsulation efficiency. It is not possible to prepare neutral liposomes composed of purified phosphatidylcholines. It may be because the presence of charge is required for the formation of ice crystals to aid in the rupture/fusion process. Similarly, sucrose (a cryo-protectant), divalent metal ions (which can neutralize the surface charge) and high ionic strength salt solutions cannot be entrapped efficiently. Nevertheless, the method is simple, rapid and mild for entrapped solutes, and results in a high proportion of large unilamellar vesicles, which are useful for study of membrane transport phenomenon.

In this method, the organic solution of lipids is dried in pyrex test tube under a stream of nitrogen, then redissolved in diethyl ether and again dried with nitrogen stream to remove traces of chloroform. The buffer solution is added to the dried lipids in the tube. The gas space is flushed with nitrogen and the top of the tube is covered with parafilm. The tube is vortexed for about 10 min until a homogeneous milky-dispersion is obtained. This sealed tube is transferred into a sonicator bath and held in a vertical position with a clamp, so that fluid levels inside and outside of the tube are equal. The dispersion is continuously sonicated for 10-15 min at room temperature until partial clarification is obtained. After sonication, the materials to be entrapped, are added either in solid form or as a small aliquot of concentrated solution and then mixed well. The tube is flushed with nitrogen, sealed and the dispersion is frozen rapidly by shaking in a bath of liquid nitrogen. After complete freezing, the tube is removed from the bath and allowed to thaw by standing at room temperature. It is sonicated again for no longer than 30 sec at room temperature. Column chromatography or centrifugation separates the unentrapped material.

The freeze thaw technique has been extended by Oku & MacDonald [36] to incorporate a dialysis step against hypo-osmolar buffer in place of final sonication. In this case, SUVs are first mixed with salt solution at concentration of several molar, followed by freeze thawing several times. During subsequent dialysis the large vesicles formed by freeze thawing swell and rupture as a result of osmotic lysis whereupon they fuse with each other to yield a large number of giant vesicles of diameter between 10 and 50 μm. The inclusion of some negatively charged lipids gives rather higher trapped volume (20μL/mg as compared to 10μL/mg for neutral phospholipids).

pH induced vesiculation

This method is contributed by Hauser & Gains [37] wherein ULVs are prepared from MLVs without sonification or high-pressure application. They are reassembled by a change in the pH. This process is called as "pH induced vesiculation", which is an electrostatic phenomenon. The transient change in pH brings about an increase in the surface charge density of the lipid bilayer, which induced spontaneous vesiculation.

The phospholipids are exposed to high pH for less than 2 min. The exposure time should not be long enough to cause detectable degradation of the phospholipid. As in the conventional MLVs, the materials that are to be entrapped inside the vesicles may be added in the water before addition to the lipid. The dispersion is completed by subjecting the dispersion to nearly six freeze thawing cycles between 15°C (ice/methanol) and 5°C. The pH of the dispersion will be 2.5-3. Sodium hydroxide solution (1M) is then added rapidly with mixing into the dispersion then the pH is reduced by addition of 0.1M HCl until a value of pH 7.5 is achieved.

Phospholipid dispersion with similar properties is obtained if concentrated NaOH solution is added directly to the dry lipid film to give dispersion without freeze thawing. The resultant dispersion consists of a relatively homogeneous population of SUVs with an average outer diameter of 20-60nm [37].

Calcium Induced Fusion

Calcium induced fusion method was developed by Papahadjopoulos et al. [38,39]. Papahadjopoulos & Vail [40] used the concept of aggregation and fusion of acid phospholipid vesicles in the presence of calcium. In this method, lipid is dried down and suspended in sonication buffer (NaCl 0.385g, histidine 31.0 mg, Tris-base 24.2 mg, EDTA 3.72 mg, water 100 mL, pH 7.4) and sonicated to prepare small liposomes. The large liposomes and lipid particles are removed by centrifugation at 100,000g. Equimolar proportion of calcium solution is added to phospholipids in the supernatant. A white flocculent precipitate is formed. It is incubated for 60 min at 37^0 C and the precipitate is separated using spinning container at 3000g for 20 min at room temperature and the supernatant is discarded. The pellet is resuspended in a buffered saline containing the material to be entrapped, and incubated at 37°C for 10 min The EDTA (170 mM) is added in buffer with mixing. A cloudy dispersion clears rapidly, which is incubated for 15 min at 37°C and further 15 min at room temperature. Finally, the Ca/EDTA complex is removed by dialysing the dispersion overnight against a litre of phosphate saline buffer.

SOLVENT DISPERSION METHODS

In solvent dispersion method, lipids are first dissolved in an organic solution, which is then brought into contact with an aqueous phase containing materials to be entrapped within the liposome. The lipids align themselves at the interface of organic and aqueous phase forming monolayer of phospholipids. Methods employing solvent dispersion fall into one of three categories.

- The organic solvent is miscible with the aqueous phase.
- The organic solvent is immiscible with the aqueous phase, the latter being in large excess.
- Organic solvent is in large excess, and is again immiscible with the aqueous phase.

Ethanol injection

This method was reported by Batzri & Korn [41]. An ethanol solution of lipids is injected rapidly through a fine needle into an excess of saline or other aqueous medium. The rate of the injection is unusually sufficient to achieve complete mixing, so that the ethanol is diluted almost instantaneously in water, and phospholipid molecules are dispersed evenly throughout the medium (Fig 5a). This procedure yields a high proportion of SUVs (dia. ~25nm), although lipid aggregates and larger vesicles may form if the mixing is not thorough enough. This method is extremely simple and has low risk of degradation of sensitive lipids. The vesicles of 100nm size may be obtained by little modification in this method, i.e. by varying the concentration of lipid in ethanol or by changing the rate of injection of ethanol solution in aqueous solution [42]. The major shortcoming of the method is the limitation of the solubility of lipids in ethanol and the volume of ethanol that can be introduced into the medium (7.5% V/V maximum), which in turn limits the quantity of lipid dispersed, so that resulting liposome dispersion is rather diluted. Another drawback is the difficulty to remove residual ethanol from phospholipid membrane.

Ether injection

Ether injection method is very similar to the ethanol injection method. It contrasts markedly with ethanol injection in many respects [43-45]. It involves injecting the immiscible organic solution very slowly into an aqueous phase through a narrow needle at the temperature of vaporizing the organic solvent (Fig. 5b). This method may also treat sensitive lipids very gently. It has little risk of causing oxidative degradation provided ether is free from peroxides. The disadvantages of the technique are the long time taken to produce a batch of liposomes and the careful control needed for introduction of the lipid solution, requiring a mechanically operated pump. If substances are degraded at elevated temperature (60°C), then the fluorinated hydrocarbons may be used instead of ether. The efficiency of encapsulation is relatively low, although the captured volume per mole of lipid is high, 8-17 L/mol. [41].

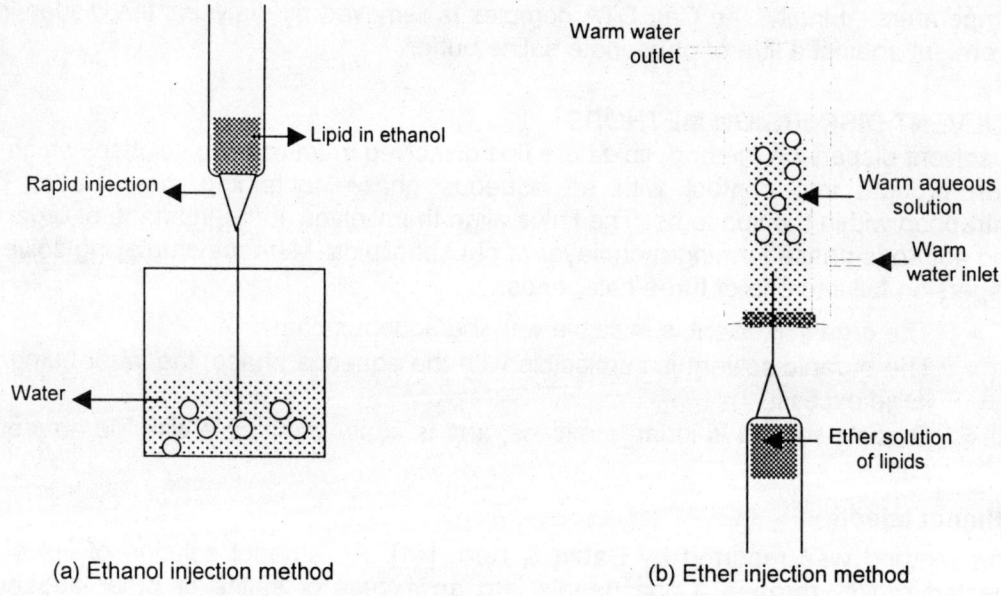

(a) Ethanol injection method   (b) Ether injection method

Fig. 5 : Solvent dispersion techniques for liposome preparation

Water in organic phase

The liposome is made up in two steps by this method, first the inner leaflet of the bilayer, then the outer half. The common feature of this method is formation of "water in oil" emulsion produced by introduction of a small quantity of aqueous medium containing material to be entrapped into a large volume of immiscible organic solution of lipid. This was followed by mechanical agitation to break up the aqueous phase into microscopic water droplets. These droplets are stabilized by the presence of phospholipid monolayer at the interface. The size of droplets is determined by the intensity of mechanical energy used to form the emulsion and amount of lipid relative to the volume of aqueous phase, since each droplet requires a complete monolayer of phospholipid covering its surface in order to prevent the coalescing with other droplets.

The aqueous solution surrounded by the monolayer of phospholipid forms the central core of the final liposome. There are number of methods for preparing droplets [46].

Double emulsion vesicles

In this method [47,48], the outer of the liposome membrane is created at a second interface between two phases by emulsification of an organic solution in water. If the organic solution, which already contains water droplets, is introduced into excess aqueous medium followed by mechanical dispersion, multi compartment vesicles are obtained. The ordered dispersion so obtained is described as a w/o/w system (i.e. double emulsion). These vesicles are suspended in aqueous medium and have an aqueous core, the two aqueous compartments being separated from each other by a pair of phospholipid monolayers whose hydrophobic surfaces face each other across a thin film of organic solvent. Removal of this solvent clearly results in an intermediate sized unilamellar vesicle. The theoretical entrapment is 100%.

The double emulsion is prepared by rapidly injecting the dispersion of microdroplets into hot aqueous solution of tris buffer with the help of 22-gauge hypodermic needle under vigorous stirring. The organic solvent is evaporated using strong jet of nitrogen thus forming double emulsion. The last traces of organic solvent are removed by evaporation and finally the volume is adjusted by adding extra-distilled water and then the product is centrifuged at 20°C for 30 min at 37,000g to remove lipid aggregates.

Reverse phase evaporation vesicles

This method was developed by Szoka & Papahadjopoulos [49]. The novel key in this method is the removal of solvent from an emulsion by evaporation. The droplets are formed by bath sonication of mixture of the two phases, then the emulsion is dried down to a semi-solid gel in a rotary evaporator under reduced pressure. At this stage, the monolayers of phospholipid surrounding each water compartment are closely opposed to each other and in some cases probably already form part of a bilayer membrane separating adjacent compartments (Fig. 6). The next step is to bring about the collapse of a certain proportion of the water droplets by vigorous mechanical shaking with a vortex mixer. In these circumstances, the lipid monolayer, which enclosed the collapsed vesicle, is contributed to adjacent intact vesicle to form the outer leaflet of the bilayer of a large unilamellar liposome. The aqueous content of the collapsed droplet provides the medium required for dispersion of these newly formed liposomes. After conversion of the gel into a homogeneous free flowing fluid, the dispersion is dialyzed in order to remove the last traces of solvent. The vesicles formed are unilamellar and have an average diameter of 0.5μm. The encapsulation percentage is found to be not higher than 50% [50].

Stable plurilamellar vesicles (SPVs)

In this method, water-in-oil dispersion is prepared as described earlier with an excess of lipid, but drying process is accompanied by continued bath sonication with a stream of nitrogen [51]. The redistribution and equilibration of aqueous solvent and solute occur during this time in between the various bilayers in each plurilameller vesicle. The internal structure of SPVs is different from that of MLV-REVs, in that they lack a large aqueous core, the majority of the entrapped aqueous medium being located in the compartment in between adjacent lamellae. The percent entrapments are normally around 30% (compared with > 60% for MLV-REVs).

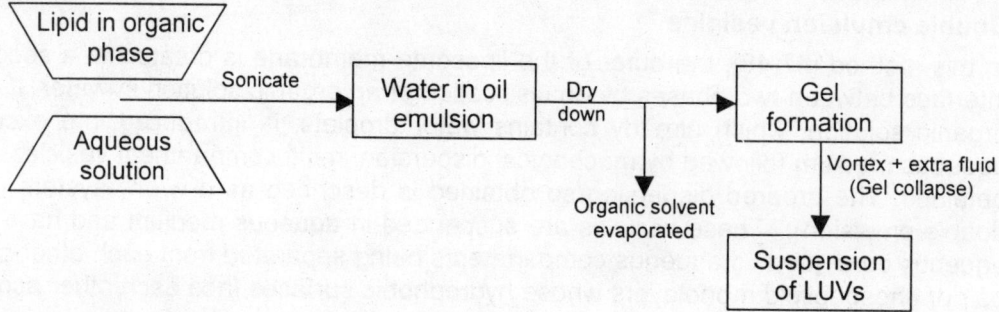

Fig. 6 : Staged in the preparation of liposomes by reverse phase evaporation

DETERGENT SOLUBILIZATION METHODS

In this method, the phospholipids are brought into intimate contact with the aqueous phase via the intermediary of detergents, which associate with phospholipid molecules and serve to screen the hydrophobic portions of the molecule from water [52,53]. The technique was originally introduced by Kagawa & Racjer [54]. The structures formed as a result of this association are known as micelles, and can be composed of several hundreds of component molecules. Their shape and size depend on chemical nature of the detergent, the concentration and other lipids involved. The concentration of detergent in water at which micelles just start to form is known as the `critical micelle concentration' (CMC). Below the CMC, the detergent molecules exist entirely in free solution. As detergent is dissolved in water in concentration higher than the CMC, micelle form in large and large amounts, while the concentration of detergent in the free form remains essentially the same as the CMC. Micelles containing components in addition to the detergent (or composed of two or more detergents) are known as "mixed micelles".

In contrast to phospholipids, detergents are highly soluble in both aqueous and organic media and there is equilibrium between the detergent molecules in the water phase, and in the lipid environment of the micelle. The critical micelle concentration can give an indication of the position of this equilibrium. Upon lowering the concentration of detergent in the bulk aqueous phase, the molecules of detergent can be removed from mixed micelle by dialysis. A higher CMC indicates that the equilibrium is strongly shifted towards the bulk solution, so that removal from the mixed membrane by dialysis is relatively easy.

As a general rule, membrane-solubilizing detergents have a higher affinity for phospholipid membranes than for the pure detergent micelles. Thus, as detergent is added in increasing amounts to the membrane preparation, more and more detergent gets incorporated into the bilayer, until a point is reached where a transition from the lamellar to the usually spherical micellar phase configuration takes place. As the detergent concentration increased further, the micelles are reduced in size until they become saturated with detergent, whereupon the concentration of free molecules equals the CMC and simple detergent micelles are seen to form. Again, it is usually found that a high concentration is advantageous for solubilizing membrane phospholipids although one might expect the converse, since a high affinity for lipid membranes should be reflected by a low CMC. Helenius and Simons [55] and Lichtenberg [56] proposed a three-stage model of the interaction of detergents with the lipid bilayers at increasing detergent/lipid radios. At low (sublytic) concentrations the detergent equilibrates between vesicular lipid and the water phase (stage-I). At this stage, the mean vesicle size increases [57,58] and functional properties of the bilayer charge [59-61]. Reaching a critical detergent concentration (`saturation' of the bilayers), the membrane structure tends to be unstable and transforms gradually into micelles (stage-II). In this stage detergent saturated bilayers coexist with lipid-saturated micelles. At stage-III, all lipid exists in mixed micelle form.

The data of Ollivon et al., [58] suggested that, at least for octyl glucoside, lamellar sheets are formed as an intermediate in the transition from vesicles to micelles. The 'vesicles-to-sheet' transition starts with the formation of large detergent stabilized pores. It is followed by the `sheet-to-micelle' transition. The morphological consequences of the incorporation of neutral detergents into liposomal bilayers at sublytic concentrations (formation of mixed bilayers) have been discussed by Lasch et al. [62].

Invariably in all methods, which employ detergent in the preparation of liposomes, the basic feature is to remove the detergent from preformed mixed micelles containing phospholipids, whereupon unilamellar vesicles form spontaneously. The detergent methods are not very efficient in terms of percentage entrapment values, on the other hand they are certainly the best general methods for preparing liposomes with lipophilic proteins inserted into the membranes. Another special feature is the ability to vary size of the liposomes by precise control of the conditions of detergent removal [63-65].

PURIFICATION OF LIPOSOMES

Liposomes are commonly purified by either gel filtration column chromatography or by dialysis or centrifugation. In column chromatographic separation Sephadex G-50 is most widely used material. In this column chromatographic separation [22,66] liposome membrane may bind or interact with the surface of the polydextran beads. There may be small amount of lipid lost resulting into destabilization of the membrane leading to permeability changes and subsequent leakage of entrapped solute. This problem can be overcome either by avoiding forming too small size liposomes or by pre-saturating the column material with empty liposomes of the same lipid composition as the test sample either before or after the packing of the column.

In dialysis method [67] any standard technique may be used. For large-scale liposome preparations, hollow fiber dialysis cartridges are preferred. It is also convenient method for studying the leakage of small molecules from liposomes [1].

Liposomes may be separated by centrifugation method [68-70]. The separation of liposomes by centrifugation is depended on the size as well as the composition of the bilayers. SUVs in normal saline may be sedimented by spinning at 200,000g for 10 to 20 hr in an ultracentrifuge. Multilamellar liposomes may be spun down much more readily, i.e. at 100,000g for less than one hr.

CHARACTERIZATION OF LIPOSOMES

The behavior of liposomes in both physical and biological systems is governed by the factors such as physical size, membrane permeability, percent-entrapped solutes, chemical composition as well as the quantity and purity of the starting materials. Therefore, the liposomes are characterized for physical attributes i.e. shape, size and its distribution, percentage drug capture, entrapped volume, lamellarity, drug release and chemical compositions (estimation of phospholipids, phospholipids oxidation and analysis of cholesterol).

Physical properties

Size and its distribution

There are number of methods reported in the literature to determine average size and size distribution of the vesicles [71-74]. The most precise method to determine size of the liposomes is electron microscopy since it permits one to view each individual liposome and to obtain exact information about the profile of liposome population over the whole range of sizes. Unfortunately, it is very time consuming and requires equipment that may not always be available immediately to hand. In contrast, laser light scattering (quasi-elastic laser light scattering) method is very simple and rapid to perform but having disadvantage of measuring an average property of the bulk of the liposomes. All these methods require very costly equipment. If only approximate idea of size range is required then gel exclusion chromatographic techniques are recommended, since only expense incurred, is for buffers and gel materials.

Microscopic Methods

Light microscopy has been utilized to examine the gross size distribution of large vesicles produced from single chain amphiphiles [75]. If the bilayers contain fluorescent hydrophilic probes, the liposomes can be examined under a fluorescent microscope. The resolution of the light microscope limits this technique for obtaining the complete size distribution of the preparation. However using negative stain electron microscopy, one can obtain an estimate of the lower end of the size distribution. For the large vesicle (5 μm), negative stain electron microscopy is not suitable because vesicle distortion during preparation of the specimen makes it difficult to obtain an estimate of the diameter of the original particle.

A technical difficulty in obtaining good negative stains of liposomes is the spreading of the vesicles on the carbon-coated grid. Treating the grid with 0.1 mg/mL solution of bacitracin [76] or coating the support films with silica by the evaporation of silicon monoxide [77], usually permits a satisfactory spreading of liposomes for negative staining. Glow discharging of the grids immediately prior to use is of considerable help to the spreading of liposomes on the grid surface.

Freeze etched and freezed fracture electron microscopy techniques have been extensively used to study vesicle size and structure. The freeze etch technique is particularly suitable for the measurement of small vesicle diameters since the effects of random cleavage that can occur through and around the vesicle, can be compensated for the each step. For populations of large size vesicles freeze fracture technique can yield a representative morphological view of the liposome and has been useful for examining the morphological changes that can occur in the bilayer surface as the phospholipids pass through the gel-liquid-crystalline transition [78-81] or through the lamellar hexagonal transition [82]. However, the freeze fracture technique has a serious drawback in estimating the size distribution and mean vesicle size of a heterogeneous population of the vesicles, the fracture plane passes through the mid planes that are randomly positioned in the frozen section resulting in non-midplane fracture. Thus, the observed profile radius depends on the distance of the vesicle center from the plane of the fracture, while the probability that a vesicle will be in the fracture plane depends on the vesicle radius. A homogeneous population of vesicles will therefore yield a distribution profile of sizes with largest being equal to the true radius of the vesicle.

Laser light scattering

Proton correlation spectroscopy (PCS) is the analysis of the time dependence of intensity fluctuation in scattered laser light due to the Brownian motion of particles in solution/dispersion. Since small particles diffuse more rapidly than large particles, the rate of fluctuation of scattered light intensity varies accordingly. Thus, the translational diffusion coefficient (D) can be measured, which in turn can be used to determine the mean hydrodynamic radius (Rh) of the particles using the Stokes-Einstein equation. Using this technique one can measure particles in the range of about 3nm to about 3μm.

$$D = kT / 6\pi\eta R_h \quad \text{---------} \quad \text{(Stokes-Einstein equation)}$$

Where, K = Boltzmann's constant, T = absolute temperature, η = solvent viscosity,
R_h = mean hydrodynamic radius

Gel permeation

Exclusion chromatography on large pure gels was introduced by Huang [22] to separate SUVs from radial MLVs. However, large vesicles of 1-3μm diameter usually fail to enter the gel and are retained on the top of the column [83]. A thin layer chromatography system using agarose beads has been introduced as a convenient, fast technique for obtaining a rough estimation of the size distribution of a liposome preparation [84]. However, it was not reported if this procedure was sensitive to a physical blockage of the pores of the agarose gel as it is more likely to be incase of conventional column chromatography.

Surface Charge

Bangham et al. [71] have developed a method which depends upon free-flow electrophoresis of MLVs. A technique has been developed that separate extruded vesicles according to their surface charge by electrophoresis on a cellulose acetate plate in a sodium borate buffer pH 8.8 [85]. The lipid samples (5 nmoles) are applied to the plate and electrophoresis is carried out at 4°C on a flat bed apparatus for 30 min at 18 V/cm. The plate is dried and the phospholipids are visualized by the molybdenum blue reagent. Liposomes up to 0.2μm in diameter can migrate on this support and with this technique as little as 2-mole % of charged lipids can be detected in a liposome bilayer. This sensitive assay should prove valuable for examining the charge heterogeneity in liposome preparation for following fusion between two populations of vesicles with different charge and for determining the presence of charge impurities, e.g. fatty acids in liposomes.

Percent capture (entrapment)

It is essential to measure the quantity of solute entrapped in liposomes before they are studied for behavior of this entrapped material in physical and biological systems, since the effects observed experimentally will usually be dose related. After removal of unincorporated material by the separation techniques, one may assume that the quantity of material entrapped is 100%, but the preparation may change upon storage. For longer-term stability test and for developing new liposome formulation or method of preparation, a technique is needed for separating free from entrapped material. In general, two methods may be used, i.e. mini column centrifugation, and protamine aggregation [86].

In mini column centrifugation method the hydrated gel (Sephadex G-50) is filled in a barrel of 1mL syringe without plunger, which is pluged with a Whatman GF/B filter pad. This barrel rested in a centrifuge tube. The tube is spun at 2000 rpm for 3 min to remove excess saline solution from the gel. After centrifugation the gel column is dried and comes away from the side of the barrel. Then, eluted saline is removed from the collection tube. Liposome dispersion (0.2 mL, undiluted) is applied dropwise on to the top of the gel bed, and column is spun at 2000 rpm for 3 min to expel the void volume containing the liposomes into the centrifuge tube. Elute is then removed and set aside for assay.

The protamine aggregate method [87,88] may be used for liposomes of any composition (both material and negative-charged). However, a preliminary test should be carried out before to check that the material entrapped does not itself precipitate in the presence of protamine after release from liposome. In this method, liposome dispersion (20mg/mL in normal saline) is placed in conical glass centrifuge tube, 0.1mL of protamine solution (10mg/mL) is added with mixing, and allowed to stand for 3 min. To this, 30mL of saline is added and then the tube is spun for 20 min at 2000g at ambient temperature. The supernatant is removed and assayed for free, unentrapped compound by standard methods. The suspended pellet is resuspended in 0.6mL of 10% triton X-100 to dissolve the material completely. The volume is made up appropriately and assayed for entrapped material.

Entrapped Volume

The entrapped volume of a population of liposomes (in μL/mg phospholipid) can often be deduced from measurements of the total quantity of solute entrapped inside liposomes. It could be assumed that the concentration of solute in the aqueous medium inside liposomes is the same as that in the solution used to start with, and no solute has leaked out of the liposomes after separation from unentrapped material. However, in many cases such assumption is invalid. For example, in two-phase methods of preparation, water can be lost from the internal compartment during the drying down step used to remove organic solvent. On other occasions, water may enter or be expelled from the liposome as a result of unanticipated osmotic differences.

The best way to measure external volume is to measure the quantity of water directly. This can be performed using a spectroscopically inert fluid as the external medium and measuring the water signal for example by NMR [89]. In this method, liposome prepared in aqueous solution consisting of ordinary water are spun at high centrifugal force (200,000g for 6 hr) to give a tight pellet, from which the supernatant is decanted off to remove every drop of excess fluid (including some liposome, if necessary). The pellet is then resuspended in deuterium oxide (D_2O). The permeability of the membrane to water is such that D_2O and H_2O equilibrate very rapidly throughout the whole volume of the medium. A small aliquot is removed for quantification of phospholipid and the remainder is used to obtain an NMR scan of H_2O, the peak height of which can be related to concentration by comparison with standards containing known amount of H_2O in D_2O.

Lamellarity

The average number of bilayers present in liposome can be found by freeze-electron microscopy and by ^{31}P-NMR. In later technique, the signals are recorded before and after the addition of broadening agent such as manganese ions, which interact with the outer leaflet of the outermost bilayers. Thus, a 50% reduction in NMR signal means that the liposome preparation is unilamellar and 25% reduction in the intensity of the original NMR signal means that there are 2 bilayers in the liposome [29].

Nowadays, freeze-fracturing electron microscopy has become a very popular method to study structural details of aqueous lipid dispersions [90-95].

Phase behavior of liposomes

An important feature of lipid membrane is the existence of a temperature dependent, reversible phase transition, where the hydrocarbon chains of the phospholipid undergo a transformation from an ordered (gel) state to more disordered fluid (liquid crystalline) state. These changes have been documented by freeze fracturing electron microscopy but most conveniently demonstrated by differential scanning calorimetery [96].

The physical state of the bilayers profoundly affects the permeability, leakage rates and overall stability of the liposomes. The phase transition temperatures (Tc) is a function of phospholipid content of the bilayers. The Tc can give good clues regarding liposomal stability, permeability and whether drug is entrapped in the bilayers or in the aqueous compartment, Tc values of some synthetic phospholipids are listed in Table 1.

Drug release

Many workers extensively studied the drug release from liposomes in recent years [98-100]. It is realized that the mechanism of drug release from the liposomes can be assessed by the use of a well-calibrated *in vitro* diffusion cell.

The liposome based formulations can be assessed by employing in vitro assays to predict pharmacokinetics and bioavailability of the drug before employing costly and time-consuming in vivo studies. The dilution-induced drug release in buffer and plasma was employed as predictor for pharmacokinetic performance of liposomal formulations and another assay, which determined intracellular drug release induced by liposome degradation in the presence of mouse-liver lysosome lysate was used to assess the bioavailability of the drug [101].

Table 1. Tc of some important synthetic phospholipid [97]

Lipids	Charge	Tc
Dipalmitoyl phosphatidylcholine (DPPC)	0	41
Dimyristoyl phosphatidylethanolamine (DMPE)	0	48
Distearoyl phosphatidylcholine (DSPC)	0	58
Dioleyl phosphatidyl glycerol (DOPG)	-1	18
Dilauryl phosphatidyl glycerol (DLPG)	-1	04
Dipalmitoyl phosphatidyl glycerol (DPPG)	-1	41
Distearoyl phosphatidyl glycerol (DSPG)	-1	58
Dilauryl phosphatidylcholine (DLPC)	0	0
Dimyristoyl phosphatidylcholine (DMPC)	0	23

Chemical properties

Quantitative determination of phospholipids

It is difficult to measure directly the phospholipid concentration, since dried lipids can often contain considerable quantities of residual solvent. Consequently, the method most widely used for determination of phospholipid is an indirect one in which the phosphate content of the sample is first measured [102]. The phospholipids are measured either using Bartlett assay or Stewart assay. In Bartlett assay [102]. The phospholipid phosphorus in the sample is first hydrolyzed to inorganic phosphate. This is converted in to phosphomolybdic acid by the addition of ammonium molybdate and phosphomolybdic acid is quantitatively reduced to a blue-colored compound by amino-naphthyl-sulphonic acid. The intensity of blue color is measured spectrophotometrically. Bartlett assay is very sensitive but is not reasonably reproducible. The sensitivity of the Bartlett assay to inorganic phosphate creates problem with measurement of phospholipid liposomes suspended in physiological buffers, which usually contain phosphate ions. This can be overcome by employing a more specific method, which is unaffected by inorganic phosphate.

Another method for determination of phospholipid is Stewart assay [103] where phospholipids form a complex with ammonium ferrothiocyanate in organic solution. The advantage of this method is that the presence of inorganic phosphate does not interfere with the assay. This method is not applicable to samples where mixture of unknown phospholipids may be present. In this method, the standard curve is first prepared by adding ammonium ferrothiocyanate (0.1M) solution with different known concentrations of phospholipids in chloroform. Similarly, the samples are treated and optical density of these solutions is measured at 485 nm and the absorbance of samples is compared with standard curve of phospholipids.

Phospholipid hydrolysis

The major product of lecithin hydrolysis is lysolecithin where one fatty acid chain is lost by deesterification. Ideally, estimation of phospholipid hydrolysis by quantitation of lysolecithin could be carried out by HPLC where the column outflow can be monitored continuously by UV absorbance to obtain a quantitative record of the eluted components. Unfortunately, many natural phospholipids have fatty acids, which are unsaturated and therefore absorb, to different extent in the 1- and 2-position. It is difficult to relate peak height accurately to absolute quantities of lysophosphatidylcholine (LPC), since one does not know the absorbance of the fatty acid species that have been retained on the glycerol bridge. Consequently, methods are preferred which permit detection of LPC via the phosphate group, after first separating the hydrolysis product (LPC) from the parent PC by TLC. The spots can either be stained with iodine, then scraped off and the phosphate content is measured directly, or they can be measured by scanning densitometry. Hydrolysis products of other phospholipids can be estimated in the same way.

Phospholipid oxidation

Oxidation of the fatty acids of phospholipids, in the absence of specific oxidants occurs via a free radical chain mechanism. The initiation step is abstraction of a hydrogen atom from the lipid chain that can occur most commonly as a result of exposure to electromagnetic radiation or due to trace amount of contamination with transition metal ions. Poly-chain-saturated lipids are particularly prone to oxidative degradation.

A number of techniques are available for determining the oxidation of phospholipids at different stages, the methods include UV absorbance [104], TBA (for endoperoxides), iodometric (for hydroperoxides) and GLC method.

Cholesterol analysis

Cholesterol is qualitatively analyzed using capillary column of flexible fused silica [105] whereas it is quantitatively estimated (in the range 0-8 µg) by measuring the absorbance of purple complex produced with iron upon reaction with a combined reagent containing ferric perchlorate, ethyl acetate and sulfuric acid at 610 nm.

STABILITY OF LIPOSOMES

Liposome stability problems are of course much more severe. Many different changes can occur in liposomes with the passage of time. Liposomal phospholipids can undergo chemical degradation such as oxidation and hydrolysis. Either as a result of these changes or otherwise, liposomes maintained in aqueous dispersion may aggregate, fuse or leak their contents.

Methods devised to overcome the problems of liposome instability fall into two categories- those designed to minimize the degradation process and, secondly, those which contrive to help liposomes survive in the conditions, which encourage these processes.

Prevention of chemical degradation

Precautions must be taken to minimize chemical degradation by using freshly purified lipids and freshly distilled solvents and should include an anti-oxidant as a component of the lipid membrane. Similarly procedure involving high temperature should be avoided and an oxygen free environment should be created or environment should be deoxygenated using nitrogen flushing.

It may also be worthwhile including an iron chelator in the formulation to prevent initiation of the free radical chain reaction. The anti-oxidant commonly used at present time is α-tocopherol (Vit-E), a common non-toxic dietary lipid, β, γ and δ-tocopherols may also be used as they are more effective as long term anti-oxidants [106]. Apart from oxidation problems, the level of oxidizable lipid in the membrane is to be reduced by using saturated lipids instead of unsaturated ones.

Hydrolysis of ester linkage proceeds most slowly at pH values close to neutral. The hydrolysis may be avoided altogether by the use of lipids, which contain ether instead of ester linkages such as found in membrane of halophilic bacteria [107]. Hydrolysis in vivo as a result of enzymatic attack can be prevented by the use of sphingomyelin, or phospholipid derivatives with the 2-ester linkage replaced by a carbomyloxy function [108,109].

There are a number of techniques to analyse liposome stability. Love et al. [110] used high performance gel permeation liquid chromatography and gel permeation chromatography to analyze stability of liposomes.

Prevention of physical degradation

Leakage and fusion of vesicles can occur as a result of lattice defects in the membrane introduced during their manufacture. It is however reported particularly in SUVs when liposomes are prepared below the membrane phase transition temperature. There is evidence for packing defects in other types of vesicles (detergent dialysis vesicle, freeze-thawed vesicles) even above the phase transition temperature. These irregularities can be dispensed by a process termed `annealing' which consists simply of incubating the liposomes at a temperature high enough above the phase transition temperature to allow differences in packing density between opposite sides of the bilayers to equalize by trans-membrane flip-flop.

Even in annealing vesicles, aggregation, fusion, etc. can take place to significant extents over a long period of time. Aggregation (and sedimentation) of neutral liposomes is brought about by Vander Waals interaction and tends to be more pronounced in large vesicles, where the increased planarity of the membrane allows greater areas of membrane to come into contact with each other. Factors such as residual solvent and trace elements can enhance the process for uncharged membranes. It is a natural and unavoidable phenomenon and the simplest way to overcome is to impart small quantities of negative charge to the lipid mixture [77].

SUVs (<40nm) are prone to fusion for relieving stress arising from the high curvature of the membrane. Since this can occur particularly at the phase transition temperature (Tc), it is advisable to store liposome dispersion at a temperature away from the Tc. It could be advantageous to include sufficient cholesterol in the membrane to reduce or completely remove the transition, particularly if it is in a temperature range close to that at which the liposomes are to be stored or handled. For liposomes, which have negative charge in the membrane, care must be taken to avoid high concentration of metal ions. It may be worth while including a metal ion chelator in the suspending buffer.

The large polar or ionic molecules are retained much more effectively than low molecular weight lipophilic compounds. In general, for both classes of compounds a rigid, more saturated membrane with a high molar ratio of cholesterol is the most stable with regard to leakage of solutes. The permeability can be increased at the Tc, particularly in the presence of high-density lipoprotein (HDL), tubulin or actin [111].

Freezing or lyophilization techniques constitute an alternative method of overcoming instability problems by transforming the liposomes into a solid or anhydrous form, where chemical degradation of lipid components or solutes is less likely to occur. However, these techniques are not yet fully perfected. Methods for cryo preservation have achieved some success [112].

The stability of liposomes may also be increased by cross-linking membrane component covalently using methods such as gluteraldehyde fixation, osmification or polymerization of alkyne-containing phospholipids [113]. These methods can increase the mechanical strength of the membrane and render them less susceptible to disruption *in vivo* by serum components.

CONCLUSION

Twenty five years of research into the use of liposomes in drug delivery have led to vastly improved technology in terms of drug capture, vesicle stability on storage, scale-up production and the design of formulations for special tasks. In parallel, remarkable advances have been made in understanding and controlling liposomes behavior in vivo. This has facilitated the application of a wide range of liposomal drugs in the treatment and prevention of diseases in experimental animals clinically. In case of sterile production of liposomes, reproducibility of preparation, pyrogen content, method of sterilization and its impact on the stability of the product, integrity of lipid, potentiality cost, quality control methods and regulatory issues, as well as acute, subacute and chronic toxicities are seldom addressed. Further, the utility of liposome formulation technology at the floor of industry is to be explored by simplifying, standardizing and optimizing methods of preparation and enhancing the storage stability of the product. The safety of liposome formulations must be specifically and categorically demonstrated. A comprehensive programme of relevant toxicity testing is required before any liposome formulation is accepted for widespread clinical investigation.

The recent research is concentrated on the use of liposome to deliver hemoglobin and act as surrogate red blood cells. These liposome-based red blood cells appear most promising as second generation delivery system. Another field where liposomes may find application in the industry is recombinant DNA technology for the synthesis of exotic chemicals, including drugs. Because, liposomes may transfer normally non-penetrating molecules into cells and organelles, they could be particularly useful for transferring fragments of genetic material from cell to cell. The scientists are also engaged in designing of liposomal prodrug, using principle of specific enzymatic cleavage and facilitated spontaneous hydrolysis.

Another field of liposomal research is producing sterically stabilized liposomes (SSL) for prolonged circulation in blood stream. These SSL have ability to reduce in vivo recognition and phagocytic uptake, resulting in prolonged circulation and localization in tumors as well as other sites of pathology. This has no doubt restored their potential as a widely useful delivery system but also has created new challenges; the need of the agent associated with the liposome during incubation and distribution followed by control of its release for activity. The pathological sites, which can be approached for selective and controlled delivery by ligand targeting must be addressed. Yet another area that continuously demands significant efforts is designing the liposome which can be used for non-invasive route of administration. This will no doubt continue to contribute significantly to more efficient use of 'old' drugs with better and established therapeutic index vis a vis minimum side effects.

REFERENCES

1. Bangham, A.D., Standish, M.M. and Watkins, J.C. (1965). **J. Mol. Biol.** 13, 238.

2. Gangemi, J.D., Nachitigal, M., Barnhart, D., Karenchi, L. and Jani, P. (1987). **J. Infect. Dis.** 155, 510.

3. Kim, S. and Howell, S.B. (1987). **Cancer Treat. Res.** 71,705.

4. Rahman, Y.E., Rosenthal, M.W. and Cerny, E.A. (1973). **Science** 180, 300.

5. Delos, R.J., Shaubinger, R.M., Brunette, E.N., Lin, J.M., Lin, E.J., Montaomery, A.B., Fried, D.S. and Papahadjopoulos, D.P. (1987). **Am. Rev. Respir. Dis.** 135, 731

6. Hirono, K. and Hunt, C.A. (1986). **J. Pharm. Sci.** 74,915.

7. Gregoriadis, G. (1976). **N. Eng. J. Med.** 295, 704.

8. Fendler, J.H. and Romero, A. (1977). **Life Sci.** 20, 1109.

9. Brockerhoft, H. and Ayenger, N.K.N. (1979). **Lipids** 14, 88.

10. Ladbrooke, B.D., Williams, R.M. and Chapman, D. (1968). **Biochim. Biophys. Acta** 150, 333.

11. Horwitz, C., Krut, L. and Kaminsky, L. (1971). **Biochim. Biophy. Acta** 239, 329.

12. Yeagle, P., Hutton, W., Huang, C.H. and Martin, R. (1975). **Proc. Natl. Acad. Sci.** U.S.A, 72, 3477.

13. Sklar, L.A., Hudson, B.S. and Simoni, R.D. (1977). **Biochemistry** 16, 819.

14. Mayer, L.D., Hope, M.J., Cullis, P.R. and Janoff, A.S. (1985). **Biochim. Biophys. Acta** 817, 193.

15. Reeves, J.P. and Dowben, R.M. (1969). **J. Cell. Physiol.** 73, 49.

16. Lasic, D.D., Belie, A. and Valentincic, T. (1988). **J. Am. Chem. Soc.** 110, 970.

17. Payne, N.I., Timmins, P., Ambroes, C.V., Klard, M.D. and Ridgeway, F. (1986). **J. Pharm. Sci.** 75,325.

18. Imperial Chemical industries ltd. (1978). Belgian Patent 866697 14.1.

19. Mahew, E., Lazo, R., Vail, W.J., King, J. and Green, A.M. (1984). **Biochim. Biophys. Acta** 775, 169.

20. Saunder, L., Perrin, J. and Gammack, D.B. (1962). **J. Pharm. Pharmacol.** 14, 567.

21. Ambramson, M.B., Katzman, R. and Gregor, H.P. (1964). **J. Biol. Chem.** 239, 70.

22. Huang, C.H. (1969). **Biochemistry** 8, 344.

23. Hauser, H. (1971). **Biochem. Biophys. Res. Comm.** 45, 1049.

24. Barenholtz, Y., Gibbes, D., Litman, B.J., Goll, J., Thompson, T.E. and Carlson, F.D. (1977). **Biochemistry** 16, 2806.

25. Barenholtz, Y., Amselem, S.and Lichtenberg, D. (1979). **FEBS Lett.** 99. 210.

26. Hamilton, R.L., Goerkc, J., Guol, S.S., Williass, M.C. and Havel, R.J. (1980). **Lipid Res.** 21, 981.

27. Friendman, J.E., Lelkes, P.I., Rosenheck, K. and Oplatka, A.(1986). **J. Biol. Chem.** 261, 5745.

28. Olson, F., Hunt, C.A., Szoka, F.C., Vail, W., Mayhew, E. and Papahadjopoulos, D. (1980). **Biochim. Biophys. Acta** 601, 559.

29. Hope, M.J., Bally, M.B., Webb, G. and Cullis, P.R. (1985). **Biochim. Biophys. Acta** 812, 55.

30. Mayer, L.D., Hope, M.J. and Cullis, P.R. (1986). **Biochim. Biophys. Acta** 858, 161.

31. Schneider, T., Sachse, A., Rossling, G. and Brandl, M. (1994). **Drug Dev. Ind. Pharm.** 20, 2787.

32. Schneider, T., Sachse, A., Rossling, G. and Brandl, M. (1995). **Int. J. Pharm.** 117, 1.

33. Kirby, C. and Gregoriadis, G. (1984). **Biotechnology** 2, 979.

34. Pick, U. (1981). **Arch. Biochim. Biophys.** 212, 186.

35. Kasahara, M. and Hunckle, P.C. (1977). **J. Biol. Chem.** 252, 7384.

36. Oku, N. and MacDonald, R.C. (1983). **Biochemistry** 22, 855.

37. Hasuer, H. and Gains, N. (1982). **Proc. Natl. Acad. Sci.** USA, 79, 1683.

38. Papahadjopoulos, D., Vail, W.J., Pangborn, W.A. and Poste, G. (1976). **Biochim. Biophys. Acta** 448, 265.

39. Papahadjopoulos, D., Vail, W.J., Newton, C., Nir, S., Jacobson, K., Postel, G. and Lazo, R. (1977). **Biochim. Biophys. Acta** 465, 579.

40. Papahadjopoulos, D. and Vail, W.J. (1978). **Ann. N.Y. Acad. Sci.** 308, 259.

41. Batzri, S. and Korn, E.D. (1973). **Biochim. Biophys. Acta** 298, 1015.

42. Kremer, J.M., Esker, M.W., Pathmamanoharan, C. and Wiersema, P.H. (1977). **Biochemistry** 16, 3932.

43. Deamer, D.W. (1978). **Ann. N.Y. Acad. Sci.** 308, 250.

44. Deamer, D.W., Bangham, A.D. (1976). **Biochim. Biophys. Acta** 443, 629.

45. Schieren, H., Rudolph, S., Fiukelstein, M., Coleman, P. and Weisman, G.(1978). **Biochim. Biophys. Acta** 542, 137.

46. Kim, S. and Martin, G.M. (1981). **Biochim. Biophys. Acta** 646, 4.

47. Matsumoto, S., Kohda, M. and Murata, S. (1977). **J. Coll. Interface Sci.** 62, 149.

48. Batelle Memorial Inst. (1979). British Patent Appl. No. 2001929A.

49. Szoka, F. and Papahadjopoulos, D. (1978). **Proc. Natl. Acad. Sci.** USA, 75, 4194.

50. Szoka, F.C., Olson, F., Heath, T., Vail, J., Mayhew, E. and Papahadjopoulos, D. (1980). **Biochim. Biophys. Acta** 601, 559.

51. Gruner, S.M., Lenk, R.P., Janoff, A.S. and Ostro, M.J. (1985). **Biochemistry** 24, 2833.

52. Korenbrot, J.I. (1977). **Ann. Rev. Physiol.** 39, 19.

53. Razin, S. (1972). **Biochim. Biophys. Acta** 265, 241.

54. Kagawa, Y. and Racjer, E. (1971). **J. Biol. Chem.** 246, 5477.

55. Helenius, A. and Simons, K. (1975). **Biochim. Biophys. Acta** 415, 29.

56. Lichtenberg, D. (1985). **Biochim. Biophys. Acta** 821, 470.

57. Alonso, A., Saez, R., Villena, A. and Goni, F.M. (1982). **J. Membrane Biol.** 67, 55.

58. Ollivon, M., Eidelman, O., Blumenthal, R. and Walter, A. (1988). **Biochemistry** 27, 1695.

59. Inoue, K. and Kitagawa, T. (1976). **Biochim. Biophys. Acta** 426, 1.

60. Prado, A., Arrondo, J.L.R. and Villena, A. (1983). **Biochim. Biophy. Acta** 733, 163.

61. Sunamoto, J., Kondo, H. and Yoshimatsu, A. (1978). **Biochim. Biophys. Acta** 510, 52.

62. Lasch, J., Hoffman, J., Richter, W. and Meyer, H.W. (1992). **J. Lipo. Res.** 2, 1.

63. Enoch, H.G. and Strittmater, P. (1979). **Proc. Natl. Acad. Sci.** USA, 76, 145.

64. Mimms, L.T., Zampigh G., Nazaki, Y., Tanford, C. and Reyolds, J.A. (1981). **Biochemistry** 20, 833.

65. Helenius, A., Frier, E. and Kortenbeek, J. (1977). **J. Cell. Biol.** 75, 866.

66. Tyrrell, D. A., Keeton, B. R. and Dubowitz, V. (1976). **Br. Med. J.** 2, 88.

67. Kinsky, S. C. (1972). **Biochim. Biophys. Acta.** 265, 1.

68. Papahadjopoulos, D., Vail, W.J., Jacobson, K. and Poste, G. (1975). **Biochim. Biophys. Acta** 394, 483.

69. Roseman, M., Litman, B.J. and Thompson, T.E. (1975). **Biochemistry** 14, 4826.

70. Johnson, S.M. (1975). **Biochem. Soc. Trans.** 3, 160.

71. Bangham, A.D., Hill, M.V. and Miller, N.G. (1974). **Methods Membr. Biol.** 1, 1.

72. Mason, J.T. and Huang, C. (1978). **Ann. N.Y. Acad. Sci.** 308, 29.

73. Bergelson, L.D. (1979). **Methods Membr. Biol.** 9, 275.

74. Meeren, P.V., Laethem, M.V., Vanderdeelen, J. and Baert, L. (1992). **J. Lipo. Res.** 2, 23.

75. Hargreaves, W.R. and Deamer, D.W. (1978). **Biochemistry** 17, 3759.

76. Gregory, D.W. and Pirie, B.J.S. (1973). **J. Microsc.** 99, 251.

77. Larrabee, A.L. (1979). **Biochemistry** 18, 3321.

78. Luna, E. and McConnell, H.M. (1977). **Biochim. Biophys. Acta** 466, 381.

79. Luna, E. and McConnell, H.M. (1978). **Biochim. Biophys. Acta** 509, 462.

80. Geurts Vankessel, W.S.M., Har, W.M.A. and Demel, R.A. (1977). **Biochim. Biophys. Acta.** 486, 525.

81. Papahadjopoulos, D., Poste, G. and Vail, W. J. (1979). **Method Membr. Biol.** 10, 1.

82. Vail, W.J. and Stollery, J.G. (1979). **Biochim. Biophys. Acta** 551, 74.

83. Sharma, P., Tyrell, D.A. and Ryman, B.E. (1977). **Biochem.Soc.Tran.** 5, 1146.

84. Van Ren Swoude, A.J.P.M., Blumenthal, R. and Weinstein, J.N. (1980). **Biochim. Biophys. Acta** 595, 151.

85. Fraley, R., Wyatt, J. and Papahadjopoulos, D. (1981). In :"Liposomes:From Physical Structure to Therapeutic Applications", (Knight, C. G. Ed.), Elsevier North Holland, Biomedical Press, Amsterdam, New York, Oxford, p.69.

86. Fry, D.W., White C. and Goldman, D.J. (1978). **Anal. Biochem.** 90, 809.

87. Rosier, R.N., Gunter, T.E., Tucker, D.A. and Gunter, K.K. (1979). **Anal. Biochem.** 96, 384.

88. Gunter, K.K., Gunter, T.E., Jarkowski, A. and Rosier, R.N. (1982). **Anal. Biochem.** 120, 113.

89. Pidgeon, C., Hunt, A.H. and Dittrich. K. (1986). **Pharma. Res.** 3, 23.

90. Zingsheim, H.P. (1972). **Biochim. Biophys. Acta** 265, 339.

91. Zingsheim, H.P. and Plattner, H. (1976). **Methods Membr. Biol.** 7, 1.

92. Sleytr, U.B. and Robards, A.W. (1977). **J. Microsc.** 110, 1.

93. Verkleij, A.J., Ververgaert, P.H.J.T. (1978). **Biochim. Biophys. Acta** 515, 303.

94. VanVenetic, R., Leunissen-Bijvelt, J., Verkleij, A.J. and Ververgaert, P.H.J.T. (1980). **J. Microsc.** 118:401.

95. Szoka, F. and Papahadjopoulos, D. (1980). **Ann. Rev. Bioeng.** 9, 467.

96. Cullins, P.R. and Hope, M.J. (1985). In : Biochemistry of lipid and membrane (Vance, D.E. and Vance, J.E. Eds.), Benzamin / Cumming Inc, p.56.

97. Weiner, N., Williams, N, Birha, G., Ramachandran, C., Shipma, C. Jr. and Flynn, G. (1989). **Antimicrob. Agents Chemother.** 1217.

98. Ganesan, M.G., Weiner, N.D., Flynn, G.I. and Ho, N.F.H. (1984). **Int. J. Pharm.** 20, 139.

99. Egbaria, K., Ramachandran, C., Kittayanod, D. and Weiner, N. (1990). **Antimicrob. Agents Chemother.** 34, 107.

100. Victoria, M., Knepp, C., Szoka, Jr., Richard, H.C. (1990). **J. Contr. Rel.** 12, 25.

101. Amselem, S., Cohen, R. and Barenholz, Y. (1993). **Chem. Phys. Lipids** 64, 219.

102. Bartlett, G.R.J. (1959). **J. Biol. Chem.** 234, 466.

103. Stewart, J.C.M. (1959). **Anal. Biochem.** 104, 10.

104. Klein, R.A. (1980). **Biochim. Biophys. Acta** 210, 486.

105. Brooks, C.J.W., Machachlan, J., Cole, W.J., Lawric, T.D.V. (1984). **Proc. Symp. Anal. Steroids**, Hungary, p.349.

106. Lambelet, P, and Loliger, J. (1984). **Chem. Phys. Lipids** 35, 185.

107. Kates, M. and Kushwaha, S.C. (1976). In: Lipids (Paoletti, R. Ed.), Raven Press, New York, Vol1, p 267.

108. Bali, A., Dhawan, S. and Gupta, C.M. (1983). **FEBS Lett.** 154, 373.

109. Agrawal, K., Bali, A. and Gupta, C.M. (1986). **Biochim. Biophys. Acta** 856, 36.

110. Love, W.G., Amos, N., Williams, B.D. and Kellaway, I.W. (1990). **J. Microencap.** 7, 105.

111. Weinstein, J.N., Klausher, R.D., Innerarity, T., Ralston, E. and Blumenthal, R. (1981). **Biochim. Biophys. Acta** 647, 270.

112. Crowe, L.M., Womersley, C., Crowe, J.H., Reid, D., Appel, L.and Rudolph, A. (1986). **Biochim. Biophys. Acta** 861, 131.

113. Leaver, J., Alonso, A., Aziz, A.D. and Chapman, D. (1983). **Biochim. Biophys. Acta** 732, 210.

5

LIPOSOMES AS VEHICLE FOR ALLERGEN PRESENTATION AND IMMUNOMODULATION IN THE IMMUNOTHERAPY OF ALLERGIC DISORDERS

S. V. GANGAL* and B. B. SHARMA

Centre for Biochemical Technology, Mall Road, New Delhi 110 007

INTRODUCTION

Vaccination has been the most successful means of protecting humans and domestic animals from infectious diseases. Most vaccines operate by limiting infections, not necessarily by preventing them; it is the host immune system that mediates control on ultimate clearance of the infectious agent. Many of the most widely used vaccines developed for use in humans is based on live replicating organisms that have been attenuated. Vaccination with these agents results in a limited infection, but measurable disease pathogenesis is usually avoided and recovery is complete. The resultant immuneresponses are protective against the fully virulent pathogens and long-term immunological memory is induced. Today, attenuated vaccines are still used and efforts to develop the next generation vaccines are active.

Inactivated vaccines differ considerably from standard attenuated vaccines since they use 'killed' pathogenic organisms, such as viral particles or bacterial cells. Subunit vaccines represent further reduction or simplification of these inactivated products since only a limited number of components from the appropriate pathogen are formulated into a vaccine. Both inactivated and subunit vaccines are considered to be much safer than their attenuated counterparts because they contain absolutely no infectious agents. The safety profile is further enhanced for subunit vaccines because of their defined physical and chemical characteristics. This is the main reason for continued research into vaccines of this type.

Vaccines involved in allergy immunotherapy consist of allergens, harmless substances for normal individuals, to which the atopic patient gets sensitized. After the discovery of pollen extraction methodology by Willian Dunbar in 1910, the allergen specific immmunotherapy was first started in 1911 by Noon and John Freeman with pollen extracts in hay fever patient. Then, in 1940, first placebo controlled clinical trial of desensitization was carried out by William Frankland. Following this, allergy immunotherapy spread all over the world and was used to treat the patient of type I allegry, asthma, hay fever, rhinitis and conjunctivitis, etc. The vaccines used for allergy immunotherapy have been aqueous extracts of the allergenic materials. Recently, attention is being paid to design vaccines, which can improve upon the limitations of conventional immunotherapy.

The design of vaccines is directed by numerous considerations that include immunogenicity, safety and stability. However, it is the qualitative and quantitative characteristics of immune responses induced by vaccination that are the most crucial aspects of modern vaccines. There are five major factors which effect immune responses.

- The nature and the dose of the immunogens/allergen
- The adjuvant or carriers used in the formulation
- The immunization schedule
- The route of administration
- The immune status of the host being immunized

LIPOSOMES

Twenty years after the discovery of the immunological adjuvant properties of liposomes [1], and the ensuing multitude of related animal immunization studies [2-4], liposomes as adjuvants have come of age [5,6], with the first liposomes-based vaccine (against hepatitis A) being licensed for use in humans. Liposomes are artificial microscopic vesicles where the lipids are arranged in a continuous bilayer configuration surrounding the aqueous compartments [7]. Liposomes are easy to prepare and can have several variations in their compositions as per the requirement of particular protein antigen.

Functionalized liposomes

Functionalized liposomes are defined as liposomes whose surface has been modified so that they exhibit a specific ability to interact actively with the biological environment, i.e. liposomes containing or exhibiting tissue-selective enzymes, (monoclonal) antibodies, and antibody fragments, surface glycoproteins, carbohydrates or haptens, all of which are being explored either to achieve tissue/cell-selective targeting for drug delivery or nonspecific immunostimulation or to elicit a specific immune response.

Liposomes are taken up by the macrophages very fast and may induce immune response in the following ways:

Nonspecific macrophage immunostimulation

As an alternative to chemotherapy, immunomodulation, e.g., activation of monocytes to a tumoricidal state using liposomes incorporated immunostimulants, has been suggested, with the rationale that liposomes are avidly taken up by macrophages. Hence, they should efficiently deliver the immunstimulating agents to their cellular targets: a unique application of the concept of "passive" targeting. Potent immunostimulants such as interleukin-2 [8], muramyl dipeptide (MDP) [9,10] and lipophilic derivatives have all been used successfully to elicit strong macrophage stimulation.

Cellular and humoral antibody response

It is generally accepted that macrophage uptake of antigen-carrying liposomes and digestion of the antigen(s) to peptides that bind to class II major histocompatibility (MHC) molecules is the mechanism responsible for enhanced T-cell-dependent humoral immune response [11]. Following lysosomal degradation, the processed antigens are presented in conjunction with class II MHC molecules, which trigger $CD4^+$ T cell and B cell response. For enhanced adjuvant effect, antigens may also be incorporated within the liposomal inner compartments.

Cytotoxic T-lymphocyte response

In addition to eliciting a humoral immune response, liposomes can be engineered so that the antigenic peptides are complexed with the class I MHC glycoproteins, resulting in the induction of $CD8^+$ cytotoxic T lymphocytes (CTL). A CTL response is triggered when instead of conventional (pH-insensitive) liposomes; pH dependent fusogenic liposomes are employed as antigen carriers. Following uptake into the phagolysosomal vacuole, pH -dependent liposomes fuse with the lysosomal membrane as a consequence of the pH drop, and peptides are released into the cytosol. This has been demonstrated *in vitro* [12,13] and *in vivo* [14,15] with ovalbumin-containing pH-sensitive liposomes in mouse EL-4 thylmoma cells that were sensitized for ovalbumin-specific CTL killing [16].

Mucosal immunity (IgA response)

Oral administration of antigen carrying liposomes may be a unique means to stimulate IgA secretion, specifically in the oral mucosa where it would aid in the generation of a salivary IgA response to sero-type specific carbohydrates of *Streptococcus mutans* and thus reduces colonization of the oral cavity by virulent bacteria and protect against caries. It is known that mucosal secretion of IgA is induced in the so-called gut-associated lymphoid tissue (GALT) or Peyer's patches in the small intestine. Specifically, the so-called M cells in the Peyer's patches phagocytic antigens from the gut lumen, providing a target for antigen-carrying liposomes in the small intestine [17].

REGULATION OF THE IMMUNE SYSTEM

There are three significant cellular interactions involved in the regulation of the immune system.

    a. macrophage-T-cell
    b. T-cell-T-cell
    c. T-cell-B-cell

Macrophage-T-cell interactions

When antigens is first encountered, it is metabolized by macrophages [18]. The product of this initial step leads to degraded peptide fragments called *processed antigen* and is presented to the helper/induce T-cell population ($CD4^+8^-$) in the framework of the MHC class II molecules. In this process a number of interleukins are generated. The processed antigen is then presented to the helper T-cell subpopulation and is recognized by the CD3/TCR complex. This clone of T-cells is than induced to expand and to produce receptors specific for antigen and for IL-2 and is also stimulated to produce IL-2 and it can interact and expand a separate clone of antigen-sensitized T -cells, which can synthesize other lymphokines such as interferon gamma. Interferon gamma can stimulate antigen-presenting cells (e.g., macrophages) to synthesize class II molecules. Thus, there exists a cascading system of intercellular communication of cellular interaction mediated through signals provided by macrophages, lymphocytes and interleukins

T-cell-T-cell interactions

This type of regulation involves the interactions of different subsets of T-cells. T-cells can communicate with other subpopulations of T-cells through IL-2 cytokine cascade CD4⁻8⁺ T-cells can also interact with target cells or with membrane-associated antigens on target cells in the context of class I antigens, found on target cells, thus providing antigen presentation to the cytotoxic T cells. Recent evidence suggests that at least two subgroup of helper T-cells exist: Th-1 and Th-2. Different patterns of cytokine reactions have been identified with these helper T-cell subgroups, the Th-1 mediating primarily delayed hypersensitivity reaction, and the Th-2 mediating IgE synthesis and eosinophilia. Although the pattern of cytokine production in atopic asthma is unknown, apredominant Th-2 like lymphocyte subpopulation has been found in bronchial biopsy specimens and bronchoalveolar lavage fluids of patients with bronchial asthma [19].

T-cell-B-cell interactions

The third type of regulation occurs between T-lymphocytes and B-lymphocytes. Two major types of communication pathways between T-lymphocytes and B-lymphocytes are involved in regulation: upregulation and downregulation. T-lymphocytes involved in the upregulation of B-cell function are regarded to as the *helper inducer T-cell population* (CD4⁺8⁺). Another subset involved in the down regulation of B-cell function is referred to as *suppressor cytotoxic* (CD4⁻8⁺) T-cells. There are other interactions of interleukins involved in the synthesis of IgE such as IL-4, IL-5, and IL-6 and inhibitory responses seen with other lymphokines such as interferon-γ.

LIPOSOMES AS IMMUNOLOGICAL ADJUVANTS

A large amount of literature exists on the various applications of liposomes in immunology, not only as potential drug carrier [20] or as tools to study phenomena underlying immune functions [21-23] but also as promising immunological adjuvants for human and veterinary uses [24,25].

The immunoadjuvanticity of liposomes, first recognized by Allison and Gregoriadis in 1974 [1] has been since repeatedly demonstrated for both, humoral and cell-mediated immunity [3,4,36], with as apparently unique and obligatory requirement a physical association between antigen and the liposomal vehicle [27-30]. Using encapsulated and covalent linked antigen, it was demonstrated that not only the association with liposomes but also the mode of antigen association influences the activation of the immune system [31-33]. Thus, in identical conditions of doses and protein:lipid ratios, encapsulated antigen was shown to stimulated preferentially the production of IgG1 and covalently linked antigen to favor a longer lasting activation characterized by increased production of IgM, IgG3, and IgG2a together with that of IgG1. In *in vitro* experiments, other differences were also noted between the two liposomal antigenic formulations such as the anti-IL-1 sensitivity of the proliferative response they elicited [34]. These overall results suggest that, besides their general immunopotentiating effect, liposomal antigens might follow different path in the immune system depending on the mode of antigen-liposome association. Therefore leading to activation of distinct Th subsets such as the Th-1 and Th-2 initially described by Mosmann et al., [35] which promote cell-mediated and humoral immunity, respectively.

Unlike other potent immunoadjuvants, e.g. Complete Freud's adjuvant, which are unacceptable for human use because of undesirable necrotic reactions at the site of injection, liposome-encapsulated antigens do not induce local granuloma formation [36]. Another advantage of using liposomes as an immunostimulator is their apparent ineffectiveness in revoking delayed hypersensitivity reactions to the encapsulated antigen [37]. Furthermore, the lipids used in the synthesis of the commonly used liposomal vesicles are not foreign to the body and no apparent ill effects have been found in injected human subjects [36,38,39]. Although liposomal vesicles may prove to be effective and safe vaccine carriers, the critical physico-chemical factors of these vesicles in stimulating an optimal response are ill defined and the cellular mechanisms mediating their immunopotentiating effects have not been established.

Such a versatile, non-toxic immunoadjuvant system, potentially capable of orienting the response according to some specific required needs, may find important clinical applications and complement advantageously aluminum hydroxide, the only currently licensed adjuvant for human use, which essentially potentiates humoral immunity [40]. Because of potential impact of liposomes in vaccine design, the interaction of liposomal antigen with immune cells has to be more deeply understood and characterized in conditions compatible with vaccination standards in vaccine design, liposomal systems may offer many advantages over more classic adjuvants such as alum or Freund's adjuvant. Freund's adjuvant, which effectively potentitates cell-mediated immunity, is associated with severe inflammatory and toxic side effects, while alum is less reactogenic but does not promote cell-mediated immunity.

Optimal adjuvanticity of liposomes can be achieved by the appropriate choice of vesicle composition [41,42], surface charge [32], and phospholipid to antigen mass ratio [43], ligand-mediated targeting of liposomes to immunocompetent cells [44] and the use of liposome-entrapped cytokines such as interleukin-2 [45,33]. Hence, the availability of liposomes with variable structural characteristics and mode of antigen accommodation suggests versatility in immunoadjuvant action and vaccine design.

LIPOSOMES IN POTENTIATION OF CELL-MEDIATED IMMUNITY

In addition to their ability to enhance antibody formation, liposomes are also effective in promoting cell-mediated immunity. Different types of cellular responses induced by liposome-associated macromolecules have been studied.

Lymphocyte proliferation response

The proliferative response of cultured lymphocytes challenged with antigen is considered as *in vitro* correlate of cell-mediated immunity [46]. The extent of cellular multiplication can be determined by measuring the incorporation of tritiated thymidine into DNA of the dividing cells. In an attempt to evaluate the efficacy of liposome-associated antigen in eliciting a primarily T-cell proliferative response, rabbits were immunized in one foot pad with liposome-encapsulated BSA and cells from the draining popliteal lymph node were subsequently cultured in the presence of the antigen. It is evident that lymph node cells primed with liposome-entrapped BSA elicited a significantly higher proliferative response than cells obtained from the control lymph node primed with free BSA. It has been demonstrated that liposomes injected via the food pad are localized predominantly in the regional lymph nodes [47]. This selective localization of liposome entrapped antigen may partly explain its apparent better efficacy in providing a higher response. In contrast, the free antigen may channel through the lymph node more rapidly in less antigen retention by the regional lymphoid cells. Since the T-cell proliferative response is facilitated by the participation of macrophages [48], liposome-encapsulated antigen, being in particular form, is more likely to enhance the uptake by phagocytic cells which in turn triggers and elevated T-cell response.

Induction of cytotoxic T-lymphocytes

Liposomes have been shown to be effective carriers of major histocompatibility complex (MHC) antigens in inducing the formation of MHC-restricted cytotoxic T lymphocytes (CTL) in murine [49] and human [50,51] systems. Previous attempts to investigate the molecular interactions in eliciting the CTL response were hampered by the necessity of using intact cells or cell membranes containing the stimulating antigens. Recent advances in liposome technology enable the incorporation of highly purified recognition molecules, e.g., MHC antigens, cell surface membrane components, and viral antigens in phospholipid vesicles that are capable of triggering the T-cell effector function. The presence of both viral and MHC antigens in liposomes is necessary for the successful stimulation of secondary CTL against specific viral targets [49,52]. The generation of the CTL response by liposome-incorporated MHC antigen requires the active participation of macrophage [53]. Macrophages are involved in processing of the liposome-associated antigen and in activating helper T cells, which promote the CTL response [54].

Macrophage activation

Cell-mediated immunity may be expressed either by the direct action of the effector cell on the target, e.g., the lytic action on the viral targets by CTL, or by the release of biologically-active soluble factors, called lymphokines, from activated lymphocytes which are predominantly T cells. One of the many lymphokines obtainable from lymphocytes stimulated by antigens or mitogens is the macrophage activating factor (MAF). Macrophages stimulated by the appropriate lymphokine are more active than resting macrophages in performing phagocytic functions. It is known that MAF-activated macrophages selectively destroy neoplastic, but not normal cell [55]. The tumoricidal activity of macrophages activated by liposome encapsulated MAF was much enhanced compared to the free factor [56]. Using a tumor model in mice, it has been demonstrated that tumor metastasis can be eradicated by activating the tumoricidal functions of macrophages with liposome-encapsulated lymphokines [57]. These studies raise hope for the clinical application of liposome-encapsulated lymphokines in the treatment of metastatic tumors.

It is clear that the versatility of phospholipid vesicles resides in the ease of altering their physico-chemical characteristics for specific needs. The lipid composition and physical structure of a liposomal carrier can be adjusted to minimize its intrinsic immunogenicity yet retains its maximal adjuvant effect. Although the cell types involved in interacting with liposome-associated antigens and lymphokines are being identified, the basic mechanisms at the cellular and molecular levels mediating the potentiated response remain ill defined. The elucidation of the relationship between the nature of liposome/antigen interaction and the potentiated immune response will facilitate a better design of vaccine carriers for human use. In view of the success, though limited, in using liposomal carriers for the delivery of labile substances via the gastrointestinal tract, the development of a suitable lipid vesicle for the delivery of oral vaccine may be on the horizon. Finally, the application of liposomal carriers for the delivery of other biological macromolecules must take into consideration the impact of potential immunological complications.

ROLE OF T-CELLS IN THE ALLERGIC RESPONSE

It is now widely believed that IgE synthesis, the accumulation of eosinophils and basophils and the increase in mast cell numbers associated with the inflammatory component of the allergic response, all depend on the production of cytokines from Th-2 type cells. These comprise IL-4, IL-10, IL-13 in mice, and IL-4, IL-5 and IL-13 in humans. Mosmann and Coffman [58] first proposed the concept of subdivision of helper (CD4+) T cells based on their cytokine profile. Th-2 type cells preferentially transcribe and translate mRNA for IL-4 and IL-5 and predominate in inflammatory responses associated with atopic allergy and helminthic parasitic infections. IL-4 is an essential cofactor for the production of IgE by B cells, a property also shared by IL-13, IL-5, together with GM-CSF and IL-3, promote eosinophil maturation from CD34 precursor cells, as well as eosinophil activation and survival. The counter part of the Th-2 type cell is the Th-1 type cells. Through the elaboration of IFN-γ and IL-2 (but not IL-4 and IL-5), Th-1 type cells regulate classical delayed-type hyper-sensitivity reactions and other effector functions usually associated with macrophage activation and T-cell mediated immunity.

Although this dichotomy of T cells is firmly established in mice, there was initial scepticism about the existence of a human counterpart of type 1 and type 2 CD4[+] cells. It was found, however, that allergen-specific T-cell clones derived from the peripheral blood of atopic donors secreted cytokines according to a Th-2 type pattern, whereas bacterial antigen-specific clones secreted cytokines according to a Th-1 type pattern [59]. Furthermore, bronchoalveolar lavage [60] and bronchial biopsy [61] specimens obtained from atopic donors challenged with a specific allergen contained inflammatory infiltrate rich in cells expressing mRNA encoding predominantly IL-4 and IL-5, rather than IL-2 and IFN-γ.

It is not clear how Th cells differentiate between bacterial and allergen antigens, since their is no evidence that such antigens have specific structural features that Th cells might recognize. In some diseases, such as leprosy and human immuno-deficiency virus (HIV) infection, Th-1 or Th-2 type responses may predominate in different persons at different stages of the disease, although the Th cells presumably recognize the same array of foreign antigens. Since the antigen specificity of a Th cell is established apparently randomly in the thymus, it is difficult to conceptualize how Th cells recognizing a particular antigen could be preprogrammed at this stage of development to secrete a particular pattern of cytokines in a subsequent encounter with this antigen. Particularly since this ability may result from permanent structural alterations in the genome of the Th cell. To accommodate these problems, it has been suggested that, at any inflammatory site, Th-1 and Th-2 type helped T cells differentiate from a common antigen-specific post-thymic precursor termed Thp' that produces IL-2. A cell intermediate between Thp and Th-1/Th-2 type helper T cells that produces both sets of cytokines (IL-4 and IL-5 as well as IL-2 and IFN-γ) has also been described. But whether this cell type (termed 'Th0') is an essential intermediate in the development of Th0 into Th-1 or Th-2 type cells is still unclear. Several factors appear to influence the development of Th-1 and Th-2 type cells. These include the nature and concentration of antigen, route of administration, the type of antigen-presenting cell (APC), and the presence or absence of cytokines secreted by other cells in the microenvironment.

It is considered that even a committed Th-1 cell can convert to a Th-2 cell and vice-versa. Under such conditions, the addition of IL-4 to Th-1 type T cell clones proliferating in response to specific antigen alters the profile of secreted cytokines away from a Th-1 type and towards a Th-2 type profile. Furthermore, IL-4 promotes the differentiation of Th-2 cells in the early stages of an antigen-specific response of Th cells and together with IL-10 inhibits the secretion of cytokines by Th-1 type cells and inhibits the responses of Th-2 type cells. IFN-γ promotes the differentiation of Th-1 type cells and inhibits the responses of Th-2 type cells. IFN-γ production is regulated by IL-12 with the balance between IL-2 and IL-4 determining the Th-type 1 or 2 response.

The alternative view is that the pattern of cytokine secretion by two subtypes is immutable and already established in Th cells before clonal expansion. In this case, the changes brought about by treatments with such cytokines as IL-4, IFN-γ and IL-12 may reflect population shifts in mixtures of irreversibly committed Th cells, rather than changes in differentiation at the clonal level. In either case there is the question of whether these alterations are imprinted on the genotype or phenotype of Th cells that proliferate at localized inflammatory sites so that they can be passed on to progeny memory Th cells and, if so, how could this be accomplished in molecular terms?

With regard to the role of APC in this process, it has been shown that Th-1 and Th-2 pathways are differentially activated by two costimulatory molecules, B7-1 (CD80) and B7-2 (CD86), expressed on APC [62, 63]. Anti-B7-1 reduce the incidence of experimental allergic encephalomyelitis (EAE) while anti-B7-2 increase disease severity. Thus, interaction of B7-1 and B7-2 with their shared counter-receptors, CD28 and CTLA-4, may result in very different outcomes in clinical disease by influencing commitment of precursors to a Th-1 or Th-2 lineage.

There are also important association between IgE responsiveness to specific allergens and the human leukocyte antigen (HLA) system. Thus, in addition to the regulatory loci, significant associations between HLA class II DR and DP phenotypes and allergic IgE and IgG responses to environmental allergens (including ragweed, pollen, ryegrass and house dust mite) have been identified [64]. Furthermore, a linkage has been observed between specific sequences on the α-chain of the T-cell receptor encoded on chromosome 14 and the allergic phenotype which increase the complexity of the genetics of atopy and asthma [65].

LIPOSOME ENTRAPPED ALLERGEN IN IMMUNOTHERAPY

The foreign substances have the capacity to evoke immunologic responses and are referred to as *antigens* or *immunogens* and all are recognized as foreign by the host. *Allergens* are a specialized class of immunogens which elicit the formation of IgE antibodies that trigger allergic reactions in certain genetically predisposed (i.e., atopic) individuals, Thus, all allergens are antigens but all antigens are not necessarily allergens.

Allergy or *hypersensitivity* may be defined as a constellation of signs and symptoms in which the altered immunologic reactions between foreign substances (antigens or allergens) and antibody or sensitized lymphocytes are thought to play a major role, resulting clinically in pathologic reactions referred to as the *allergic reactions*.

The hypersensitivity reactions are broadly categorized into four types. The *type I reaction* is initiated by allergen or antigen reacting with tissue cells passively sensitized by antibody produced elsewhere, leading to the release of pharma-cologically active substances. These *analphylatic reactions* include both general anaphylaxis in humans and other animals and local manifestations of anaphylaxis, such as that observed in the skin following diagnostic skin-prick tests, as well as local responses in the respiratory and gastrointestinal tracts. A further example is the instances of sudden death in infancy in which anaphylactic hypersensitivity to cows milk proteins was a proposed mechanism [66].

Type II reactions (cytolytic or cytotoxic) are initiated by antibody reacting either with an antigenic component of a tissue cell or with an antigen or hapten intimately associated with these cells. Complement is usually but not always, necessary to effect the cellular damage.

Type III reactions (Arthus reactions and immune complex or toxic complex syndrome) occur when antigen and antibody, reacting in antigen excess, form complexes which, possibly with the aid of complement, are toxic to cells.

Type IV reactions refer to situations where specifically sensitive cells react with allergen or antigen deposited at the local site, as in delayed-or tuberculin-type hypersensitivity.

In allergy a Th-2 response is dominated to basically harmless substances (nonpathogenic) therefore through immunotherapy it is beneficial to change the response from Th-2 to Th-2 type. Immunotherapy is one of the most frequently administered treatments for *type I* hypersensitive reactions. In this approach, a series of injections of the offending allergen, to which the patient is sensitive, is administered until a maintenance level reached at which the symptoms are controlled. The exact mechanism of immunotherapy is poorly understood but is often attributed to the following proposed mechanisms:

1. Decrease in allergen specific IgE over time
2. Ablation of expectant post-seasonal rise in allergen specific IgE
3. Increase in allergen specific IgG, the blocking antibodies
4. Increase in allergen specific IgG and IgA antibodies in nasal secretions
5. Decrease in allergen induced basophil histamine release in some patients
6. Generation of antigen specific suppressor T cells

Conventional immunotherapy leads to initial increase in serum IgE that may cause severe systemic reactions on repeated doses. To overcome this problem, allergens have been modified by polymerization to reduce the allergenicity without sacrificing the immunogenicity, however, this can alter the native characteristics of the allergenic proteins. The past 10 years have seen intense research activity directed towards the understanding the regulation of immune response in allergy immunotherapy. Recent work indicates that liposomes as adjuvants can be helpful to overcome many of these problems. Allison and Gregoriadis first demonstrated liposome-mediated enhancement of antibody formation in 1974 [1]. Since then, the effectiveness of liposomes in potentiating the immune response of a variety of antigens in numerous independent studies has been documented. In immuno-prophylaxis the aim is to direct the immune response from Th-2 to Th-1 pathway. Since liposomes possess a natural tendency to localize in reticuloendothelial cells, including macrophages, it may be argued that encapsulation of allergens into liposomes could selectively increase the Th-1 response. This will certainly be helpful to overcome the problems associated with conventional immunotherapy. It has been reported from the previous work done by our group that liposome-entrapped allergen induces specific IgG and diminishes specific IgE level in mice and modulates the immune response from Th-2 to Th-1, which may be useful in immunotherapy of allergic disorders [67-70]. The dual effect of liposomes in immune response, i.e. immunoadjuvanticity and immunomodulation, appears to reinforce the likelihood that the liposomes may well become the next generation vaccine carriers.

Allergenic extracts used in immunotherapy comprise a large group of products such as pollens, fungi, house dust mite, food, etc. They are unique compared to other biological and conventional pharmaceuticals. The present form of aqueous extract used, needs to be replaced by better modified vaccines to increase the efficacy and safety in the treatment of allergic disorders. Allergens entrapped into liposomes have been reported to show a great promise in this field.

Immunotherapy is one of the most frequently administered treatment for type I hypersensitivity reaction. In this approach, a series of injection of the offending allergen to which the patient is sensitive, are administered until a maintenance level is reached at which the symptoms are controlled. Conventional immunotherapy leads to initial increase in serum IgE that may cause severe systemic reaction on repeated doses. To overcome this problem, allergens have been modified by polymerization to reduce the allergenicity without sacrificing their immunogenicity, however, this can alter the native characteristics of the allergenic proteins. It has been reported from the previous work done by our group that liposome entrapped allergen induces specific IgG and diminishes specific IgE level in mice and modulate the immune response [67-70]. This may be useful in immunotherapy of allergic disorders.

In the present study, liposome entrapped mite allergen preparation was formulated with the aim of utilizing adjuvant property of liposomes in allergy immunotherapy. To study the immunoadjuvanticity of liposome entrapped mite allergen and to compare it with alum (which is an adjuvant licensed for human use), Balb/c (halotype H-2d) (NIN, Hyderabad) were immunized with different doses and the antibodies IgG, its subclass and IgE were measured in the sera. To elucidate the way, in which liposomes confer protection, IgG subclasses were also studied. Further, cytokine induction by allergen entrapped liposomes were studied.

Immunization protocol

Animals	-	Balb/c mice
Group I	-	Control mice injected with PBS
Group II	-	Free antigen (FA)
Group III	-	Alum adsorbed antigen (AAA)
Group IV	-	Liposome entrapped antigen (LEA)

Dose and route

Different groups of mice were divided into subgroups and were injected PBS or 2.5 or 25 or 50 µg allergen either as free allergen (crude mite extract) or adsorbed on 5 mg alum per animal or as LEA (made of crude lecithin; cholesterol, 7:3) per animal intraperitoneally (i.p.)

Immunization schedule

Days	Immunization protocol
Zero day	Priming
9th day	First booster
16th day	Serum separation
25th day	Second booster
32nd day	Serum separation
36th day	Third booster
44th day	Serum separation
62nd day	Fourth booster
70th day	Serum separation

Sampling

Blood was drawn from the retro-orbital plexuses, predilated with infra red lamp on the 7th or 8th day after each booster and separated sera were tested for specific antibodies by enzyme linked immunosorbent assay (ELISA).

RESULTS AND DISCUSSION

It has been reported earlier that immunization of mice with liposome entrapped allergen after second booster results in the induction of an IgG response with a concomitant decrease in IgE response as compared to mice treated with free *Artemesia* pollen allergen (65-70). The protection conferred by LEA may be due to the ability of liposomes to selectively induce appropriate immunoglobulin isotypes. We have taken these studies a step further to elucidate the mechanism of adjuvanticity of liposome entrapped allergen and hence ubiquitous allergen mite. *Dermatophagoides farinae* was incorporated into liposomes and the effect on the induction of antibody response was seen by determining serum antibodies such as IgM, IgG and its subclasses and IgE.

Our results show that as compared to mice injected with FA and AAA, mice injected with LEA induced higher antibody response of IgM, IgG and all the IgG subclasses except for IgG1 levels, which in LEA mice were higher than FA treated mice. AAA treated mice showed the maximum levels of IgG1 (Fig. 3). In the AAA group, there was consistent increase in IgG1 and IgM response with the increase in dose. As expected, LEA group showed the maximum IgM levels and the response was highest with the 25 μg dose (Fig. 1).

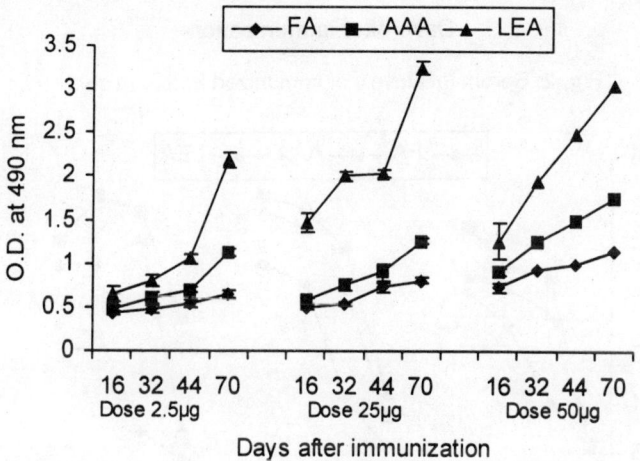

Fig.1 : Serum IgM levels of immunized Balb/c mice

As indicated in respective figures (Fig. 4 and 5), among other IgG subclasses, IgG2a, IgG2b levels were very high in the mice treated with LEA but there was only slight increase in these antibodies levels in AAA injected mice as compared to FA immunized group. Also, IgG2a levels in LEA group were maximum with 25μg dose but remained same for all the doses of FA and AAA groups whereas IgG2b levels increased with the increase in dose in all the cases.

IgG3 levels in LEA group were much higher than FA treated group whereas there was almost no difference in levels of FA and AAA treated mice against all the doses. Induction of serum IgE levels in mice injected with LEA was low as compared to FA and AAA injected mice (Fig. 4). Increase in IgG (blocking antibodies) reduces the access of (whatsoever available) specific IgG to the mast cells. This decreases the degranulation of mast cells resulting in lowering of the release of inflammatory mediators responsible for causing discomfort to the patient during conventional immunotherapy which results in failure to achieve the required maintenance dose for the effective treatment. Hence, by achieving the increase in specific IgG with concurrent decrease in IgE antibodies using allergen entrapped in liposomes, it may be possible to reduce the risk of systemic reactions and increase the safety and efficacy of the immunotherapy.

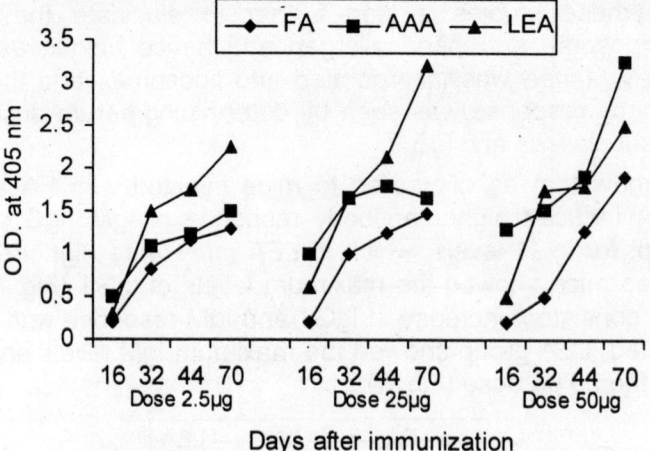

Fig. 2: Serum IgG levels of immunized Balb/c mice

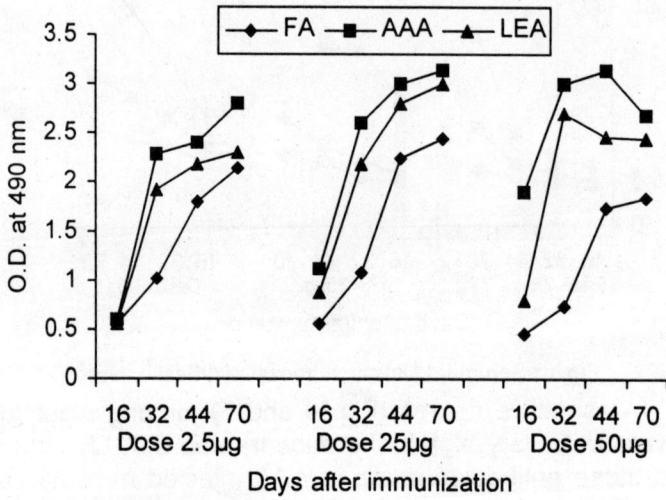

Fig. 3: Serum IgG1 levels in immunizaed Balb/c mice

It has been reported [71] that the ration of specific IgG to specific IgE was found to correlate significantly with symptomatic improvement. Therefore, IgG to IgE ratios was calculated. Our results showed that there was a significant increase in the ratio of specific IgG to IgE in mice given allergen entrapped in liposomes over that in mice injected with free allergenic protein or AAA (Fig. 5). Since 25µg dose showed the maximum increase in the ratio in both the strains of mice, therefore, all further studies on cytokine pattern to see the correlation with the above antibody subclasses response were carried out with 25 µg dose. In conclusion, it can be stated that the entrapment of allergen in liposomes could be effective for immunotherapy of Type I allergic disorders.

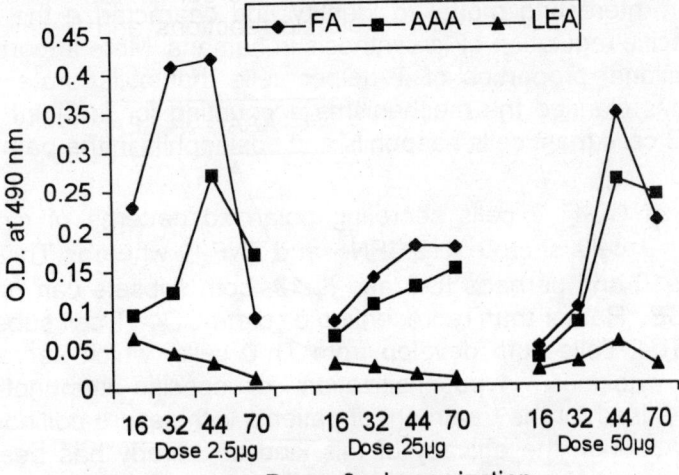

Fig. 4: Serum IgE levels in immunized Balb/c mice

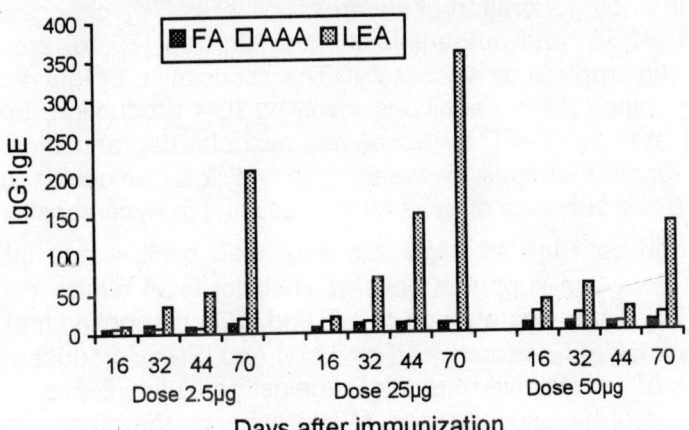

Fig. 5 : Serum IgG:IgE of immunized Balb/c mice

CYTOKINES AND ALLERGY IMMUNOTHERAPY

In the 1970s, evidence accumulated that some of the active molecules produced by cells of the immune system other than immunoglobulins were also involved in the network of intercellular communication. These substances are now referred to as **cytokines** rather than lymphokines. Many research groups have focussed on the role of cytokines in regulating IgE production and in controlling, the downstream effector cells such as mast cells, basophils and eosinophil. Simultaneously, there has been increasing interest in the role of T-lymphocytes in allergy.

The cellular basis of IgE regulation has actively been investigated to gain an insight into the pathogenesis of a condition, which affects a considerable proportion

The cellular basis of IgE regulation has actively been investigated to gain an insight into the pathogenesis of a condition, which affects a considerable proportion of the population. The investigation of molecular events underlying IgE synthesis has provided an interesting model to identify and characterize the signals involved in isotype-specific regulation of Ig synthesis in humans. More importantly, intense study of the functional properties of T helper cells that collaborate with B cells for Ig synthesis has clarified the mechanisms accounting for the joint involvement of IgE producing B cells mast cells/basophils and eosinophils in the pathogenesis of allergic reactions.

Clones of CD4[+] T cells secreting polarized patterns of cytokines have been identified Th-1 cells secrete IL-2, IFN-γ and TNF-β, whereas Th-2 cells secrete IL-4, IL-5 and IL-10 and perhaps IL-9 and IL-13; both subsets can produce IL-3, TNF-α and GM-CSE. Rather than representing discrete CD4[+] T cell subsets, it appears that Th-1 and Th-2 cells both develop from Th-0 cells, which secrete an intermediate pattern of cytokines. Hyposensitization, or specific immunotherapy, has been successfully used for the treatment of patients with severe pollinosis and other type I allergens. Although the efficacy of this kind of therapy has been shown for many allergies, the underlying mechanism is still a matter of controversy [72,73]. Several physiologic responses, including blocking antibodies, modulation of specific IgE by restoration or by generation of suppressor T cells [74], changes in cells sensitivity or activation [72,73] and autoanti-idiotype antibodies [75,76] are potentially important for immunotherapy to be successful. The association of IgG 4 and IgE responses is especially important in conditions involving IL-4 production, because both isotypes are stimulated by IL-4 [77]. Moreover, basophil degranulation can be initiated not only by forming bridges between adjacent IgE molecules but also by bridging molecules of a subclass of IgG thereby resulting in hypersensitivity reactions.

Although both IgE and IgG are enhanced by IL-4 and inhibited by IFN-γ, low levels of IFN-γ can suppress only IgE, but not IgG4 (which corresponds to IgG1 in mouse) [78]. Thus, segregation of IgE and IgG4 responses that might be dependent on the balance of IL-4 (produced by Th-2) and IFN-γ (produced by Th-2) could result in the loss of a protective role of IgE against parasitic infections on the one hand and the success of hyposensitization of allergens on the other. Their development into Th-1 or Th-2 cells is most likely determined by the precise spectrum of cytokines encountered during activation. It may therefore be possible to modulate the immune response from Th-2 to Th-1 by changing the cytokine profile or it may be possible to determine the Th-1 or Th-2 modulation from the cytokine production before and after immunotherapy.

Immunization protocol

Animals	-	Balb/c mice (NIN, Hyderabad)
Group I	-	Control mice injected with PBS
Group II	-	Free antigen (FA)
Group III	-	Alum adsorbed antigen (AAA)
Group IV	-	Liposome entrapped antigen (LEA)
Group V	-	Empty liposomes (EL)
Dose	-	25µg allergen
Route	-	Intraperitoneal (i.p.)

Immunization schedule

Days	Immunization protocol
Zero day	Priming
3rd day	Blood drawn
10th day	First booster
13th day	Blood drawn
24th day	Second drawn
27th day	Blood drawn
36th day	Third booster
62nd day	Fourth booster
70th day	Mice sacrificed

Bleeding of animals

In our laboratory, it was observed that the maximum serum cytokine levels appear on the 3rd day after each booster, hence blood was drawn from the retroorbital plexuses on the 3rd day after each booster and sera were separated and tested for cytokine levels.

RESULTS AND DISCUSSION

The difference in IFN-γ levels in various groups became clear only after second booster (Fig. 6). In LEA treated mice, IFN-γ levels were approximately six times higher than FA injected mice. IFN-γ levels in the sera of AAA were lower than in LEA injected mice. As compared to FA group. IFN-γ levels in AAA immunized mice (Fig. 7) were higher in both the strains of mice. IL-4 levels in FA and AAA group were more than LEA treated mice after each booster (Fig. 8). This correlates well with the higher IgE levels in FA and AAA immunized mice and lower IgE levels in LEA injected mice.

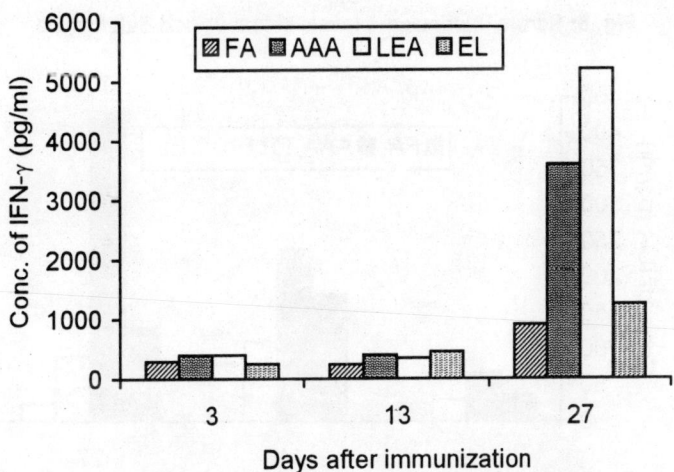

Fig. 6 : Serum interferon-γ levels of immunized Balb/c mice

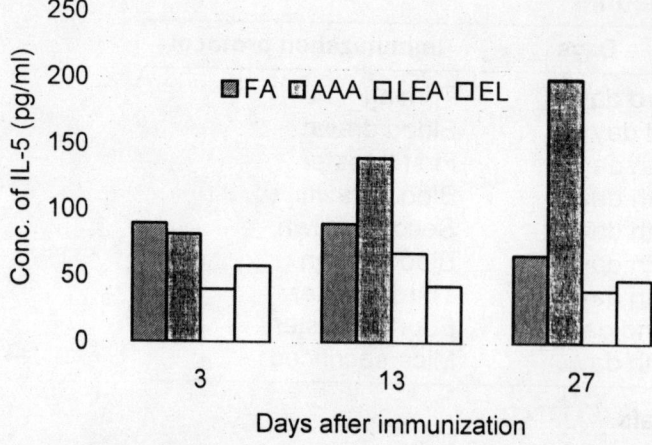

Fig. 7: Serum interleukin-4 levels of immunized Balb/c mice

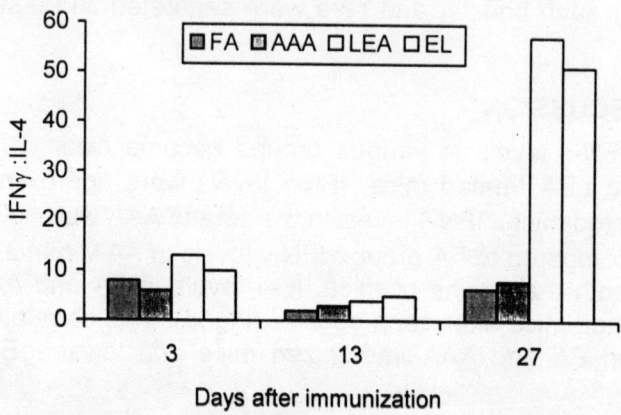

Fig. 8: Serum interleukin-5 levels of immunized Balb/c mice

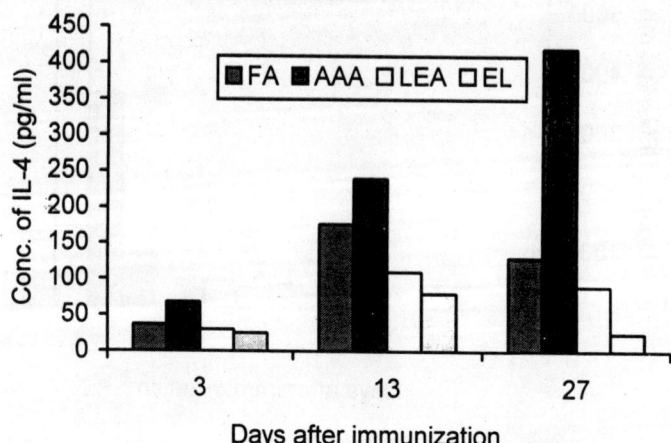

Fig. 9 : IFN-γ: IL-4 in serum of immunized Balb/c mice

In alum treated group, IL-5 levels in both the strains of mice increased after each, priming dose, indicative of Th-2 type of immune response. After second booster, IL-5 levels in LEA group was lower as compared to FA and AAA groups (Fig. 8) which favour Th-1 immune response by LEA.

The observations reported here show the potential of liposomes to become authorized human adjuvants, since very few adjuvants have been shown to boost cell-mediated immunity potentially, and moreover, Th-1 type response has been associated with protective immunity and successful immunotherapy.

REFERENCES

1. Allison, A.C. and Gregoriadis, G. (1974). **Nature** 252, 252.

2. Gregoriadis, G., McCormack, B., Allison, A.C. and Poste, G. Eds. (1993) New Generation Vaccines: The role of basic immunology, Plenum Press.

3. Gregoriadis, G. (1990). **Immunol. Today** 11, 89-97.

4. Alving, C.R. (1991). **J. Immunol. Methods.** 140, 1-13

5. Kay, A.B. Ed. (1997). Allergy and allergic diseases, Blackwell Science Ltd., USA.

6. Gluck, R. (1995) In: Vaccine design: The subunit and adjuvant approach (Ed. Powell, M.F. and Newman, M.) Plenum Press, 325-345.

7. Bangham, A.D., Standish, M.M. and Watkins, J.C. (1965). **Mol. Biol.** 13, 238-252.

8. Bergers, J.J., Denotter, W., Dullens, H.F.J., Kerkvliet, C.T.M. and Crommelin, D.J.A. (1994). **Pharm. Res.**

9. Fidler, I.J., Some, S. Fogler, W.E. and Barrus, Z.L. (1981). **Proc. Natl. Acad. Sci. USA** 78, 1680-1684.

10. Schroit, A.J. and Fidler, I.J. (1982). **Cancer Res.** 42, 161-167.

11. Szoka, F.C. Jr. (1992). **Res. Immunol.** 42, 161-167.

12. Reddy, R., Zhou, F., Huang, L., Carbone, F., Bevan, M. and Rouse, B.T. (1991). **J. Immunol. Methods** 141, 157-163.

13. Nairs, S., Zhou, F., Reddy, R., Huang, L., and Rouse, B.T., (1992). **J. Exp. Med.** 175, 609-612.

14. Reddy, R., Zhou, F., Nair, S., Huang, L. and Rouse, B.T. (1992). **J. Immunol.** 148, 1585-1589.

15. Zhou, F., Rouse, B.T. and Huang, L. (1992). **J. Immunol.** 149, 1599-1604.

16. Huang, L., Reddy, R., Nair, S.K., Zhou, F. and Rouse, B.T. (1992). **Res. Immunol.** 143, 192-196.

17. Michalek, S.M., Childers, N.K., Katz, J., Denys, F.R., Berry, A.K., Eldridge, J.H., McGhee, J.R. and Curtiss, R. (1989). **Curr. Top. Microbiol. Immunol.** 146, 51-58.

18. Skurkovich, S., Skurkovich, B. and Bellanti, J.A. (1987). **Clin. Immunol. Immunopathol.** 43, 362.

19. Robinson, D.S. et al. (1992). **New Engl. J. Med.** 36, 298.

20. Bakker-Woundenberg, I.A.J.M., Lokerse, A.F., Tne Kate, M.T., Melissen, P.M.B., Van Vianen, W. and Van Etten, E.W. M. (1993). **Eur. J. Clin. Microbiol. Infect. Dis.** 12, 61-67.

21. Walden, P. (1988). **Eur. J. Immun.** 18, 1851-1854.

22. Bakouche, O. and Lachman, L.B. (1990). **Lymphokin Res.** 9, 259-281.

23. DalMonte, P. and Szoka, F.C. Jr. (1989). **J. Immun.** 142, 1437-1443.

24. Alving, C.R. and Richards, R.L. (1990). **Immun. Lett.** 25, 275-280.

25. Phillips, N.C., Loutfi, A., A-Kareem, A.M., Shibata, H.R. and Baines, M.G. (1990). **Cancer Detect. Prev.** 14, 491-496.

26. Van Rooijen, N. (1990). Liposomes as carrier and immunoadjuvant of vaccine antigensIn: Bacterial Antigens Allan, R. Liss, New York, 225-279.

27. Shek, P.N. and Sabiston, B.H. (1981). **Immunology** 45, 349-356.

28. Therien, H.M. and Shahum, E. (1989). **Imm. Lett.** 22, 253-258.

29. Verma, J.N., Rao, M., Amselem, S., Krzych, V., Alving, C.R., Green, S.J. and Wassef, N.M. (1992). **Infect. Immun.** 60, 2438-2444.

30. Brewer, J.M. and Alexander, J. (1992). **Immunology** 75, 570-575.

31. Therien, H.M. and Shahu, E., (1991). **Cell. Immun.** 136, 402-413.

32. Latif, N.A. and Bacchawat, B.K. (1987). **Immun. Lett.** 15, 45-51.

33. Van Rooijen, N. and Su, D. (1989). In: Immunological adjuvants and vaccines (Eds. Gregoriadis, G., Allison, A.C. and Poste, G.) Plenum Press, New York, 95-106.

34. Shahum, E. and Therein, H.M. (1994). **Vaccine** 12, 1125-1131.

35. Mosmann, T.R. Cherwinski, H., Bond, M.W., Giedlin, M.A. and Coffman, R.L. (1986). **J. Immun.** 13, 2348-2357.

36. Allison, A.C. and Gregoriadis, G. (1976) In: Recent Results in cancer research (Eds. Mathe, G., Florentin, I. And Simmler, M.C) Springer-Verlag, Heidelberg, 58.

37. Gregoriadis, G. and Allison, A.C. (1974) **FEBS Lett.** 45, 71.

38. Richardson, V.J. Ryman, B.E., Jewkes, R.F. Jeyasingh, K., Tattersall, M.H.N., Newlands, E.S. and Kaye, S.B. (1979). **Br. J. Cancer** 40, 35.

39. Bekhetz, P.E., Braidman, I.F., Crawley, J.C.E. and Gregoriadis, G. (1977). **Lancet** 1, 116.

40. Bomford, R. (1980). **Clin. Exp. Immun.** 39, 435-441.

41. Gregoriadis, G., Davis, D. and Davies, A. (1987). **Vaccine** 5, 143.

42. Van Rooijen, N. (1988). In: Liposomes as drug carriers: Recent trends and progress (Ed. Gregoriadis, G.) Wiley, Chichester, 145-165.

43. Davis, D. and Gregoriadis, G. (1987) **Immunology** 61, 229.

44. Garcon, N., Gregoriadis, G., Taylor, M. and Summerfield, J. (1988). **Immunology** 64, 743.

45. Tan, L. and Gregoriadis, G. (1989). **Biochem. Soc. Trans.** 17, 693-694.

46. Bloom, R.R. (1977). **Adv. Immunol.** 13, 101.

47. Ryman, B.E., Jewkes, R.F., Jeyasingh, K., Osborne, M.P., Patel, H.M., Richardson, V.J. Tattersall, M.H.N. and Tyrell, D.A. (1978). **Ann. N.Y. Acad. Sci.** 308, 281.

48. Suzuki, K. and Tomasi, T.B. Jr. (1980). **Cell Immunol.** 49, 317.

49. Finberg, R., Mescher, M. and Burakoff, S.J. (1978) **J. Exp. Med.** 148, 1620.

50. Engelhard, V.H., Strominger, J.L., Mescher, M. and Burakoff, S. (1978). **Proc. Natl. Acad. Sci. USA** 75, 5688.

51. Burakoff, S.J., Engelhard, V.H., Kaufman, J. and Strominger, J.L. (1980). **Nature** 283, 495.

52. Hale, A.H., Ruebush, M.J. and Harris, D.T. (1980). In: Liposomes and Immunobiology (Eds. Tom, B.H. and Six, H.R.) Elsevier, New York, 211.

53. Weinberger, O., Herrmann, S.H., Mescher, M.F., Benacerrag, B. and Burakoff, S.J. (1980). **Proc. Natl. Acad. Sci. USA.** 77, 6091.

54. Weinberger, O., Herrmann, S.H., Mescher, M.F., Benacerrag, B. and Burakoff, S.J. (1981). **Proc. Natl. Acad. Sci. USA.** 78, 1796.

55. Fidler, I.J. (1978) **Is. J. Med. Sci.** 14, 17.

56. Poste, G., Kirsh, R., Raz, A., Sone, S., Cora, B., Fogler, W.E. and Fidler, I.J. (1980). In: Liposomes and Immunobiology (Eds. Tom, B.H. and Siz, H.R.) Elsevier, New York, 93.

57. Fidler, I.J. Flart, I.R., Raz, A., Fogler, W.E., Kirsh, R. and Poste, G. (1980). In: Liposomes and Immunobiology (Eds. Tom, B.H. and Siz, H.R.) Elsevier, New York, 109.

58. Mosmann, T.R. and Coffman, R. L. (1987). **Immunol. Today** 8, 223-227.

59. Parronchi, P., Macchia, D., Piccinni, M.P. et al. (1991). **Proc. Natl. Acad. Sci. USA** 88, 4538-4542.

60. Robinson, D.S., Hamid, Q., Ying, S. et al., (1992). **New Engl. J. Med.** 326, 298-304.

61. Ying, S., Durham, S.R., Corrigan, C.J., Hamid, O. and Kay, A.B. (1995). **Am. J. Res. Cell. Mol. Biol.** 12, 477-487.

62. Kuchroo, V.K., Das, M.P., Brown, J.A. et al., (1995). **Cell** 80, 707-18.

63. Thompson, C.B. (1995). **Cell** 81, 979-982.

64. Young, R.P., Dekker, J.W., Wordsworth, B.P. et al. (1994). **Clin. Exp. Allergy** 24, 431-439.

65. Moffatt, M.F., Hill, M.R., Cornelis, F. et al. (1994). **Lancet** 343, 1597-1600.

66. Parish, W.E., Barrett, A.M., Coombs, R.R.A., Gunther, M. and Camps, E.E. (1960). **Lancet** 11, 1106-1110.

67. Arora, N. and Gangal, S.V. (1990). **Int. Arch. Allergy App. Immunol.** 91, 22-29.

68. Arora, N. and Gangal, S.V. (1990). **Mol. Cell. Biochem.** 97, 173-179.

69. Arora, N. and Gangal, S.V. (1991). **Allergy** 46, 386-392.

70. Arora, N. and Gangal, S.V. (1992). **Clin. Exp. Allergy** 22, 35-42.

71. Dijurp, F. (1985). **Allergy** 40, 469-486.

72. Bousquet, J. and Michel, F.B. (1988) **Allergy** 43 (Supp. 8), 16.

73. Ewan, P.W. **Curr. Opin. Immunol.** 1, 672.

74. Tamir, R., Castracane, J.M. and Rocklin, R.E. (1987) **J. Allergy Clin. Immunol.** 79, 591.

75. Castracane, J.M. and Rocklin, R.E. (1988). **Int. Arch. Allergy. Appl. Immunol.** 86, 288.

76. Castracane, J.M. and Roclkin, R.E. (1988). **Int. Arch. Allergy Appl. Immunol.** 86, 295.

77. Lundgren, M. (1989). **Eur. J. Immunol.** 19, 1311.

78. Ishizaka, A., et al. (1990). **Clin. Exp. Immunol.** 79, 392.

6

MACROPHAGE TARGETING AND COLLOIDAL DRUG CARRIERS

S. P. VYAS

Department of Pharmaceutical Sciences
Dr. Harisingh Gour Vishwavidyalaya, Sagar (M.P.) INDIA

- Introduction
- The macrophage system
- Objectives of targeted delivery to macrophages

- Drug-carrier targeting to macrophages
- Approaches and carriers for macrophages targeting
- Future perspectives

INTRODUCTION

Significantly high costs and expenses involved in the development of new drug molecules have compelled scientists all over the world to search for the alternative ways of administering the existing drug molecules with enhanced effectiveness and minimized toxic/side effects. Efforts directed to achieve this aim have resulted in the development of site specific drug delivery. Recent years have seen the development of various strategies for selective delivery of drug molecules to the desired organ/tissue or cells. Macrophages and related cells have been the major focus for attention of drug delivery scientists because they play important role in pathogenic disorders, immunological consequences and lysosomal storage diseases. Diverse objectives and desired effects have been achieved by delivering the bioactives selectively to the macrophages. Present review is an attempt to give comprehensive account of targeted drug delivery to the macrophages, it's rationales and means of macrophage activation. It is customarily that the role of macrophages in host defence in brief should be understood so that targeting to and stimulation of macrophages be realized and rationalized.

THE MACROPHAGE SYSTEM

Macrophages are phagocytic cells present either in circulating plasma (wandering macrophages) or in endothelial lining and the reticular spaces of the connective tissues of the mammals (fixed or tissue macrophages). They have a pivotal role in protecting the host against a wide variety of invading microorganisms and developing neoplasms through initialization of humoral and cell mediated immune responses as well as intracellular oxidative or hydrolytic activity [1]. The combination of monocytes, mobile macrophages and a few specialised endothelial cells in the bone marrow, spleen and lymph nodes is also referred to as the *reticuloendothelial system*. Various tissue macrophages which form integral part of RES include Kupffer cells in liver, langerhans cells In epithelium, macrophages in spleen and lymph nodes, alveolar macrophages and interstitial macrophages in lungs, osteoblasts in bone tissues, astrocytes in brain; microglias in CNS and histiocytes in skin and subcutaneous tissue [2]. Macrophages are well investigated as a system in the field of immunology, biotechnology and drug delivery owing to their appreciation for receptor mediated disposition of the endogenous ligands and macrophage mediated activation and immunological consequences.

Phagocytosis by macrophages

Phagocytosis is the main cellular activity involved in the internalization of the colloidal and macromolecular carriers and is defined as the internalization of plasma membrane with concomitant engulfment of extracellular material and extracellular fluid. Phagocytosis in classical sense is the engulfment of the endogenous and exogenous particulate materials, such as bacteria, erythrocytes, latex beads and colloidal particles. It is often performed by the phagocytic cells of the RES including the Kupffer cells of the hepatic sinusoids, the tissue fixed macrophages (histocytes) and the blood macrophages or monocytes. The process completes involving sequential steps of **recognition** (mediated by coating of blood components, mainly opsonin and high density lipoproteins), **adhesion** (attachment of the particle to the macrophage cells of the RES) and **digestion** (whereby the particles are transferred to phagosome, phago-lysosome and finally to digestive vacuoles) (Fig. 1). Multiple attachment of particle associated ligands with membrane receptors is an essential stimulus for phagocytic capture of particles (Zippering).

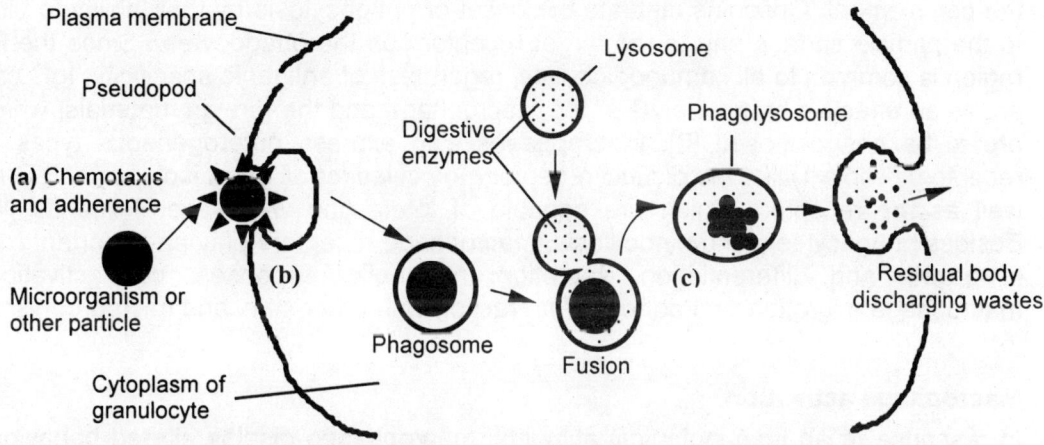

Fig. 1 : Schematic representation of phagocytosis and subsequent events

The phagocytosis by macrophages is governed and regulated by certain factors, which prevent the engulfing of endogenous structures and at the same time selective phagocytosis of only foreign non-self particles takes place. Extent of particle capture and clearance by macrophages is determined primarily by the physicochemical nature of the surface, however, other factors, such as nature of the particle matrix, particle stability and physiological state of the species can be important. Macrophages possess high phagocytic propensity towards rough surfaces, which are typical characteristic of dead tissues or particles of foreign origin. Endogenous structures escape the phagocytosis because of their smooth surfaces and protective protein coats [2].

Macrophage associated receptors

The phagocytosis of certain particles like latex particles and carbonyl iron is affected by intrinsic surface properties like hydrophobicity or surface charge; but in most parts, phagocytic processes occur via specific interaction with receptor molecules. *Receptors* are membrane-associated proteins having specific affinity for a variety of molecules such as polypeptides, polysaccharides, glycolipids or proteins. The latter smaller molecules, which bind to the receptors specifically are referred to as *ligands*. The macrophages express several specific receptors for a spectrum of ligands. The ligands as known to have specific receptor could be utilised in controlled and targeted drug delivery to the macrophages. The receptors commonly present or expressed under stimulated conditions on the macrophage; and able to negotiate endocytosis upon interaction with ligands are given in table 1. Macrophages do not express clonal idiotypic receptors like lymphocytes but they express receptor molecules, which are selective for a category of ligands e.g., Sugar specific recognition of glycoconjugates or the common Fc fragments of IgG subclasses [3]. The phagocytosis of particulates by macrophages in culture is mediated via the adsorption of plasma protein by a process known as opsonization. The opsonized particles adhere to the phagocytic cell membrane and are subsequently internalised by phagocytes. The surface of macrophages bears over thirty receptors, including those corresponding to the Fc portion of immunoglobulins and the C3b component of the complement. Opsonins mediate the onset of phagocytosis by their ability to bind to the particle surface and to the target receptors on the phagocytes. Since the Fc region is common to all immunoglobulins, regardless of antigenic specificity, IgG can act as an effective bridge between the macrophage and the foreign materials, which are to be phagocytosed [2]. Macrophages also express heterogeneous types of receptors (Table 1) like the distinct receptor molecules for different isotypes of IgG as well as the receptors which are capable of interacting with several ligands [4]. Besides phagocytosis and pinocytosis, macrophage receptors play an important role in growth and differentiation, secretion, metabolic responses, cell activation, macrophage migration and adhesive interaction with other cells and microorganisms [5].

Macrophage activation

In response to an immunological stimulus, macrophages display altered behaviour and this phenomenon is referred to as the activation of the macrophages. Activated macrophages acquire the ability to kill a number of obligate intracellular bacteria and parasites, which are not killed by non-immunologically stimulated inflammatory macrophages [14,15]. They also exhibit augmented tumoricidal activities and play an important role in an early destruction of neoplastic cells [16-18].

Altered behaviour of these macrophages has been described in literature in terms of increased adherence to glass, increased mobility, increased phagocytic capabilities, increased enzymatic activities and altered secretory profile. Activated macrophages possess enhanced capability to produce reactive oxygen intermediates (ROI) and can effectively kill tumor cells. *In vivo* stimulation experiments have revealed that interferon-γ and muramyl di-peptide and its lipophilic analogue (muramyl tripeptide phosphatidylethanolamine) [14] can induce macrophage activation. Presence of low concentrations of bacterial lipo-polysaccharides (LPS) has been found to have synergistic effects [19]. Interleukin-1 (IL-1) [20] and tumor necrosis factor (TNF) [15] have also been found to have an effect identical to bacterial LPS.

After appropriate stimulation, macrophages participate in antigen processing, antigen presentation and production of IL-1 concomitantly with class II antigen expression. Histo-compatibility antigens HLA-DR (DQ & DP) have been found to be processed in macrophages [21]. Besides most of the macrophages can produce and secrete; although with variable efficiency various products like interleukins, prostaglandins, leukotrienes which are effective and decisive modulators of immune response. Products secreted by macrophages including interferon gamma and interleukins have been realised to regulate the immune response of macrophages [20-22].

Table 1. Various receptors, which trigger phagocytosis and subsequent events in receptor mediated endocytic pathways

Receptors	Ligands	Cells	Ref.
Fc Receptors			3,6
(i) FcR1	Monomeric and complexed IgG	Monocytes and macrophages	
(ii) FcR2	Complexed IgG	Monocytes, macrophages, Granulocytes	
(iii) FcR3	Complexed IgG	Mature macrophages, Natural Killer-cells	
Complement receptors			
(i) CR1	C3b	Macrophages	
(ii) CR2	C3b1	Macrophages	7,8
(iii) CR4	C3b1	Macrophages	
Mannose/Fucose receptors	Mannose/ fucose residues	Mature macrophages and hepatic endothelium	5,9
Glucan receptor	Glucan residues	Mature macrophages and monocytes	10
∝-Macroglobulin	Protease complex	Macrophages	11
Scavenger receptor	Modified Lipo-proteins, polysaccharides & polynucleotides	Macrophages	12
Galactosyl particle receptor	Galactose	Kupffer cells	13
WGA receptor	Wheat germ agglutinins	Macrophages	5

OBJECTIVES OF TARGETED DRUG DELIVERY TO MACROPHAGES

Targeted drug delivery to the macrophages has been realised as a rationalised strategy which offer opportunities for the treatment of various diseases of varied aetiology as summarised in the table 2. The objectives generally sought in targeting bioactives to the macrophages include effective eradication of intracellular pathogens, treatment of lysosomal storage diseases, targeting of immunomodulators for macrophage activation, cell deactivation, cell or cell product depletion and blocking the macrophages.

Table 2. List of diseases associated with macrophages

Etiology	Diseases
Protozoal	Leshmaniasis, toxoplasmosis, trypanosomiasis
Bacterial	Tuberculosis, leprocy, salmonellosis, listerosis, legionella infections, brucella infections
Neoplastic	Monocytic leukemia, Histiocytosis, Metastases
Viral	Dengue Measles, AIDS, Japanese encephalitis, Herpes simplex infections, Rift valley fever virus
Metabolic	Gaucher's disease, Rheumatoid Arithritis, Iron over doses, Xanthomatoses, gangliosidoses
Rickettsial	Rickettsia rickettssii infection, Rickettsia prowazeski infection
Fungal	Cryptococcus neoformans infections

Adapted and modified from [5,28,29]

Effective eradication of intracellular pathogens

Effective eradication of pathogens localised intracellularly in the macrophages requires sufficiently high concentrations of the drugs within the cell or in even cell organelle (as lysosomes). This condition is difficult to achieve due to poor diffusion of the available antimicrobial agents in to the cells with subsequent poor retention. Another reason is reduced activity of antimicrobial agents at the lysosomal pH. Conventional drug therapy thus requires relatively higher doses of drugs in order to obtain such higher concentrations in to the interior of macrophages. However, excessively high drug concentration levels unnecessarily expose the normal body tissues for undesirable side effects, which are often unacceptably severe. The scarcity of antibiotics for greater intracellular efficacy led to the development of endocytosable drug carriers such as liposomes and nanoparticles, which mimic the entry path of bacteria by penetrating the macrophages into phagosomes or lysosomes. This type of selective and effective transport of bioactives in to the interior of macrophages seems to be the most logical approach in the treatment of such diseases [25].

Treatment of lysosomal storage diseases

Targeted delivery of certain bioactives like enzymes to macrophages is often desired to correct or modify the metabolic disorders associated with lysosomes of mature macrophages, particularly in the therapy of lysosomal storage diseases like Gaucher's disease, Pompe's disease etc.[5]. Treatment of lysosomal storage diseases, which originate from congenital deficiency of enzymes requires enzyme to reach the lysosomes in it's intact form; which entails for third order targeting with the help of carriers like liposomes or other cellular carrier systems. Macrophage targeting has also been attempted in the treatment of iron overdoses and heavy metal poisoning for sequestering and removal of cellular metal deposits.

Targeting of immunomodulators for macrophage activation

Systemic activation of macrophages for augmented tumoricidal and microbicidal properties, have been achieved by targeting immunomodulators like lymphokines [26], interferon γ [14,27], muramyl dipeptide and its lipophilic analogue muramyl tripeptide phosphatidylethanolamine (MTPPE) [14,17], bacterial endotoxin or lipopolysaccharide[19] to the macrophages [28,29]. Further the targeting of immunomodulators is required because the systemic administration of such agents may crop up severe adverse effects. The lymphokines have been realised to elicit pharmacological effects on other non-target sites including endothelium and as a result often lead towards unacceptably severe contraindication manifestations.

Cell deactivation, cell or cell product depletion

These are desirable priori per se in pathophysiological conditions including chronic inflammation and delayed type hypersensitivity associated with tissue destruction by activated macrophages and their products (rheumatoid arthritis or graft rejection) [30-32]. Depletion of macrophages or a sub-population level of macrophages is experimentally also desired for the immunological studies on the role of macrophages *in-vivo*. In such studies, a liposomally encapsulated toxic compound (e.g. Dichloro-methylene diphosphonate) which does not penetrate cells in the free state is selectively targeted to the macrophages [33], which subsequently renders various levels of macrophage deactivation and immunological consequences are recorded.

Blockade of macrophages

The rationale substantiating the principle of macrophage blockade is that preloaded macrophage system with a saturating dose of material allows successive doses of the same (or different) material to freely access other target tissues. Dextran sulphate, aggregated albumin, colloidal gold stabilised with gelatin, latex beads and liposomes have been used to explore this phenomenon. It is understood that macromolecules as dextran sulphate aggregate with plasma proteins in order to generate a complex that is avidly sequestered by macrophages. This approach however is not clinically viable as it may lead to inactivation of the important host defence cells [34].

DRUG-CARRIER TARGETING TO MACROPHAGES

The selective and effective delivery and localisation of bioactives in the vicinity of pre-selected targets in therapeutic concentrations is referred to as targeting [35]. Various orders of targeting on the basis of anatomical levels of target like organ or tissue level targeting (first order), cellular targeting (second order) or intracellular organelle targeting (third order) have been proposed and discussed [36]. Approaches for targeting bioactives to macrophages are mainly based on the methods involving carrier systems, which carry desirable bioactives encapsulated or entrapped.

Carriers investigated for targeting in general may be exogenous (liposomes, nanoparticles, microspheres, micro or multiple emulsion, polymeric micelles etc.) or endogenous (resealed erythrocytes, and lipoproteins). After i.v. administration, carriers like liposomes, microspheres and resealed erythrocytes are rapidly intercepted and taken up by tissue macrophages, mainly of liver and spleen. Such carriers are degraded in lysosomes and entrapped material is released in lysosomes, which subsequently diffuses into the cytoplasm. The bioactives may escape to the exterior of macrophages via diffusion (Fig. 2). During the above process, macrophages may migrate to a different site, thereby broadening the spectrum of distribution of the drug in the body. The macrophages co-ordinated distribution of carrier contents is referred to as "co-ordinated cellular drug delivery system" and it has been proposed for the treatment of infectious diseases. Targeting through intrinsic affinity of carriers towards the macrophages is known as passive targeting.

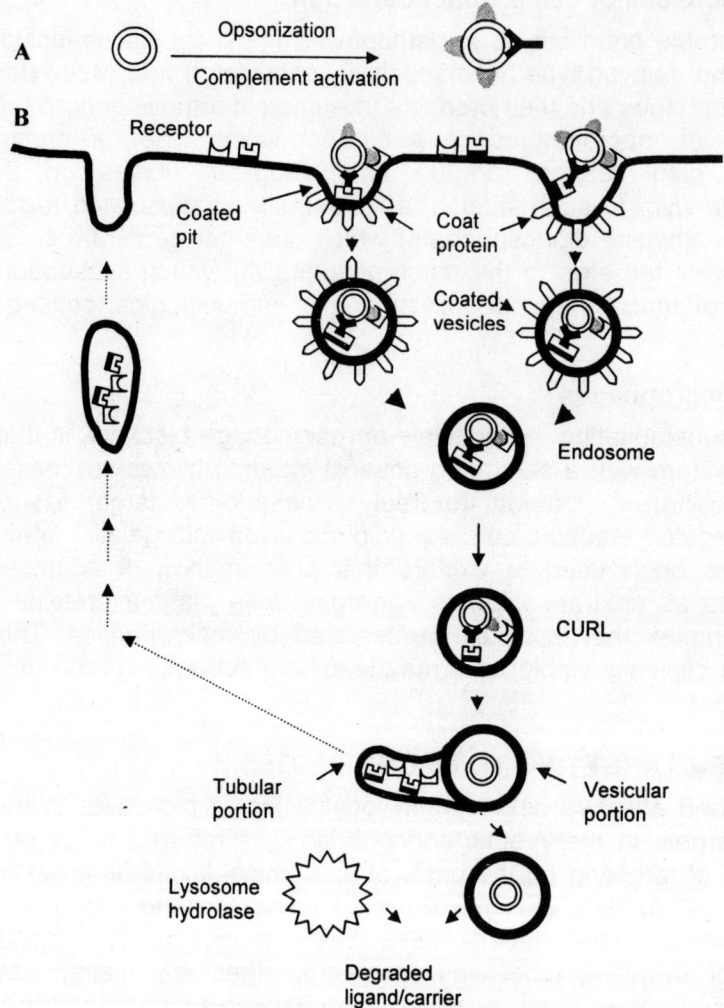

Fig. 2 : Fate of drug carriers in the receptor-mediated macrophage targeting. A. Opsonization by complement components and Fc. B. Receptor mediated phagocytosis. Role of *CURL* (clathrin or non-clathrin mediated pathway) and lysosomal apparatus in the release of the system in the vicinity of target

Further enhancement in the rate and extent of targeting involves the use of recognition elements present on the surface of target cells like cell surface antigens or receptors which recognise the navigator molecules (ligands) appended carriers. Ligands together with carrier components are internalised after binding to the receptors via receptor mediated endocytosis. The process leads to cellular targeting referred to as active targeting. The ligands can be anchored on to the carrier system or can be conjugated to the drug molecules and the resultant conjugate system as a whole undergoes receptor mediated endocytosis, selectively by cells, which express corresponding receptor(s).

APPROACHES AND CARRIERS FOR MACROPHAGES TARGETING

The drug substances or the macrophage activators or both are generally delivered through carrier(s), irrespective of order or type of targeting. This carrier(s) should customarily be colloidal in size, long circulatory, inert, nonimmunogenic, stable and amenable to surface modifications. The most often and widely studied and employed carrier systems include liposomes, nanoparticles and cellular carriers.

Liposomes

Liposomes have exclusively been studied for passive targeting of bioactives to the macrophages. Liposomes are easy to prepare and exhibit versatility in entrapping drugs of varying physico-chemical nature. They are non-immunogenic and are known to possess natural affinity towards the macrophages. Some of the important applications of the liposomes in the passive and active targeting of bioactives are summarised in the Table 3. It has been realized that certain classes of phospholipids are preferentially recognised by macrophages. The negatively charged phospholipids such as phosphatidylserine (PS) and phosphatidylglycerol (PG) in liposomes consisting of phosphatidylcholine (PC) greatly enhance their binding to macrophages and subsequently phagocytosed by them. The fate of the carrier is influenced, however, by the vesicle size, vesicles of $\geq 7\mu m$ are mechanically filtered by the alveolar macrophages. Thus the rate and extent of macrophagic interception and uptake can be modulated by the manipulation of the lipid composition, vesicle size and carrier surfacial disposition.

Receptor mediated targeting

Liposomes demonstrate natural affinity towards the macrophages where they are sequestered and cleared from the circulation (passive targeting); however their uptake can further be enhanced via receptor mediated endocytosis and possibly selective uptake can be negotiated in favour of the compartments predominant of these cells. This hypothesis has been substantiated and proven with the help of the experiments, which revealed that the uptake of liposomes by macrophages could significantly be facilitated by inclusion of receptor specific appropriate ligands [38-44]. Ghosh and Bacchawat [38] reported that the rate and extent of uptake of liposomes (containing [125]I γ-globulin as marker) by liver macrophages is significantly increased on appending mannopyranoside onto the liposomal surface. Similarly, Barrat et al [42] demonstrated that liposomes containing mannose-terminated glycolipids are taken up more avidly by peritoneal macrophages.

Table 3. Applications of passive and active targeting approaches to macrophages using liposomes

Bioactives	Applications
Passive targeting approaches	
Amphotericin B	Candidiasis [56,57], Leishmaniasis [58,59], Experimental cryptococcal meningitis [60], Cryptococcosis [61], Murine Histoplasmosis [62]
MTPPE/ IFN-γ	Macrophage activation for protection against Klebesiella pneumoniae [18]
MTP-PE	Macrophage activation for tumoricidal properties against spontaneous metastases [63, 21]
Dichloromethylene diphosphonate	Macrophage depletion [38]
Praziquantel	Macrophage activation [64]
Sparfloaxacin	M.avium-M. intracellularlae complex infection in mice [65]
Gentamycin	Staphylococcal pneumoniae [66]
Active targeting approaches	
Pentamidine	Leishmaniasis [67]
Antisense oligonucleotide	Leishmaniasis [68]
Hamycin	Leishmaniasis [69]
Idoxyuridine/ acyclovir	Herpes simplex virus [54]
Asiaticoside	Tuberculosis and leprosy [70]
Rifampicin	Tuberculosis [71]

The most frequently utilised receptor for macrophage targeting is considered to be mannose/fucose receptors, which are expressed over the cellular membrane of liver, spleen and alveolar macrophages. The receptor categorically triggers and facilitates endocytosis of glycoproteins terminated with mannose, fucose and glucosamine. Mannose residues have been appended onto the liposomes in the form of mannosylated albumin [39], palmitoylated derivatives of carbohydrates like pullulan, amylopectin and mannan [40], mannobiose arachidonic esters [41], mannose terminated glycolipids of natural and synthetic origin [42], manno-pyranoside [43], mannose terminated glycoproteins [44]. These have been reported to be critical molecular modules in initiation of endocytosis and subsequently leading to cellular (phagocytic) uptake of carrier-drug composite. Vyas and Sakthivel [114] have reported pressurised pack-based liposomes for pulmonary targeting of isoprenaline in an *in vitro* study and indicated that the delivery towards macrophages could also be a function of the route of administration. To further improve the pulmonary targeting of tuberculosis, ligand (maleylated albumin and stearoylated amylopectin) appended pressurised packed liposomes were studied and the roles of receptor mediated macrophage targeting of appended ligands and the route of administration were established (Vyas et al., unpublished).

Antibody mediated targeting

Liposomes appended with antibodies or their fragments, as receptor/antigenic site(s) oriented moieties on the cell surface, referred to as immunoliposomes is a well-established strategy of functional cellular targeting competence. Many approaches have been tried in order to obtain the quantitative targetability through immunoliposomes in drug delivery including antimicrobial and cancer therapy, enzyme delivery (lysosomal storage therapy) and gene delivery (gene transfection therapy). The surface modifier and key ligands in so far used include heat aggregated cell specific antibodies and covalently or noncovalently associated polyclonal or monoclonal antibodies. Liposomes coated with heat aggregated isologous IgM containing Horse radish peroxidase (HRP) have been found to be taken up and processed in lysosomes of peroxide deficient macrophages [45]. Fc receptors on the cells have been found to be involved in the active uptake of such liposomes. A marked liposomal uptake by murine macrophhages was practically achieved by pretreatment of liposomes with relevant antibodies [46,47]. Heath et al [48] described a method for the covalent linking of immunoglobulins to large unilamellar liposomes. The method involved the periodate oxidation of glycosphingolipids of the liposomal membrane.

Anti target monoclonal antibody with specific avidity directed to carbohydrate containing antigens were anchored on liposomes (immunoliposomes) and investigated to deliver the drugs like Iodoxyuridine/Acyclovir selectively to the cell lines infected with Herpes simplex virus [49]. Instead of using complete IgG portion, immunologically active fragments [F(ab)$_2$ and Fab'] could effectively improve the access of monoclonal antibodies to the receptor bearing cells [50] (Fig. 3).

Microspheres

Microspheres are intrinsically prone for passive targeting of bioactives to the macrophages. The well founded course of their passive biofate has been realised and explored to facilitate selective accumulation of these carrier components in to the cells of RES following intravenous administration. Study on bio-distribution of gelatin nanoparticles of mean diameter 280nm and microspheres with mean diameter 14.9 μm revealed that most of the nanoparticles were accumulated in organs of RES predominance while 95.4% of the microspheres were found in the lungs [67]. It has been proposed that particles larger than 250 nm can be used for targeting to spleen macrophages [68]. Hoffman et al.[69] demonstrated an avid uptake of gelatin microspheres by macrophages and subsequent release of biologically active streptomycin within the cells following phagocytic uptake, and intracellular degradation of microspheres.

Malaise et al. [70] showed that particles bearing adsorbed IgG on their surface was phagocytosed more rapidly than the naive particles. The uptake proceeds mainly via recognition by the specific Fc macrophage receptors. Tabata and Ikada [71] also observed an increased uptake of IgG, tuftsin, fibronectin or gelatin coated polymeric microspheres. Knepp and co-workers [72] reported a rapid uptake of fluorescein labeled albumin microspheres of size less than 5 μm by mouse myelomonocyte leukemia cells (a macrophage related cell line). The biodegradable microspheres prepared using copolymers of lactic acid and glycolic acid, crystallised carbohydrates, human serum albumin and poly (d,l-lactide) containing antigens and immunomodulators have been shown to be of great therapeutic potentials [73].

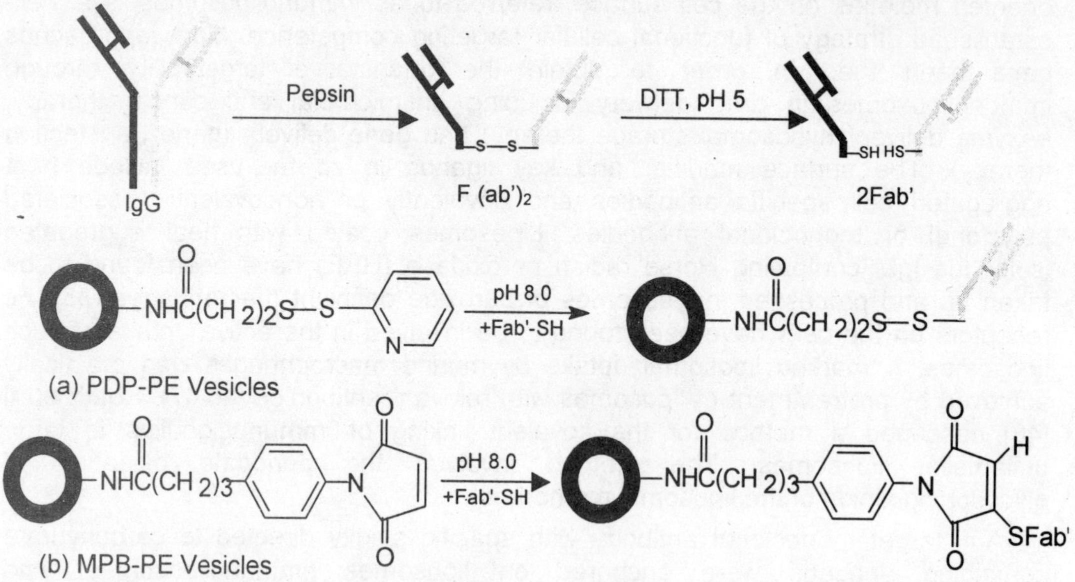

Fig. 3: Immunoliposomes with Fab' fragments as targeting ligands (a) Conversion of IgG to Fab' fragments containing free endogenous thiol groups, and (b) Fab' fragments with free sulfhydral groups react with liposomes containing 3-(2-pyridyldithio) propionate-PE (PDP-PE) OR with liposomes containing 4-(p-maleimidophenyl) butyrate-PE (MPB-PE)

Nanoparticles

Biodegradable polymeric nanoparticles especially polyalkylcyanoacrylate nano-particles and their contents thereby are passively targeted to the macrophages. The selective targeting is advocated to be of therapeutic significance in treatment of tumors and intracellular infections.

Couvreuer et al. [74] reported an increased uptake of the radioactivity in liver, spleen and lungs when ^3H vinblastin or dactinomycin was coupled to polymethyl cyanoacrylate (PMCA) or polyethyl cyanoacrylate (PECA) nanoparticles. Exceptionally higher accumulations in liver and spleen are reported with dactinomycin loaded polybutyl cyanoacrylate (PBCA) nanoparticles resulting into 44 and 64 fold higher drug concentrations in spleen and liver respectively upon intravenous injection [75]. Kreuter and Hartmann [76] observed similar results with 5-flurouracil containing PBCA nanoparticles. *In vitro* studies using mouse peritoneal macrophages in culture revealed that the uptake of ^2H dactinomycin (anticancer drug) from PACA based nanoparticles by peritoneal macrophages was nearly three times higher than that of the free drug. Fattal et.al. [78] observed and reported an increased effectiveness of ampicillin loaded polyhexyl cyanoacrylate (PHCA) nanoparticles in the treatment of experimental salmonellosis. This reflected in effective reduction in mortality suppressing dose, which was reduced from 3 doses of 32 mg each (of free drug) to 0.8 mg of ampicillin (when bound to nanoparticles) and bacterial count of liver and spleen was reduced down to 1000 to 10000 times.

Similarly, at least 20-fold increase in the therapeutic index of ampicillin for liver and spleen bacterial counts was observed when the nanoparticles bound drug was administered in athymic mice induced with experimental listerosis. Even complete liver sterilization was observed after two injections of 0.8 mg of nanoparticles bound drug, where as no such sterilization was achieved with free ampicillin. Spleen bacterial counts were less affected by the treatment with free or bound ampicillin [79]. These results are further supported by the *in vitro* studies involving mouse peritoneal macrophages infected with *Listeria monocytogenes*, where 1μg/ml of ampicillin bound to nanoparticles effectively decreased the intracellular bacterial load by 99% in 30 hrs, whilst the same concentration of free drug could not inhibit the bacterial growth [80].

Fourage et al. [81] have reported the accumulation of dehydroemetine (antileishmanial agent) in liver and spleen, when it is administered contained in PACA nanoparticles with reduced cardiac side effects. Chiannilkulchai et al. [82] while attempting the targeting of doxorubicin using polyisohexyl cyanoacrylate (PIHCA) nanoparticles carrier systems to murine hepatic metastases demonstrated highly promising results as compared to the treatment based on administration of free drug. It was observed that the concentration of doxorubicin in tumor was significantly (2.5 times) high, following the administration of PIHCA nanoparticles loaded doxorubicin. It was suggested that this higher concentration probably resulted from the dramatic permeation of the healthy tissues mediated through selective uptake by kupffer cells. It was subsequently confirmed by the histological observations, which reveals considerable accumulation of the nanoparticles (30-50 particles/cell) in lysosomal vesicles of Kupffer cells, while almost negligible to nil number of nanoparticles was observed in the neoplastic cells. Thus liver macrophages serve to be as an efficient reservoir of drug able to induce a gradient of drug concentration favorable for massive and prolonged diffusion of free drug towards neighboring malignant cells.

PIHCA nanoparticles have also been used as carrier for primaquine intracellular delivery against cellular *Leishmaniasis donavani* and as a result 21 fold increase in the activity of primaquine was recorded [83]. Interestingly, the unloaded PIHCA nanoparticles, also exhibited a significant anti-leishmanial activity probably to induction of respiratory burst after phagocytosis; which was more pronounced in infected cells than non-infected cells [84]. Schaffer et al. [85] studied the phagocytosis of three types of nanoparticles [Poly(alkyl cyanoacrylate), Poly (methyl methacrylate) and Human serum albumin] by gamma interferon-activated and non activated macrophages. It was found that PIHCA nanoparticles or human serum albumin nanoparticles with average diameter 200 nm were the most useful tool capable of negotiating an efficient targeting of anti-viral substances to macrophages. They also demonstrated that all HIV infected macrophages demonstrated a satisfactory phagocytic activity. It was concluded that successful drug targeting seems to be a possible event using nanoparticles. Chavany et al. [86] found that the antisense oligonucleotides (Thymidinate) entrapped in poly (alkyl cyanoacrylate) nanoparticles were stable *in vivo* and displayed 8 times greater intracellular levels than conventional levels which are often attained on free oligonucleotide administration. Some representative examples of the macrophage targeting through nanoparticles have been summarized in Table 4.

Table 4. Approaches of macrophage targeting using nanoparticles

Bioactive	Polymers	Target site	Ref.
[3H] dactinomycin	PBCA	Murine peritoneal macrophage	92
[3H] vinblastin	PMCA/PECA	Murine tissue macrophage	79
[3H] dactinomycin	PBCA	Rat tissue macrophages	80
5-Flourouracil	PBCA	Murine resident macrophages	81
Doxorubicin	PIHCA	Murine hepatic metastases	87
Ampicillin	PHCA	Experimental salmonellosis	83
Ampicillin	PIHCA	Experimental listeriosis in mice	84
Dehydroemetine	PACA	Experimental leishmaniasis in mice	86
Primaquine	PIHCA	Experimental leishmaniasis in mice	90
AmphotericinB	PMMA	Experimental leishmaniasis in mice	93
Antisens oligonucleotide oligo(thymidinate)	PIBCA/PIHCA	Anti-HIV	91

PBCA polybutyl cyanoacrylate; PMCA polymethyl cyanoacrylate; PECA polyethyl cyanoacrylate; PIHCA polyisohexyl cyanoacrylate; PHCA polyhexyl cyanoacrylate; PACA polyalkyl cyanoacrylate; PMMAPolymethyl methacrylate; PIBCA polyisobutyl cyanoacrylate

Resealed Erythrocytes

Drug loaded resealed erythrocytes have been used for targeting of bioactives to the macrophages. The systems are developed following osmotic lysis of erythrocytes followed by their resealing in the presence of the drug solution; which results in the exchange of intracellular and extracellular solutes leading to drug encapsulation within the membrane envelope of reseales/reannealed erythrocytes.

After intravenous injection such drug loaded resealed erythrocytes are rapidly sequestered and cleared from the circulation by macrophages mainly of liver and spleen. Relative contributions of macrophages of liver and spleen in clearing the resealed erythrocytes depend upon the surfacial modification or damage; which are caused during the process of drug loading. It has been demonstrated that slightly damaged resealed erythrocytes are dumped into spleen, while heavily altered ones removed by liver. Obviously, resealed erythrocytes can be used for delivering drugs or bioactives selectively to the macrophages.

Surface manipulations of the erythrocytes could alter the event of opsonization and subsequent macrophage uptake qualitatively as well as quantitatively. The mild chemical treatment of erythrocytes in vitro with N-ethyl maleiamide results in to their splenic extraction after intravenous administration. More severe treatment with glutaraldehyde triggers Fc-mediated clearance specifically by liver. Differences can however, be noted in selectivity to cell populations within the liver. The removal of sialic acid from red blood cells exposes the terminal galactosyl residues, which results in the enhanced hepatocyte uptake, where as the sequential removal of galactose residues exposes N-acetylglucosamine or mannose leading to the enhanced uptake of erythrocytes by kupffer cells [89]. Some important applications of resealed erythrocytes in the targeting of bioactives to the macrophages are summarized in the Table 5.

Table 5. Resealed erythrocytes exploited for macrophage targeting

Bioactives	Applications	Ref.
Glucocerebrosidase	Treatment of Gaucher's disease	95
β-Glucouronidase, βGalactosidase and βglucosidase	Lysosomal storage diseases	96
Pentamidine	Treatment of leishmaniasis	97
Desferrioxamine	Treatment of RES overload	98
Homidium Bromide	Trypanocidal activity	99
Tricothecene mycotoxin (T-2 toxin)	Study of toxic action of T-2toxin	100
Isometanidium	Trypanocidal activity	101
β-Glucouroxidase	Lysosomal storage disease	102
Metronidazole	Liver targeting	103
Ricin-a chain	RES targeting	104

Bio-conjugates and soluble carriers

The particulate carriers permit the loading of large amount of drug without covalent linkage however, they have poor permeability across endothelial lining and as a result poor extravasation too. They may also lead to the blockade of mononuclear phagocytes system and chronic toxicity on repeated administration if the phagocytosed material is not degraded rapidly enough.

Therefore, soluble drug carrier systems utilising macromolecules have been proposed as better alternatives by many workers. Molecules of the bioactives are coupled to the endogenous ligands specific for receptors present over the cell surface. Such conjugates have been termed as the 'bioconjugates'. When the ligands coupled to drug molecules interact with the specific receptor present over the cell membrane; the conjugate is internalised, after which the bioactive molecules are released in the interior of the cell [23,101].

The receptor most widely exploited for this purpose is the charge scavenger receptor system of macrophages, which recognizes a number of structurally diverse polyanionic macromolecules. These include modified proteins (e.g. acetylated or oxidized LDL, Maleylated bovine serum albumin), certain polysaccharide (e.g. fucoidin, dextran sulphate), polynucleotide (polyinosinic and polyguanylic acid), certain phospholipids (phosphatidylserine), polyvinyl sulphate and bacterial poly-saccharides. Other receptor systems, which are specific for endogenous ligands like proteins, growth factors, enzymes, hormones, antibodies, and sugar specific recognition elements (lectins)are also being explored for the probable potentials in targeting as bioconjugates [23,100].

Immunoconjuates

The use of monoclonal antibodies in drug(s) targeting to specific cell types is a promising approach in view of their spectrum of the tissue specificity. Drugs are coupled to antibody, thereby creating a hybrid molecule with the specificity of the immunological ligand that retains the therapeutic activity of the drug.

Conjugates of antibody and toxins (immunotoxins) in which the cell-binding moiety of toxin is replaced by the binding specificity of an antibody are reported to have significantly higher yet selective toxicity towards the target cells. Immunotoxin consisting of deglycosylated ricin-a-chain or pseudomonas exotoxins and mono-clonal antibody directed against gp41 (an antigenic substance present on the HIV-1 envelope have selective and potent toxicity towards HIV-1 infected H-9 and U-937 cells [102]. A novel strategy involving prodrug activation by antibody enzyme conjugate has been developed. Here enzymes targeted are chosen for their ability to convert relatively non-toxic drug precursors in to their active form [103].

Haisma et al. [104] described a monoclonal antibody-B glucouronidase conjugate as an activator of the prodrug epirubicin for the treatment of the cancer. This approach can be utilised for the treatment of diseases arising from the congenital deficiency of the enzymes and for achieving cell deactivation, and cell and/or cell product depletion of any sub population of the macrophages.

Conjugates with modified proteins and glycosylated polymers

Identification of the receptors, which facilitate the endocytosis of glycoproteins, on the surface of macrophages and monocytes has initiated a series of targeting approaches based on the glycoproteins. Neoglycoproteins, which consist of the protein backbone may be chemically modified with sugars so as to mimic the geometric organization of the sugar groups of naturally occurring glycoproteins (Fig.4). Such neoglycoproteins are further substituted with drug molecules and the resulting neoglycoprotein-drug conjugate can be used for targeting drug molecules to the macrophages [100,101].

Conjugates of mannosyl derivative of poly-L-lysine macromolecule and antiviral drug PMEA (Phosphonomethoxy-ethyladenine) are more potent in inhibiting Herpes simplex virus type 1 replication in vitro in human macrophages than the freely administered drug [105]. Conjugates of N-acetylmuramyl dipeptide (MDP), a macrophage activating agent with mannosylated BSA exhibits significant macrophage activating property. The conjugated MDP induces eradication of lung metastases in 70% of the mice where as free MDP is pharmacodynamically inactive [106]. MDP conjugated to poly-L-lysine substituted with mannosyl or gluconoyl residues is also nearly as efficient as MDP-mannosylated BSA conjugate in activating macrophages. Glycoconjugates of MDP with mannosylated BSA or with gluconoylated or mannosylated poly-L-lysine induce active antiviral effect against Herpes simplex virus type 1 whereas free MDP has no such effects [100,107].

Similarly, conjugates of allopurinol-riboside with gluconylated or mannosylated poly-L-lysine were found to be 80 times more active than free drug *in vitro* in activating leishmania infected macrophages [108]. Succinyl-5'azidothymidine (succinyl AZT) conjugated via glycyl-glycyl spacers to mannosylated poly-L-lysine has been reported to be more efficient than free AZT or free succinyl AZT against HIV multiplication in human macrophages [109].

The conjugates of oligonucleotides with glycoproteins also demonstrate an efficient targeting potential. *In vivo* biodistribution studies have shown that conjugates of oligonucleotides of mannnosylated BSA exhibit significantly higher selective accumulation in macrophages of liver and spleen [100]. Glycoconjugates can also be used to increase the efficiency of gene transfer. Various authors have prepared poly-lysine plasmid complexes exploiting recognition elements like transferrin, insulin or asialo-orosomucoid; which have been used for effective gene delivery [101]. Galactosylated poly lysine-plasmid complex is efficiently taken up by hepatoma line HepG2 cells and expression of related protein (Luciferase) was observed by these cells [100]. The technique when mastered fully could be of immense importance in solving problems arising from congenital deficiency of enzymes.

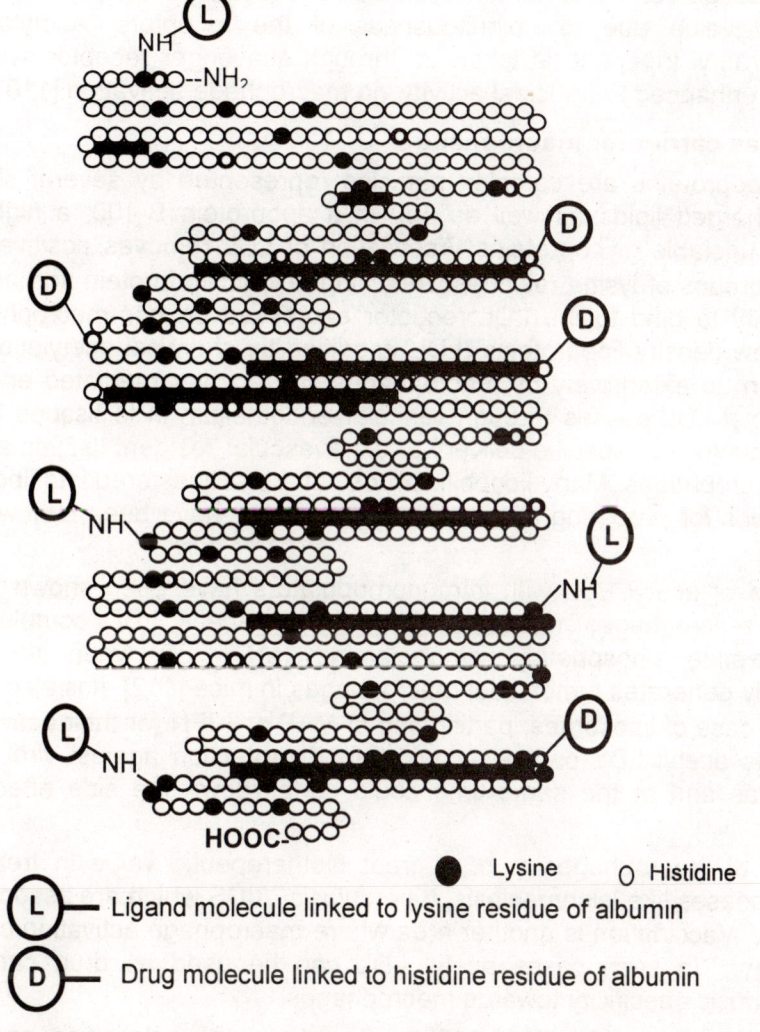

● Lysine   ○ Histidine

Ⓛ — Ligand molecule linked to lysine residue of albumin

Ⓓ — Drug molecule linked to histidine residue of albumin

Fig. 4 : Schematic representation of a neoglyco-protein. Ligand and drug molecules are linked to albumin backbone

Basu et al. [23] used the chemical conjugates of methotrexate with maleylated bovine serum albumin for the treatment of Leishmaniasis and found the drug conjugate to be 100 times more effective then the free drug in eliminating the intracellular amastigotes of *L. donavani* and *L. mexicana amazonesis*. Maleylated bovine serum albumin has also been shown to significantly improve the delivery of para-aminosalicylic acid (in the treatment of tuberculosis) and daunomycin (anticancer drug used in the treatment of histiocytosis) and better therapeutic results have been obtained. The system has been reported to demonstrate advantages in regard to ease of preparation, longer shelf life, ease of sterilization and formulation in to apyrogenic preparation. Similar approach using altered low density lipoproteins, mannosylated neoglycoproteins and yeast mannan have also been reported.

Other receptor system for lipoproteins, growth factors, cytokines are also being intensively investigated. These carrier systems have shown some potential but they are of limited value due to ubiquitousness of the receptors. Acetylated LDL containing muramyl tripeptide is taken up through scavenger receptor system and has shown an enhanced tumoricidal activity via macrophage activation [110].

Lipoproteins as carrier for macrophage

Low-density lipoproteins are complex particles represented by several classes of neutral and charged lipids as well as 500 kDa apoprotein B-100, a highly water insoluble and unstable glycoproteins. Acetylation of LDL removes positive charges from ε amino groups of lysine residues. Resulting anionic lipoprotein and acetyl LDL losses its ability to bind to the LDL receptor expressed on non-macrophage cells [111]. Thus, low-density lipoproteins (LDL) modified by chemical acetylation (Acetyl LDL) are taken up extensively by macrophages via receptor mediated endocytosis [110,111]. Acetyl LDL passes through vascular endothelium in to tissues therefore, they are suitable for site specific delivery to extravascular resident tissues and tumor associated macrophages. Many lipophilic drugs can be sequestered into lipoproteins. Several methods for preparing lipoprotein drug complex have been reviewed in the literature [110].

Complexes of acetyl LDL with immunomodulators have been shown to initiate activation of macrophages for tumoricidal action. Acetyl LDL complexed with muramyl tripeptide phosphatidyl ethanolamine (MTP-PE); when administered intraperitonealy generates tumoricidal macrophages in mice [112]. It is also expected that; as in the case of liposomes; partitioning of MAF or γ-IFN (or their active peptide fragments) into acetyl LDL particles could impart protection against viral diseases and carcinomas and at the same time could curtail down the side effects to the minimum.

Activation of macrophages is of a great biotherapeutic value in treatment of pathogenic diseases like leishmaniasis, tuberculosis, AIDS which are associated with macrophages. Vaccination is another area where macrophage activation could be a useful strategy. In such cases acetyl LDL can be used as drug carrier as it possesses intrinsic specificity towards macrophages.

Vyas and his associates [115,116] have categorically classified endogenous lipoproteins and systems derived from them as self-assembling supramolecular systems having high association number (degree of association). The degree of association is defined as a number of associating molecules combining in order to achieve better thermodynamic stability so as to behave as a single large association unit. However, these endogenous carriers suffer from major problems, which limit their use as drug carriers, and entail for semi-synthetic and synthetic mimics of endogenous lipoprotein particles. The most important of them is the inability to entrap hydrophilic drugs without their conversion to lipophilic prodrugs and subsequently altered receptor-mediated uptake by different liver cells.

However, Samain and co-workers [117] developed synthetic mimics of natural endogenous particles (mainly LDL) and named them as "Supramolecular Biovector (SMBV)". These synthetic mimics incorporate bio-components as one of the construction element. SMBVs are lipoprotein-based carriers appended with polymerized polysaccharide with exterior coat layer of endogenous low-density lipoproteins (LDL). Vyas and co-workers reviewed the composition and structure of these synthetic mimics of LDL (Fig. 6) and their possible role for the site-specific drug delivery towards macrophages [115, 116]. The SMBVs are composed of a basic skeleton of cross-linked natural polysaccharides which is surface acylated using fatty acids to constitute a hydrophobic domain (mimic of lipoprotein lipidic core). This hydrophobic skeleton is eventually stabilized using an external phospholipid shell, onto which apolipoproteins are anchored to endow the system site specificity.

Synthesis of SMBV essentially involves cross-linking and derivatization step of polysaccharides followed by a homogenization, a drying followed by a regioselective acylation step. The structures of SMBV allow the entrapment of wide spectrum of drugs, i.e., lipophilic, hydrophilic or amphiphilic. Furthermore, The system is versatile enough to entrap a drug that is ionic in nature, either by grafting of ionic ligands in fatty acid layer or on to the polysaccharide nucleus thus allowing retention of the drugs by an ion exchange phenomenon. Both neutral SMBVs (Type I) and ionic ligand grafted SMBVs (Type II) are reported in the literature [115-117].

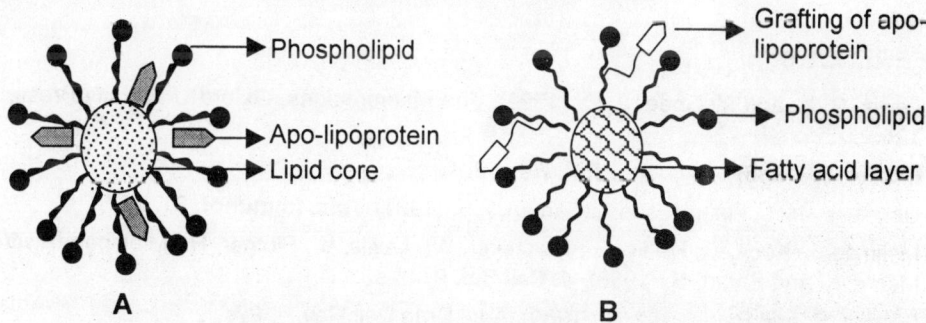

Fig. 5 : Structure of (A) lipoprotein and (B) supramolecular biovectors based upon the skeleton of a lipidic core surrounded by apo-lipoprotein anchored phospholipidic shell

FUTURE PROSPECTS

Macrophage targeting of bioactives especially of biological response modifiers and antibiotics holds great potential in combating the complications arising in patients suffering from immune disorders or immuno-compromised patients due to chemotherapy or some other etiological reasons. Besides, it can also provide a novel way of treating age-old epidemics like leishmaniasis.

Elimination and ablation of toxic side effects from biological response modifiers by targeting them to macrophages has opened the vistas of possibility of their use in the chemotherapy of cancer and in the treatment and prophylaxis of infectious diseases. The safety and efficacy of macrophage targeting of one such agent, muramyl-tripeptide-phosphatidylethanolamine (MTP-PE) by incorporating it in the liposomes has been already established in adults and children through phase-I and phase-II clinical trials [17]. The approach of macrophage targeting is likely to be developed as an effective method of vaccination in recent future.

Treatment of autoimmune and inflammatory diseases by selectively depleting the macrophages or their sub-populations is being attempted and considered which will definitely set up new hopes in the management of such diseases. Macrophage depletion has now become a most promising stratagem for studying the role of macrophages in the host defense related mechanisms and many complex questions are likely to be answered by this approach.

The concepts of inverse targeting and macrophage depletion are also being attended immensely as powerful tools for facilitating gene transfer which would definitely open up an altogether new area for the possible applications of the macrophages [113]. It is concluded that apart from the therapeutic site, macrophage targeting will also play a significant role in investigating and explaining various phenomena which fall within the domains of immunology, cell biology, biotechnology and human physiology. Thus selective masking, drug targeting and activation of macrophages as a concerted event or activity in isolation is a rationalized approach which offers distinctive diagnostic, biological and therapeutic advantages.

REFERENCES

1. Lewis, C. E. and McGhee, J. O. (1992). The Macrophages, Oxford University Press, Oxford, 126.

2. Becker, S. (1988). **Adv. Drug Del. Rev.**, 2, 1.

3. Unkeless, J. C., Fleit, H. and Mellaman, I. S. (1981). **Adv. Immunol.** 31, 247.

4. Mellman, I., Koch, T., Healy, G., Hunzeker, W., Lewis, V., Plutner, H., Miettinen, H., Vaux, D., Moore, K. and Stuart, S. (1988). **J. Cell Sci.** 9, 45.s

5. Gordon, S. and Rabinowitz, S. (1989). Adv. Drug Del. Rev. 4, 27.

6. Duncan, A., Woof, J. M., Patridge, L. J., Burton, D. R. and Winter, G. (1988). **Nature** 332, 563.

7. Sanchez-Madrid, F., Nagy, J. A., Robbins, E., Simmon, P. and Springer, T. A. (1983). **J. Exp. Med.** 158, 826.

8. Ross, G. D. and Atkinson, J. P. (1985). **Immunol. Today,** 6, 115.

9. Stahal, P. D., Wileman, T. E. and Shepard, V. L. (1985). **Op. Lit. Ref.** 2, 59.

10. Ross, G. D., Clain, J. A, and Lachmann, P. J. (1985). **J. Immunol.** 134, 3307.

11. Kaplan, J. (1980). **Cell**, 19,197.

12. Fogelman, A. M., Vanlenten, B. J., Warden, C., Haberland, M. E. and Edwards, P. A. (1988). **J. Cell Sci.** 9, 135.

13. Kolb, H. and Kolb-Bachofen, V. (1978). **Biochim. Biophys. Res. Commun.**, 85, 678.

14. Ben-Hagen, T. L., van-Vianen, W. and Bakker-Wonderberg, I. A. (1995). **J. Infect. Dis.** 171, 385.

15. Curfs, J. H., Hermen, C. C., Kremsner, P., Neifer, S., Menwissen, J. H., van Rooijen, N. and Eling, W. M. (1993). **Parasitol.** 107, 125.

16. Kleinerman, E. S. (1995). **Hematol. Oncol. Clin. North Am.** 9, 927.

17. Kleinerman, E. S., Maedi, M. and Jaffe, N. (1993). **Cancer Treat. Res.** 62, 101.

18. Asano, T. and Kleinerman, E. S. (1993). **J. Immunother.** 14, 286.

19. Brisseau, G. F., Kresta, A., Schouten, D., Bohnen, J. M., Shek, P. N., Fok, E. and Rotstein, O. D. (1994). **Antimicrob. Agents Chemother.** 38, 2671.

20. Shi, F., Kurzman, I. D. and MacEwen, E. G. (1995). **Cancer Biother.** 10, 317.

21. Zhau, F. and Huang, L. (1995). **J. Drug Target.** 3, 91.

22. Dieter, P., Ambs, P., Fitzke, E., Hidaka, H., Hoffman, R. and Schwende, H. (1995). **J. Immunol.** 55, 2595.

23. Basu, S. K., Mazumdar, S., Mukhopadhyay, B. and Mukhopadhyay, A. (1984). **Proc. Ind. Natl. Acad. Sci.** 60, 345.

24. Alving, C. R. (1988). **Adv. Drug Del. Rev.** 2,107.

25. Bakker-Wounderberg, I. A., Storm, G. and Woodle, M. C. (1994). **J. Drug Target.** 2, 363.

26. Pretzer, E., Flasher, D. and Duzgunes, N. (1997). **Antiviral Res.** 34, 1.

27. Saravolac, E. G., Kournikakis, B., Gorton, L. and Wong, J. P. (1996). **Antiviral Res.** 29, 199.

28. Thomas, K., Nijenhuis, A. M., Dontje, B. H., Daeman, T. and Sherphof, G. L. (1995). **Clin. Exp. Metastasis** 13, 328.

29. Goldbach, P., Dumont, S., Kessler, R., Poindron, P. and Stamm, A. (1996). **Am. J. Physiol.**, 270, 429.

30. Ushio, Y., Yamamoto, M., Sanchez-Bueno, A. and Yoshida, R. (1996). **Microbiol. Immunol.** 40, 489.

31. Huitinga, I., Ruuls, S. R., Jung, S., Van Rooijen, N., Hartung, H. P. and Dijkstra, C. D. (1995). **Clin. Exp. Immunol.** 100, 344.

32. Jung, S., Huitinga, I., Schmidtt, B., Zielasek, J., Dijkstra, C. D., Toyka, K. V. and Hortung, H. P. (1993). **J. Neurol. Sci.** 119, 195.

33. Kuzmin, A. I., Finegold, M. J. and Eisensmith, R. C. (1997). **Gene Ther.** 4, 309.

34. O'Mullane, J. E., Artursson, P., Tomlinson, E. (1987). In: Biological Approaches to the Controlled Delivery of Drugs (Edt. by R. L. Juliano) Ann. New York Acad. Sci., 120.

35. Meije, D. K. F., Jansem, R. W. and Molema, G. (1992). **Antiviral Res.** 18, 215.

36. Widder, K. J., Senyei, A. E. and Ranney, D. F. (1979). **Adv. Pharmacol. Chemother.** 16, 216.

37. New, R. R., Chance, M. L., Thomas, S. C. and Peters, W. (1975). **Nature** 272, 55.

38. Ghosh, P. and Bacchawat, B. K. (1980). **Biochim. Biophys Acta** 632, 562.

39. Garcon, N., Gregoriadis, G., Taylor, M. and Summerfield, J. (1988). **Immunol.** 64, 743.

40. Sunamoto, J., Goto, M., Iida, T., Hara, K., Saito, K. and Tomonaga, A. (1985). In: Receptor Mediated Targeting of Drugs (G. Gregoriadis, J. Senior, A. Tronet) Plenum Press, New York, 3591.

41. Yachi, K., Kikuchi, H., Yamauchi, H., Hirota, S. and Tomikawa, M. (1995). **J. Microencap.** 12, 377.

42. Barrat, G. M., Tenu, J. P., Yapo, A. and Petit, J. F. (1986). **Biochim. Biophys. Acta** 862, 153.

43. Bacchawat, B. K., Das, P. K. and Ghosh, P. (1984) In: Liposome Technology (Edt.by G. Gregoriadis), CRC Press, Boca Raton, FL, 95.

44. Russel, D. G. and Wilhelm, H. (1986). **J. Immunol.** 136, 2613.

45. Weissmann, G., Bloomgarden, D., Kalpan, R., Hoffstein, S., Collins, T., Gottliet, A. and Nagle, J. (1975). **Proc. Natl. Acad. Sci. USA** 72, 88.

46. Geiger, B., Carlos, G., Calef, E. and Arnon, R. (1981). **Eur. J. Immunol.** 11, 710.

47. Hsu, M. J. and Juliano, R. L. (1982). **Biochim. Biophys. Acta** 720, 411.

48. Heath, T. D., Macher, B. A. and Papahadjopoulos, D. (1981). **Biochim. Biophys. Acta** 6, 66.

49. Norley, S. G., Huang, L. and Rouse, B. T. (1986). **J. Immunol.** 136, 68.

50. Roerdink, F., Wassef, N. M., Richardson, E. C. and Alving, C. R. (1986). **Biochim. Biophys. Acta** 734, 33.

51. Gokhale, P. C., Barapatre, R. J., Advani, S. H., Kshirsagar, N. A. and Pandya, S. K. (1993). **J. Cancer Res. Clin. Oncol.** 119, 569.

52. Van Etten, E. W. M., Otte-Lambillion. M., Van Vianen. W., Ten Kate, M. T. and Bakker-Wounderberg, I. A. J. M. (1995). **J. Antimicrob. Chemother.** 35, 519.

53. Davidson, R. N., Di Martino, L., Gradoni, L., Giacchino, R., Russo, R., Gaeta, G. B., Pempinello, R., Scolt, S., Raimondi, F. and Cascio, A. (1994). **Q. J. Med.** 87, 75.

54. Yardley, V. and Croft, S. L. (1997). **Antimicrob. Agents Chemother.** 41, 752.

55. Perfect, J. R. and Wright, K. A. (1994). **J. Antimicrob. Chemother.** 33, 73.

56. Viviani, M. A., Rizzardini, G., Tortorano, A. M., Fasan, M., Capetti, A., Roverselli, A. M., Gringeri, A. and Suter, F. (1994). **Infection** 22, 137.

57. Graybill, J. R. and Bocanegra, R. (1996). **Curr. Top. Microbiol. Immunol.** 210, 159.

58. Kleinerman, E. S., Gano, J. B., Johnstone, D. A., Benzamin, R. S. and Jaffe, N. (1995). **Am. J. Clin. Oncol.** 18, 93.

59. Hrovokova, G. and Velebny, S. (1997). **Parasitol.** 114, 475.

60. Duzgunes, N., Flasher, D., Reddy, M. V., Luna Herreia, J. and Gangadharam, P. R. (1996). **Antimicrob. Agents Chemother.** 40, 2618.

61. Perepelkin, A., Rotov, K. A., Tikhonov, N. G., Petrov, V. I. and Andreev, D. A. (1996). **Antibiot. Khimioter.** 41, 28.

62. Banerjee, G., Nandi, G., Mahto, S. B., Pakrashi, A. and Basu, M. K. (1996). **J. Antimicrob. Chemother.** 38, 145.

63. Chaudhari, G. (1997). **Biochem. Pharmacol.** 53, 385.

64. Kole, L., Sakar, K., Mahato, S. B. and Das, P. K. (1994). **Biochim. Biophys. Res. Commun.** 200, 351.

65. Medda, S., Das, N., Mahato, .S. B., Mahadevan, P. R. and Basu, M. K. (1995). **Ind. J. Biochem. Biophys.** 32, 147.

66. Agarwal, A., Kandpal, H., Gupta, H. P., Singh, N. B. and Gupta, C. M. (1994). **J. Antimicrob. Agents Chemother.** 38, 588.

67. Yoshioka, T., Hashida, M., Muranishi, S. and Sezaki, H. (1981). **Int. J. Pharm.** 81, 131.

68. Davis, S. S., Illum, L., Maghimi, S. M., Davies, M. C., Porter, C. J. H., Muir, I. S., Brindley, A., Christy, N. M., Norman, M. E., Williams, P. and Dunn, S.E. (1993). **J. Contrl. Rel.** 24, 157.

69. Hoffman, E. M., Longo, W. E. and Goldberg, E. P. (1984). In: 11th Int. Symp. Cont. Rel. Soc. (W. D. Meyer, R. L. Dunn Eds.) Control Release Society, London, 27.

70. Malaise, M. G., Franchimont, P. and Mahien, P. R. (1989). **J. Immunol. Methods** 119, 231.

71. Tabata, Y. and Ikada, Y. (1989). **Pharm. Res.** 6, 296.

72. Knepp, W. A., Jayakrishnan, A., Quigg, J. M., Silren, H. S., Bagnall, J. J. and Goldberg, E. P. (1993). **J. Pharm. Pharmacol.** 45, 887.

73. Vyas, S. P. and Dixit, V. K. (1998). In: Pharmaceutical Biotechnology. CBS Publishers and Distributors, New Delhi, 589.

74. Couvreur, P., Kante, B., Leenaerts, V., Scailteus, V., Roland, M. and Speiser, P. (1980). **J. Pharm. Sci.** 69, 199.

75. Kante, B., Couvreur, P., Lenaerts, V., Scailteur, V., Roland, M. and Speiser, P. (1980). **Int. J. Pharm.** 7, 45.

76. Kreuter, J. and Hartmann, H. (1983). **Oncol.** 40, 363.

77. Guiot, P. and Couvreur, P. (1983). **J. De. Pharmacie. De. Belgique.** 38, 130.

78. Fattal, F., Youssef, M., Couvreur, P. and Andremont, A. (1989). **Antimicrob. Agents Chemother.** 33, 1540.

79. Youssef, M., Fattal, F., Alouso, M. J., Roblot Treupei, L., Sauzieres, J., Tancrde, C., Omnes, A., Couvreur, P. and Andremont, A. (1988). **Antimicrob. Agents Chemother.** 32, 1204.

80. Forestier, F., Gerrier, P., Chaumard, C., Quero, A. M., Couvier, P. and Labarre, C. (1992). **J. Antimicrob. Chemother.** 30, 173.

81. Fourage, M., Dewulf, M., Couvreur, P., Roland, M. and Vianckx, H. (1989). **J. Microencap.** 6, 29.

82. Chiannilkulchai, N., Driouich, Z., Benoit, J. P., Parodi, A. L. and Couvreur, P. (1989). **Selective Cancer Ther.** 5, 1.

83. Gaspar, R., Opperdoes, F. R. and Preat, V., Roland, M. (1992). **Annal. Trop. Med. Parasitol.** 86, 41.

84. Gaspar, R., Opperdoes, F. R., Preat, V. and Roland, M. (1992). **Pharm. Res.** 9, 782.

85. Schaffer, V., von Briesen, H., Andreasen, R., Steffan, A. M., Royer, C., Froster, S., Kreuter, J. and Robsamen-Waigman, H. (1992). **Pharm. Res.** 9, 541.

86. Chavany, C., Le Doan, T., Couvreur, P., Puisieux, F. and Helene, C. (1992). **Pharm. Res.** 9, 441.

87. Couvreur, P., Lenaerts, V., Kante, B., Roland, M. and Speiser, P. (1980). **J. Pharm. Sci.** 69, 220.

88. Vennier-Julienne, M. C., Vouldokis, I., Monjour, L. and Benoit, J. P. (1992). Proceedings of the International Conference on Biotechnology 5, 4249.

89. Wagner, H. N., Razzak, M. A., Gaertner, R. A., Caine, N. P. and Feagin, O. T. (1962). **Arch. Int. Med.** 110, 90.

90. Dale, G. L., Kuhl, L. W. and Bentler, E. (1979). **Proc. Natl. Acad. Sci. USA**, 76, 473.

91. Thorpe, S. R., Fidler, M. B. and Desnick, R. K. (1975). **Biophys. Res. Com.** 61, 146.

92. Berman, A. and Aikawa, M. (1984). **Am. J. Trop. Med. Hyg.** 33, 1112.

93. Fiorelli, G., Fargion, S., Piperno, A., Cappellini, M. D., Rossi, F., Sabbioneda, L. and Zanella, A. (1987). In: Advances in Biosciences (Edt. by C. Ropers, M. Chassaigne, C. Nicolau) Pergamon Press, NewYork, 47.

94. Deloach, J. B., Wagner, G. G. and Craig, I. M. (1981). **J. Appl. Biochem.** 3, 254.

95. Deloach, J. B., Andrew, S. A. and Shaffield, C. (1988). **Biotechnol. Appl. Biochem.** 10, 183.

96. Deloach, J. B. and Wagner, G. G. (1988). **Biotechnol. Appl. Biochem.** 10, 447.

97. Fidler, J. B. (1987). **Method Enzymol.** 149, 245.

98. Talwar, N. and Jain, N. K. (1992). **J. Contrl. Rel.** 20, 133.

99. Chestier, N., Kravtzoff, R. and Ropers, C. (1991). In: Advances in Biosciences (Edt. by R. Green, J. B. Deloach), Pergamon Press, New York, 29.

100. Monsigmy, M., Roche, A. C., Midoux, P. and Mayer, R. (1994). **Adv. Drug Deliv. Rev.** 14, 1.

101. Molema, G. and Meizer, D. K. F. (1994). **Adv. Drug Deliv. Rev.** 14, 25.

102. Till, M. A., Zolla-Pazner, S., Gorny, M. K., Patton, J. S., Uhr, J. W. and Vitetta, E. S. (1989). **Proc. Natl. Acad. Sci. USA** 86, 1987.

103. Senter, P.D. (1993). **FASEB J.** 4, 188.

104. Haisma, H. J., Boven, M., Van Muijen, M., De Jong, J., Van der Vijgh, W. J. F. and Pinedo, H. M. (1992). **Br. J. Cancer** 66, 474.

105. Midoux, P., Negre, E., Roche, A C., Mayer, R., Monsigny, M., Balzarani, J., De Clerque, E., Mayer, E., Ghaffar, A. and Gangemi, J. D. (1990). **Biochim. Biophys. Res. Commun.** 167, 1044.

106. Roche, A.C., Bailly, P. and Monsigny, M. (1985). **Invasion Metastasis**, 5, 218.

107. Derrien, D., Midoux, P., Petit, C., Negre, E., Mayer, R., Monsigny, M. and Roche, A. C. (1989). **Glycoconjugate J.** 6, 241.

108. Negre, E., Chance, M. L., Hanboula, S.Y., Monsigny, M., Roche, A. C., Mayer, R. and Homel, M. (1992). **Antimicrob. Agents Chemother.** 36, 2228.

109. Richman, D. D., Kornbluth, R. S. and Carson, D. A. (1987). **J. Exp. Med.** 166, 1144.

110. Shaw, J. M., Shaw, K. V., Yanowich, S., Iwanik, M., Futch, W. S., Rosowsky, A. and Schook, L. B. (1987). **Ann. N. Y. Acad. Sci.** 507, 252.

111. Brown, M. S. and Goldstein, J. L. (1983). **Ann. Rev. Biochem.** 52, 223.

112. Yanovich, S., Prestion, L. and Shaw, J. M. (1984). **Cancer Res.** 44, 3377.

113. Wolff, G., Worgall, S., Van Rooijen, N., Song, W. R., Harvey, B. G. and Crystal, R. G. (1997). **J. Virol.** 71, 624.

114. Vyas, S. P. and Sakthivel, T. (1994). **J. Microencap.** 11, 373.

115. Jaitely, V., Kanaujia, P. and Vyas, S.P. (1997). **Indian J. Exp. Biol.** 35, 212.

116. Vyas, S.P., Jaitely, V. and Kanaujia, P. (1997). **Pharmazie** 52, 259.

117. Peyrot, M., Sautereau, A.M., Rabanel, J.M., Nguyen, F., Tocanne, J.F. and Samain, D. (1994). **Int. J. Pharm.** 102, 25.

7

SITE-SPECIFIC GENE DELIVERY THROUGH VIROSOMES

DEBI P. SARKAR, KOMAL RAMANI and SANDEEP K. TYAGI

Department of Biochemistry,
University of Delhi South Campus,
Benito Juarez Road, New Delhi - 110021.
Tel : 011- 6881967 / 6112159; Fax : 011- 6885270 / 6886427
E.mail : dpsarkar@hotmail.com / dps@dusc.ernet.in

- Introduction
- Preparation & Characterization of DNA loaded virosomes
- Conclusion
- References

INTRODUCTION

Crossing of the permeability barrier imposed by the cellular plasma membrane is the major problem in delivering DNA and other biological macromolecules into the cytosolic compartment of a living cell. Liposomes have been very much in use for this purpose [1]. In this method the loaded liposomes are taken up by endocytosis and are localized in lysosomes where the enclosed material suffers extensive degradation by various hydrolytic enzymes [2]. In fact, this remains a serious limiting factor in gene transfer by liposomes. Another delivery system exploits the retroviral entry mechanism, either alone or in conjunction with cationic liposome [3]. Although this mode leads to efficient and stable transformation of non-dividing cells, this system suffers from undesirable side effects and non-specific targeting to normal cell [4]. The most popular Adenovirus-based gene transfer vectors suffer from similar problem [5]. Despite improvements in viral and nonviral vector systems for gene therapy, current clinical trials have had limited success, mainly due to the lack of appropriate targeted DNA delivery systems [6].

Reconstituted Sendai viral envelopes (F,HN - Virosomes) containing two glyco-proteins, F (fusion protein) and HN (hemagglutinin-neuraminidase), are known to fuse efficiently with the plasma membrane of target cells and are excellent carriers for fusion-mediated microinjection of biologically active macromolecules *in vitro*. This delivery system exploits the binding of HN to the sialic acid moiety of the membrane, followed by the F-protein-mediated fusion of the viral envelopes with the host cell plasma membrane at neutral pH [7]. However, this powerful system of gene delivery lacks cell type specificity because of the presence of HN protein, which is known to bind to various cell types through the cell surface sialoglycoconjugates [8]. In spite of all recent developments in gene therapy since 1989, the formulation of a targeted gene delivery "vector" is still far from ideal [9]. It has been recently demonstrated in our laboratory that F- Virosomes (devoid of HN glycoprotein) can specifically bind and fuse with HepG2 cells. The target specificity of F-Virosomes has been ensured by the strong interaction between the terminal β-galactose moiety of F-protein and the asialoglycoprotein receptor (ASGP-R) on the membrane of HepG2 cells [7]. In further studies, F-Virosomes has been successfully used for the delivery of biologically active macromolecules into the cytoplasm of liver cells both *in vitro* and *in vivo* [8,10-13]. Liver is known to be a model organ for somatic gene therapy. Hence, F-Virosomes by virtue of their specific interaction and fusion with liver cells should be an ideal vector for gene delivery both *in vitro* and *in vivo*. The F-Virosome-mediated delivery of reporter genes and its expression in liver cells (both *in vitro* and *in vivo*) have been discussed in this presentation.

PREPARATION AND CHARACTERIZATION OF DNA LOADED F-VIROSOMES

The plasmid, pCIS3CAT (6.7 Kb) containing chloramphenicol acetyl transferase (CAT) gene under the control of cytomegalovirus (CMV) promoter, was constructed [12]. Plasmid pBVluc, (6.38 Kb) containing the firefly luciferase gene under control of CMV promoter, was derived from pCEP4-X2 luc (Stratagene). In brief, the TritonX-100 solubilized fraction of Sendai virus was mixed with plasmid DNA (75 µg of DNA/ mg of viral protein) and reconstituted by stepwise removal of detergent using SM2 biobeads. Two to 5 µg of intact DNA was found to be encapsulated in 1 mg of F-Virosomes [12,13].

Microinjection of DNA to liver cells through membrane fusion and it's quantitation in various subcellular compartments

F-Virosome-mediated internalization of pCIS3CAT DNA by HepG2 cells in culture was examined prior to checking CAT gene expression. After 2 h of fusion followed by 24 h of incubation of HepG2 cells, the amount of plasmid DNA delivered by F-Virosomes, was found to be maximum in the nuclear fraction. The amount of DNA delivered to nucleus by the corresponding heat-treated F-Virosomes was 2 times less than that delivered by untreated F-Virosomes [12]. Heat- treated F-Virosomes being fusion-inactive, are likely to be taken up by endocytosis leading to their accumulation in lysosomes. This results in significant degradation of pCIS3CAT DNA. Under similar conditions loaded F-Virosomes fail to deliver pCIS3CAT DNA to Chinese hamster ovary (CHO) cells that lack the ASGP-R. These results strongly support the target specific, fusion-mediated delivery of DNA by F-Virosomes and efficient transport of intact DNA to the nucleus of HepG2 cells. The F-Virosome - mediated, targeted cytosolic gene delivery in vivo to liver parenchymal cells (of Balb/c mouse) is apprehended from the cytosolic localization of plasmid DNA at 2 h after injection and it's absolute nuclear localization 6 h after intravenous injection onward. This is additionally substantiated from the lysosomal accumulation of plasmid when delivered through heat-treated F-Virosomes. The overall efficiency of this delivery mode is reflected from the absence of any detectable PCR signal upon i.v. administration of free DNA. This is probably the first report of intracellular trafficking of a foreign gene under *in vivo* conditions [13].

Expression of CAT and luciferase gene after fusion-mediated DNA delivery

The amount of CAT protein expressed in HepG2 cells after F-Virosome-mediated delivery was 3-4 times more than that of the corresponding heat controls. It is interesting to note that 1 μg of DNA delivered by the Lipofectin method of transfection did not express any detectable level of CAT protein. However, 15μg of DNA delivered by Lipofectin transfection expressed 300 pg of CAT protein which is comparable to the protein expressed (0.06 fg of CAT protein/cell) when 1μg of DNA was delivered by F-Virosomes. The amount of CAT protein expressed was found to be persistent till a period of 192 h, thereby indicating the overall efficiency of this delivery system [12]. The CAT gene expression was assessed *in vivo* (Balb/c mouse) both at the level of mRNA and of protein [13]. Maximum CAT gene expression was achieved in the liver. CAT gene expression was not detected in the other tissues. The relative expression of CAT protein in the liver was comparable with mRNA levels. The expression of both mRNA and protein in mouse liver persisted over a period of 180 days with no F-specific humoral antibody response from 10 days onwards. Moreover, the animals remained healthy and active during the experiments. In an another experiment, the luciferase activity was found to be 8-10 times greater in parenchymal cells compared with the non-parenchymal counterparts. Moreover, the luciferase expression in parenchymal cells was 3-4 times more than that of corresponding heat controls. This points towards another strong evidence of membrane fusion-mediated targeted gene delivery. The F glycoprotein is known to possess Le^x- ($Gal\beta1-4[Fuc\alpha1-3]GlcNAc-$) terminated biantennary oligosaccharides [14]. The Le^x moiety possesses much higher affinity for ASGP-R present on parenchymsal cells. This property is considered to be a prerequisite of targeted delivery systems with special reference to *in vivo* conditions [15]. The liver is an ideal organ for transfection of a gene whose product is secreted into the circulation and is important for systemic gene therapy for several inherited diseases. Moreover, the nonpathogenicity of Sendai virus to humans and its poor immunogenecity have together increased the prospects of F-Virosomes in gene therapy [16,17].

Integration status of the delivered DNA in the chromosome of liver cells

To determine the state of targeted DNA in hepatocytes after i.v. injection of loaded F-Virosomes, purified chromosomal DNA was hybridized to P^{32} labeled 1.5-kb CAT gene fragment derived from pCIS3CAT. No hybridization signal was detected from purified chromosomal DNA 1 day after injection [13]. However, chromosomal DNAs from hepatocytes 15, 30, and 60 days after injection, contain high molecular weight sequences that hybridized with the CAT gene probe. Chromosomal DNA from mock-injected mice and Herring sperm DNA and DNA from non-parenchymal cells failed to show any hybridization signal. To establish the nature of integration of the DNA in mouse chromosome, purified genomic DNA from mouse liver 60 days after injection, was digested with various sets of restriction enzymes and the resulting fragments were analyzed after hybridization with 1.5-kb CAT gene probe. Purified chromosomal DNA, isolated from CAT-injected-animals and restricted with different sets of enzymes, generated CAT-positive fragments of lower size than that of the linearized plasmid (6.7 kb) and a few hybridizable fragments greater in size than the linearized plasmid. Since these band patterns do not correspond to those obtained after digestion of pCIS3CAT, this suggests the possibility of random insertion of the delivered plasmid in the mouse chromosome. The integration status was further confirmed by PCR analysis of the purified chromosomal and episomal fractions by using CAT-specific primers. Twenty four hours after injection, amplified CAT gene fragment (633 bp) was detected only from the episomal fraction but no such product was obtained from the corresponding chromosomal fractions. On the other hand, 15, 30, and 60 days after injection, amplified products were detected only from the chromosomal fractions but not from the corresponding episomal fractions. The possibility of nonspecific PCR amplification was ruled out from appropriate negative controls. The copy number of the plasmid integrated in the genome was found to range from $\approx$ 100 to 300 copies per cell as calculated from slot blot hybridization of chromosomal DNA from hepatocytes 60 days after injection.

CONCLUSION

Based on interaction with ASGP-R, viral and nonviral hepatotropic gene transfer systems have been used both *in vitro* and *in vivo*. Although partial targeting to hepatocytes was achieved, the efficiency of these vectors was found to be seriously affected because of the lysosomal degradation of endocytosed DNAs [18]. Interestingly, in case of F-Virosomes, the F protein acts in a bifunctional way, i.e., binding to hepatocytes followed by membrane fusion-mediated direct release of the virosomal aqueous contents to the cytoplasm of target cells [8]. The probable reason of this efficient and persistent expression could be attributed to the delivery of large amount of functional DNA into the nuclear compartment of the liver cells. The persistent nature of transgene expression in hepatocytes may be explained from the stable integration of CAT gene in the mouse chromosome. It is relevant to note that sustained gene expression does not appear to be influenced by the random nature of integration of foreign DNA. The F-Virosomes, being at the interface of viral and nonviral vectors, are safe enough in comparison to their nonhybrid counterparts [6]. These attributes highlight the potential of this gene carrier for targeted delivery of genes of therapeutic importance *in vivo*.

ACKNOWLEDGEMENTS

This work is dedicated to our beloved "**Guruji**", *the late Prof. B.K. Bachhawat.* We are grateful to the Department of Biotechnology (DBT), council of Scientific and Industrial Research (CSIR) and University Grants Commission (UGC), Government of India for financial support. We thank Dr. S.E. Hasnain of National Institute of Immunology, New Delhi for valuable suggestions and active collaboration.

REFFERENCES

1. Szoka, F.C. Jr. (1991). In : Membrane Fusion (Wilschut, J. and Hoekstra, D. Eds.), Marcel Dekker, New York, pp. 845-890.

2. Chowdhury, N.R., Wu, C.H., Wu, G.Y., Yerneni, P.C., Bommineni, V.R. and Chowdhury, J.R. (1993). **J. Biol. Chem.** 268, 11265-11271.

3. Hodgson, C.P. and Solaiman, F. (1996). **Nature Biotech.** 14, 339-342.

4. Nilson, B. H. K., Morling, F.J., Cosset, F.L. and Russell, S.J. (1996). **Gene Ther.** 3, 280-286.

5. Crystal, R.G. (1995). **Nature Med.** 1, 15-17.

6. Verma, I.M. and Somia, N. (1997). **Nature** 389, 239-242.

7. Bagai, S., Puri, A., Blumenthal, R. and Sarkar, D.P. (1993). **J. Virol.** 67, 3312-3318.

8. Bagai, S. and Sarkar, D.P. (1994). **J. Biol. Chem.** 269, 1966-1972.

9. Marshall, E. (1995). **Science** 269, 1050-1055.

10. Bagai, S. and Sarkar, D.P. (1993). **FEBS Lett.** 326,183-188.

11. Bagai, S. and Sarkar, D.P. (1993). **Biochem. Biophys. Acta** 1152, 15-25.

12. Ramani, K., Bora, R.S., Kumar, M., Tyagi, S.K. and Sarkar, D.P. (1997). **FEBS Lett.** 404, 164-168.

13. Ramani, K., Hassan, M.Q., Venkaiah, B., Hasnain, S.E. and Sarkar, D.P. (1998). **Proc. Natl. Acad. Sci. USA**, 95, (In Press).

14. Kumar, M. and Sarkar, D.P. (1996). **FEBS Lett.** 391, 17-20.

15. Chiu, M.H., Thomas, V.H., Stubbs, H.J. and Rice, K.G. (1995). **J. Biol. Chem.** 270, 24024-24031.

16. Welling, G. W., Nijmeijer, J. R., Derzee, R.V., Groen, G., Wilterdink, J.B. and Welling-Wester, S. (1984). **J. Chromatogr.** 297, 101-109.

17. Tomita, N., Morishita, R., Higaki, J.,Tomita, S., Aoki, M., Ogihara, T. and Kaneda, Y. (1996). **Gene Ther.** 3, 477-482.

18. Perales, J.C., et al (1997) **J. Biol. Chem.** 272, 7398-7407.

8

LIPOSOMES AS A CARRIER FOR DERMAL AND TRANSDERMAL DRUG DELIVERY

A.N. MISRA

Faculty of Technology and Engineering
M. S. University of Baroda, Vadodra - 390 001, INDIA.
Tel: (0265) 434187, Fax: (0265) 423898.

LIPOSOMES AS A CARRIER FOR DERMAL AND TRANSDERMAL DRUG DELIVERY

Ever since the introduction of vesicles (liposomes and niosomes) as dermal or transdermal drug delivery systems, strong debates have continued concerning the mechanisms behind their effects. It is still unclear whether there is need to use vesicular structure (Fig.1) to exert the desired effect or whether it is sufficient to administer simultaneously the drugs and the amphiphilic compounds of which the vesicles are composed [1]. The latter may in this case act as a penetration enhancer. One of the most disputed question is whether intact vesicles are able to penetrate into the stratum corneum [2] or even into the deeper layers of the skin [3,4].

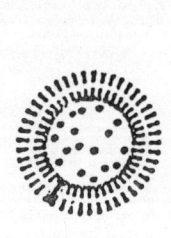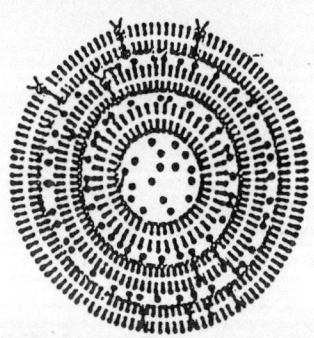

- Hydrophilic active or drug molecule, - lipophilic active or drug molecule, >O amphilic active or drug molecule

Fig. 1 : Schematic representation of a unilamellar and multilamellar vesicular structure

Mezei et al reported that topical application of liposomal triamcinolone acetonide for 5 days resulted in a drug concentration in the epidermis and dermis four times higher than that obtained using control ointment. The urinary excretion of the drug was diminished [3]. They also compared the deposition of topically applied gels of free and liposomally-entrapped triamcinolone on rabbit skin and found that application of the liposomal gel resulted in a concentration of triamcinolone acetonide approximately five times larger in the epidermis and three times higher in the dermis, than application of the free drug gel [4]. In another study, the superiority of liposomal formulation of hydrocortisone, betamethasone, and triamcinolone was confirmed where the skin lipid liposomes showed a 6 and 1.3 times blanching effect than that obtained with control formulation ointment and phospholipid based liposome formulation respectively [5]. The increased effect of dithranal on the skin by liposomes has also been reported by Gehring et al [6]. Clinical evaluation of the liposome encapsulated econazole (Pervaryl lipogel-Cilag AG, Switzerland, marketed since 1988) and the Pervaryl cream indicated that the 0.2% liposomal form was just as active as 1.0% cream form. The presently recommended therapy with pervaryl cream is a twice a day treatment for 2 weeks, while once a day treatment for 1 week is recommended with the pevaryl lipogel. The results of these studies suggested to them the inherent potential of liposomes as a potential drug delivery system for cutaneous application [7-10].

Vermorker et al. [11] reported that the systemic absorption of dihydro-testosterone from liposomal system was negligible, whereas significant absorption was observed form the acetone solution. They reported no advantage of liposomes system in systemic absorption. Ganesan et al [12], performing *in vitro* diffusion experiments with hairless mouse skin using liposomal formulation, found that neither intact liposomes nor the phospholipid of which they are comprised diffuse across the skin. Rowe et al [13] found that topically applied liposomal progesterone reduced the rate of hair growth in idiopathic hirsutism.

Patel et al. [14] suggested that liposomes can be used for the sustained release of drugs into epidermis when applied topically. For example when free and liposomally entrapped 3H-methotrexate was applied to the skin of nude mice, percutaneous absorption of drug was greatly reduced by liposomal encapsulation. Further more, the retention of 3H-methotrexate in the skin was two to three fold higher from the liposomal formulation than from the solution, again suggesting a localization of the liposomes in the epidermis, where a sustained release of methotrexate takes place. Few other studies [15,16] demonstrated targeted and sustained delivery of the drugs within the skin.

The advantage of the liposomal form over the conventional dermatological form was particularly striking when the activity of local anesthetic agents was evaluated in cream, ointment or lotion form versus liposomal form. A liposomal product containing 0.5% tetracaine produced more intensive activity (6-8 folds) than 1.0% tetracaine in cream form, which was a commercial preparation, i.e., pentocaine cream. Similar results were obtained with liposomal forms of other local anesthetic agents, e.g. lidocaine, dibucaine, benzocaine. Initial clinical investigations with hydrocortisone indicated that the 0.5% liposomal form was more effective than the 1.0% cream form. Liposomal encapsulation of "irritant" drugs have shown to reduce irritation drastically and hence can enhance patient complaince [10].

This presentation is a review of topically applied liposomal formulation, with emphasis on the interaction of liposomes with skin involved in dermal and transdermal drug delivery.

PHYSICO - CHEMICAL PROPERTIES OF LIPOSOMES

The following physico-chemical properties of liposomes influence their performance:

Size: The size of the liposomal vesicles is shown to affect the skin penetration behavior of the drug caffeine. Small vesicles exhibited lower skin permeation; higher accumulation in the skin, and a longer lag time before steady-state permeation was reached. Large vesicles showed low skin permeation with low accumulation in the skin and a shorter lag time than for small vesicles [17].

Surface Charge: The data indicated that application of positively charged liposomes resulted in almost twice the amount of lipids deposited in deeper layers of the skin compared to application of the negatively charged liposomes. Net positive charge formulation may result in marked irritation [18].

Fluidity: The composition of the lipid bilayer is critically important in determining the pharmaceutical properties of liposomes through influences on membrane fluidity, permeability, surface properties, and stability. Membrane fluidity refers to the existence of thermal phase transitions in phospholipid aggregates. As temperature increases these lipids move from a relatively ordered gel state to a more disordered fluid-like liquid crystalline state. In the gel state, liposomal membranes are more stable, less permeable to solutes and less likely to interact with destabilizing macromolecules than in the liquid crystalline state. Loading and leakage of drug from liposomes are affected at phase transition temperature(Tm). The maximum bilayer permeability occurs at the Tm [19]. In contrary to this finding, Ykomizo and Sagitani [20] suggest that phospholipid containing unsaturated fatty acids as lipophilic group (decrease in Tm value) are strong penetration enhancers of the percutaneous delivery of indomethacin.

Percutaneous absorption promoters: Percutaneous absorption promoters such as limonene and other hydrocarbon terpenes may distribute, in the presence of ethanol in the intercellular double - layered lipid membrane in the stratum corneum where cholesterol is present. It influences the membrane structure in the gel state on the basis of its affinity for cholesterol, enhances the fluidity of the membrane, and accordingly results in good absorption enhancement [21-24]. Azone, 1-dodecanol, and dodecyl-2-(N,N-dimethylamino) propionate demonstrated the importance of stratum corneum lipid interaction in the penetration enhancement activity of the enhancers employed [25].

MECHANISM OF INTERACTION OF LIPOSOMES WITH SKIN

Two types of vesicle - skin interactions (adsorption at interface and ultrastructural changes) were observed *in vitro*.

Adsorption at interface: Interaction of vesicles at the suspension-skin *interface* involving adsorption and fusion of the vesicles at the surface of stratum corneum was seen. These interactions were found for all liposome and niosome formulations that were investigated in the study. They occur even under optimal conditions under which vesicle stability in the bulk was maintained (i.e. no dehydration). It appears to be thermodynamically favorable for vesicles that are near the stratum corneum to aggregate, fuse and adhere to the stratum corneum surface in stacks of lamellar sheets. The interlamellar repeat distance (i.e. the length of the lipid molecule plus that of the water layer that separates the hydrophobic layers of the liposome), within the liposomes also decides the adherance of vesicles to the stratum corneum [26]. In literature, several groups [27-30] have described spontaneous adsorption of liposomes to different cell types. Adsorption and fusion of drug loaded vesicles (Fig. 2) onto the surface of the skin leads to a high thermodynamic activity gradient of the

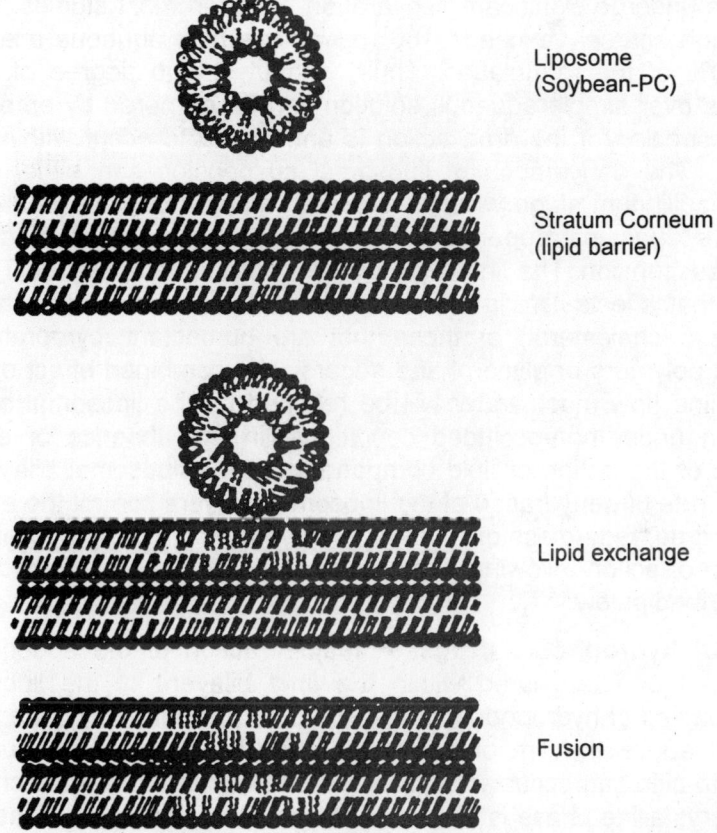

Liposome
(Soybean-PC)

Stratum Corneum
(lipid barrier)

Lipid exchange

Fusion

Fig. 2 : Model demonstrating the interaction of liquid-crystalline liposomal bilayers with the lipid barrier of the skin

drug at the suspension - stratum corneum interface, which is driving force for penetration of the (lipophilic) drug across the stratum corneum. The exact mechanisms underlying the adsorption of vesicles onto cell surfaces, and the parameters influencing vesicle -cell interactions, are not yet fully understood.

Ultrastructral changes: Interactions in deeper layers of the stratum corneum involving changes of the ultrastructure of the intercellular lipid regions were seen.

The effects of vesicles on deeper layers of the stratum corneum may lead to changes in drug permeation kinetics due to an impaired barrier function of the stratum corneum for the drug [31-33]. Hofland et al [34-36] indicated that there is relationship between the penetration - enhancing abilities of niosomes and the effect that they have on the ultra structure of human stratum corneum.

MECHANISM OF LIPOSOMAL ACTION

The mode by which liposomes facilitate transfer of drug into living skin strata and beyond has been a topic of much interest. They propose a simple hypothesis of liposomal action that accounts for a majority of the effects observed. For a liposomal formulation to be effective, especially for hydrophilic drugs, it is essential that the suspension undergo significant dehydration. Since in most studies reported the lipid concentration scarcely exceeds 100 mg/ml, the bulk aqueous medium constitutes roughly 90% of the formulation. Thus, without a high degree of dehydration, no advantages over simple aqueous solution can be garnered by employing liposomal systems, especially if the drug action is anticipated to occur within few hours after application. The dehydration of liposomal suspension can either be complete or reach an equilibrium stage wherein a certain amount of water is always held within the bilayers. Two interdependent factors control the extent of dehydration of a liposomal suspension. The first is the phase transition temperature(Tm). The second, often one that affects Tm, is the presence of components that either affect bilayer packing (e.g. cholesterol) or those that are humectants/cyroprotectants, such a hydrophilic polymers or glycerol and sugars. The combined effect of the two factors will determine how much water will be retained by the liposomal bilayers following dehydration under non-occluded conditions. In the absence of enhancer effects arising out of the action of lipid components of the liposomal bilayers on skin, the extent and rate of dehydration of the liposomal bilayers control the extent and rate of transfer of drug, regardless of whether it is hydrophobic or hydrophilic, into skin. The mechanism of action following dehydration for hydrophobic and hydrophilic drugs is been described below [37].

Transfer of hydrophobic drugs: A major fraction of the added drug would be encapsulated or intercalated within the lipid bilayers of the liposomes. Further, optimum loading of hydrophobic drugs would be possible only if the lipid bilayers are maintained above the Tm of the major lipid. The transfer of drug from the lipid bilayers into skin can occur as long as the bilayers are in a liquid crystalline state. If the liquid crystalline phase is altered to the gel state, transport of the drug will cease or be negligibly low. Dehydration of liposomal suspensions has been shown to induce transitions from the liquid crystalline phase to the gel state [38]. Thus, the extent of dehydration will determine if changes in the state of the liposomal bilayers from a liquid crystalline phase to the gel state are possible. If dehydration is complete and the bilayers are transformed from the liquid crystalline state to the gel state, then transfer of drug from the bilayer to the skin ceases. If dehydration to an equilibrium stage wherein a constant amount of water is always retained in the bilayers occurs, then transport of drug would be continuos and steady. A second consequence of dehydration involves the formation of a strong adhesive patch of liposomal bilayer on the skin. The formation of such patches maximizes the intimacy of contact between the drug - laden bilayer and the skin and probably is medicated via calcium bridges.

Transfer of hydrophilic drugs: The mode of action for liposomal transport of hydrophilic drugs parallels that for hydrophobic drug in qualitative manner. This is strictly because of major role of the water associated with the bilayers upon dehydration of the liposomal suspension. Thus, for liposomal systems that retain a constant amount of water within the bilayers following dehydration to an equilibrium state, drug transport would continue over extended periods of time. A major consequence of dehydration for hydrophilic drugs involves the enhancement or enrichment of drug concentration in the aqueous phase of the bilayers leading to an enhancement in flux of drug into and across skin.

The follicular option: The mechanism described above occurs regardless of the presence or absence of follicles in the skin specimen. However, when a follicular pathway is available, upon dehydration the liposomal bilayers can partition and pack into the follicular or hair ducts. This partitioning is favorable since the follicular ducts contain lipids. The filling of the follicular opening with the liposomal bilayers not only results in entrapped drugs being carried into the follicles but also allows partitioning of unentrapped drugs into the bilayer matrix within follicles.

The physico-chemical properties of the drug influence the transport within the skin. An antiandrogen is a slightly hydrophobic drug (water solubility, 0.44 mg/ml) with a low molecular weight (369.4) and an octanol-water partition coefficient (log K octanol-water of 1.76). Therefore, drug is a good candidate for a transdermal delivery and it appears that lipid regions (intercellular and sebaceous lipids) constitute the main pathways for the cutaneous transport of drug, as reported by Bernard et al [39]

Ethanol and propylene glycol are enhancers for the skin permeation of lipophilic drugs [40,41]. These solvents may favor drug dissolving in the sebum and open a passageway within the sebaceous glands. Inspite of the favorable action of the alcoholic solution to transport such drug into the lipidic areas such as the sebaceous glands, liposomes targeted the sebaceous glands best. Several investigations demonstrated that liposomes allow a higher accumulation in the sebaceous glands compared with non-liposomal formulations [42,43]. Dissociation between drug and phospholipids in the dermis is been reported recently. It indicates that intact liposomes do not penetrate intact into the sebaceous glands as it is still maintained by Mezei [44].

CONCLUSIONS

Liposomal vesicles fuse onto the skin surface and the intimacy of contact between the drug loaded bilayers and the skin is probably mediated via calcium bridges. Topically applied liposomal formulation particularly those prepared form lipid mixtures of composition similar to the stratum corneum may be an delivery system for the treatment of skin disorders [45]. Liposomal deposition into the stratum corneum results in substantial reservoir effect. Penetration enhancers, size, charge and membrane fluidity play important role in transport of drug from bilayers to deeper layers of skin. Hence, liposomes may be used in cosmetics and dermatological preparations to increase their beneficial properties ranging from skin lipid replacement to increasing skin moisturization by improving skin barrier properties or perhaps used as novel carrier system with non toxic penetration properties for suitable drugs. Recent reports also suggest that liposomes favors localization in the sebaceous glands, site of dermatological disorders such as acne and androgenetic alopecia.

REFERENCES

1. Mahjour, M., Mauser, B., Rashidbaigi, Z. and Fawzi, M.B., (1990). **J. Control. Rel.** 14, 243.

2. Lasch, J., Laub, R. and Wohlrab, W. (1991). **J. Control. Rel.** 18, 55.

3. Mezei, M. and Gulasekharam, V. (1980). **Life Sci.** 26, 1473.

4. Mezei, M. and Gulasekharam, V. (1982). **J. Pharm. Pharmacol.** 34, 473.

5. Massimo, F. and Giovanni, P. (1997). **J. Control. Rel.** 44, 141.

6. Gehring, W., Ghyczy, M., Gloor, M, Scheer, T. and Roding, J. (1992). **Arzneim. Forsch.**, 42, 983.

7. Mezei, M. (1990). **U.S. Patent 4,897,269**.

8. Mezei, M. (1998). **U.S. Patent 4,761,288**.

9. Mezei, M. (1990). **European Patent 0,177,233, B1**.

10. Mezei, M. (1994). **J. Pharm. Sci.** 83, 1202.

11. Vermorken, A.J., Hukkelhoven, M.W., Vermeesch, A.M., Goos, C.M. and Wirtz, P. (1983). **J. Pharm. Pharmacol.** 36, 334.

12. Ganesan, M. G., Weiner, N. D., Flynn, G. L. and Ho, N.F.H. (1984). **Int. J. Pharm.** 20, 139.

13. Rowe, T. C., Mezei, M. and Hilchie, J. (1984). **Prostate** 5, 346.

14. Patel, H. M., (1984). **U. K. Patent GB2, 143,433 A**.

15. Kim, M. K., Chung, S. J., Lee, M. H., Cho, A. R. and Shim, C. K. (1997). **J. Control. Rel.** 46, 243.

16. Hwang, Y., Jung, B. H., Chung, S. J., Lee, M. H. and Shim, C. K. (1987). **J. Control. Rel.** 49, 177.

17. Touitou, E., Alhaique, F., Dayan, N., Riccieri, F. and Levi-Schaffer, F. (1994). **J. Pharm. Sci.** 83, 1189.

18. Egbaria, K. and Weiner, N. (1991). **Cosmet. Toil.** 106, 79.

19. Fielding, R. M. (1991). **Clin. Pharmacokinet.** 21, 155.

20. Yokomizo, Y. and Sagitini, H. (1996). **J. Control. Rel.** 42, 37.

21. Takayama, K., Kikuchi, K., Obata, Y., Okabe, H., Machida, Y. and Nagai, T. (1991). **S.T.P. Pharma. Sci.** 1, 83.

22. Obata, Y., Takayama, K., Machida, Y. and Nagai, T. (1991). **Drug Des. Delivery**, 8, 137.

23. Takayama, K. and Nagai, T. (1991). **Int. J. Pharm.** 74, 115.

24. Nagai, T., Sato, M. and Takayama, K. (1994). **J. Pharm. Sci.** 83, 1199.

25. Suhonen, T. M., Pirskanen, L., Raisanen, M., Kosonen, K., Rytting, J. H., Paronen, P. and Urtti, A. (1997). **J. Control. Rel**. 43, 251.

26. Watkinson, A. C., Hadgraft, J., Street, P. R. and Richards, B. W. (1997). In: Mechanism of Transdermal Drug Delivery (Potts, R. O. and Guy, R.H. Eds.), Marcel Dekker Inc., New York, USA, 242.

27. Pagano, R. E. and Weinstein, J. N. (1978). **Annu. Rev. Biophys. Bioeng.**, 7, 435.

28. Cecooli, J., Rosales, N., Tsimis, J. and Yarosh, D. B. (1989). **J. Invest. Dermatol.** 93, 190.

29. Abraham, W. and Downing, D. T. (1990). **Biochim. Biophys. Acta.** 1021,119.

30. Callaghan, T. M., Metezeau, P., Gachelin, H., Redziniak, G., Milner, Y. and Goldberg, M. E. (1990). **J. Invest. Dermatol.** 94, 58.

31. Hoogstraate, A. J., Verhoef, J., Brussee, J., IJzerman, A. P., Spies, F. and Bodde H. E. (1991). **Int. J. Pharm** 76, 37.

32. Foldvari, M., Gesztes, A. and Mezei, M. (1990). **J. Microencapsulation**, 7, 479.

33. Bodde, H. E., Holman, B. P., Brussee, J. and Spies, F. (1988). **Proceed. Int. Symp. Control. Rel. Bioact. Mater.**15, 276.

34. Hofland, H.E.J., Bouwstra, J. A., Bodde, H. E., Spies, F., VanderGeest, R. and Junginger, H. E. (1991). **Proceed. Int. Symp. Control. Rel. Bioact. Mater.** 18.

35. Hofland, H.E.J., Bouwstra, J. A., Verhoef, J. C., Buckton, G., Chowdhary, B. Z., Ponec, M. and Junginger, H. E. (1992). **J. Pharm. Pharmacol.** 44, 287.

36. Hofland, H.E.J., Bouwstra, J. A., Spies, F., Gorris, G., Nagelkerke, J., F., Cullander, C. and Junginger, H.E. (1994). **J. Pharm. Sci.** 83, 1192.

37. Weiner, N. D., Ramachandran, C., Lieb, L. M. and Egbaria, K. (1994). **J. Pharm. Sci.** 83, 1196.

38. Crowe, L., Crowe, J., Rudolph, A., Womersley, C. and Appel, L. (1985). **Arch. Biochem. Biophys.** 242, 240.

39. Bernard, E., Dubois, J. L. and Wepierre, J. (1997). **J. Pharm. Sci.** 86, 573.

40. Berner, B. and Liu, P. (1995). In: Percutaneous Penetration Enhancers (Smith, E. W., Maibach, H. I., Eds.) CRC : Boca Raton, F. L., p.45.

41. Bendas, B.; Neubert, R.; Wohlrab, W. (1995). In: Percutaneous Penetration Enhancers (Smith, E. W., Maibach, H. I. Eds.) CRC ; Boca Raton, p.61.

42. Lieb, L. M., Ramchandran, C., Egbaria, K. and Weiner, N. (1992). **Follic. Deliv. Liposomes** 99, 108.

43. Niemiec, S. M., Ramchandran, C. and Weiner, N. (1995). **Pharm. Res.** 12, 1184.

44. Mezei, M. (1994). In : Drug Permeation Enhancement : Theory and Applications (Hsieh, D. S. Ed.), Marcel Dekker, Basel, 171.

45. Fresta, M. and Puglisi, G. (1997). **J. Control. Rel.** 44, 141.

9

PROSPECTS OF TEMPERATURE SENSITIVE LIPOSOMAL DELIVERY OF DRUG TO TUMOR

K.P. MISHRA**, A.R. GOPAL*, DIPTI MARATHE and B.N. PANDEY

Radiation Biology and Biochemistry Division
Bhabha Atomic Research Center
Trombay Mumbai 400 085.

* Present Address : Department of Mechanical Engineering and Material Science, School of Engineering, Duke University, Durham, North Carolina, USA
** Corresponding author

- Introduction
- Materials and Methods
- Results and Discussion

- Acknowledgement
- References

INTRODUCTION

Cancer treatment is generally impaired due to similar toxicity of anti-tumor drugs to normal and tumor cells. The medical challenge for directing the administered drug preferentially to tumor cells can be achieved by the use of appropriate vehicle system. Towards this objective, considerable pharmaceutical and pharmacological research has therefore been devoted to develop a variety of drug carrier systems. Liposomes offer a sustained release and reduced toxicity of drugs and have potential to efficiently deliver the drugs to diseased sites [1]. However, commonly observed rapid clearance of liposomes from blood circulation and their unwanted accumulation in RES organs present major limitations in the realization of liposome mediated targeted drug delivery [1,2]. In an attempt for localized delivery of administered liposomal drug to tumor sites, the design and use of liposomes with ability to release the entrapped drug in response to external temperature was suggested [3]. These liposomes popularly called temperature sensitive liposomes (TSL) can be designed by selecting phospholipid compositions, which display phase transition in suitable temperature range. Studies have been shown that vesicles prepared from mixtures of DPPC and DSPC become leaky and allow release of their content at a temperature above the physiological temperature [3]. This report describes studies on preparation of liposomes from DPPC, DSPC and cholesterol and their sensitivity to release encapsulated agents on incubation in hyperthermic range of temperature (e.g. 43°C). Optimizations were carried out for temperature and time dependent *in vitro* release of doxorubicin (DOX) from liposomes which is an anthracycline drug widely used for treatment of cancer patients. Furthermore, the effectiveness of temperature responsive liposomes loaded with doxorubicin was determined on the growth of transplanted fibrosarcoma solid tumor in Swiss mice in combination with application of local hyperthermia. The results have shown a significant enhancement in tumor cure in animals.

MATERIALS AND METHODS

Chemicals

DPPC, DSPC and cholesterol were purchased from Sigma Chemical Co., USA and Doxorubicin (DOX) was obtained from Meiji, Japan. 6-Carboxyfluorescein (CF) was procured from Kodak Co., USA and was further purified to remove the polar contaminants [4].

Liposome preparation and loading of CF/DOX

a. Encapsulation of CF: Liposomes were prepared by thin film hydration method using DPPC, DSPC and cholesterol at molar ratio of 5:4:2. The lipids and cholesterol were dissolved in chloroform in round bottom flask and the solvent was evaporated under vacuum depositing a thin film on the inner wall of flask. The film was adequately dried with a stream of nitrogen gas to remove traces of organic solvent followed by further overnight drying under vacuum. The film was hydrated properly with 50 mM CF dissolved in phosphate buffer saline (20 mM, 0.85% NaCl, pH 7.4) using glass beads. Multilamellar vesicles (MLVs) obtained after hydration were sonicated at 45°C for 7 min. (cycle of 30 s sonication and 30 s cooling) using titanium probe sonicator. The liposomal suspensions obtained after sonication were centrifuged at 2000g for 10 min. to remove undesired titanium particles. The supernatant was passed through Sephadex G-50 minicolumn to remove unencapsulated CF. The liposomal suspension was further dialyzed against PBS and dialyzing medium was periodically changed until dialyzing buffer showed negligible to no fluorescence. Fluorescence intensity of released CF from liposomes was measured using Hitachi Fluorimeter at λex = 390 nm and λem = 420 nm.

b. Encapsulation of DOX: Encapsulation of DOX into liposomal aqueous volume was carried out using pH gradient driven protocol [5]. The dried DPPC, DSPC, and cholesterol (5:4:2) film was hydrated with 300 mM citrate buffer (pH 4.0) and the multilamellar vesicles formed after vortexing were subjected to freeze and thaw cycles for 7 times. The resulting liposomal suspension was sonicated at 45°C and the samples were allowed to cool at room temperature. pH of suspension was raised to 7.5-8.0 using 0.5 M Na_2CO_3 solution. The sonicated liposomes were incubated at 60°C for 5 min. before adding preheated DOX solution to the suspension. Samples were further heated for 10 min. at 60°C with intermittent vortexing. The unencapsulated drug was removed by Sephadex G-50 minicolumn centrifugation. Mostly, drug:lipid ratio was 0.05 molar. The concentration of DOX in liposomal suspension was determined by measurement of its fluorescence intensity (λex = 470 nm and λex = 580 nm).

Liposomal DOX delivery to transplanted tumor in mice

Solid fibrosarcoma tumor cells were grown in hind leg of 8-10 weeks old Swiss mice weighing about 20-25 g. The free or liposomal drug was administered intravenously through tail vein of tumor bearing mice at a dose of 5 mg drug/Kg body weight. Tumors were locally heated the knee joint for 10 min. at 43°C after 5 min. of intravenous injection of free or encapsulated drug.

Tumor volume (V) was determined by measuring the diameter in cross perpendicular directions by using the relation

$$V = 4/3 \, \pi \, \{(D_1+D_2)/4\}^3$$

Where, D_1 and D_2 are diameters of the tumor in 2 perpendicular directions. The tumor growth ratio (TGR) was calculated from tumor volume and percentage cure represents the ratio of TGR values between control and treated animals.

RESULTS AND DISCUSSION

Temperature dependent leakage of CF or DOX from TSL

The *in vitro* stability of TSL at different temperature was determined by measuring the leakage of 6-CF and DOX from the vesicle into the supernatant phosphate buffer solution (pH 7.4). The fluorescence intensity of CF and DOX released from liposomes was measured as a function of incubation temperature between 20 and 45°C (Fig.1).

The per cent fluorescence intensity was calculated by comparison with the total release of the entrapped probe of drug from liposomes obtained by mixing 20 µl of liposomes with 20µl of 10% Triton X-100. These samples were diluted 100 times before measuring the fluorescence. It is seen that the release of CF was negligibly small (<15%) for incubation up to 40°C. However, a rapid increase in release of CF from liposomes was observed with the increase in temperature of incubation. As can be seen, the 73% per cent release was obtained after incubation at 43°C. On the other hand, incubation of liposomes entrapped with DOX showed a release of 34% up to 40°C reaching a saturation value of 53% at 43°C. The observed significant difference in percentage release of DOX and CF at 43°C suggests that the temperature at which liposomes became leaky was same for both the solutes but the extent of release was dependent on the nature of the entrapped molecule. The relative lower per cent release of DOX compared with CF may be ascribed to a greater lipophilic nature of DOX. A possibility also exist that although a fraction of DOX leaked out from liposomal aqueous interior but it may have remained preferably associated with the lipid bilayer than to stay free in the aqueous supernatant [6].

Time course of CF or DOX release from TSL at 43°C

The liposomes entrapped with CF or DOX were incubated in PBS at 43°C and the release kinetics of the entrapped agent was monitored as a function of incubation period (Fig.2). Liposomes containing CF were found to release about 70% of the cargo within 5 min. of incubation at 43°C which remained constant on further incubation. But, liposomes containing DOX resulted in release of 53% of the drug

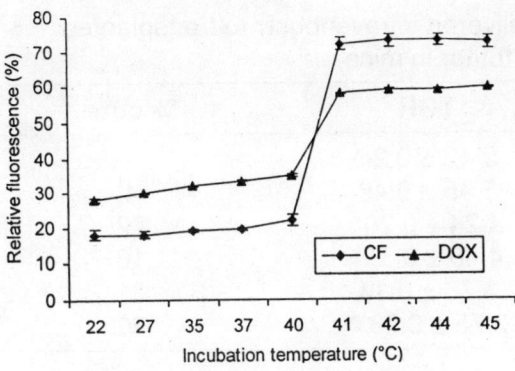
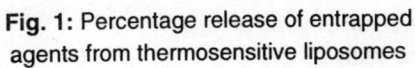
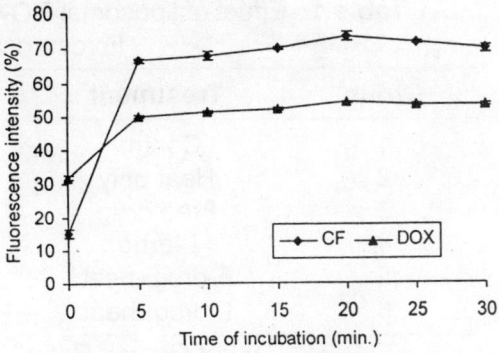

Fig. 1: Percentage release of entrapped agents from thermosensitive liposomes

Fig.2 : Rate of release of entrapped CF/DOX at 43°C for various time intervals upto 30 minutes

within 5 min. of incubation at the same temperature. These results indicate that the leakage characteristics of liposomes containing entrapped CF or DOC at hyperthermic temperature of 43°C was rapid and sharp. The observed difference in extent of release of entrapped CF and DOX may be ascribed to relative difference in the nature of hydrophobicity. It is well known that bilayer structure of liposomes becomes loose and porous at gel-to-liquid crystalline phase temperature. The present results on release of entrapped CF or DOX confirm that the designed liposomes have expected sensitivity to hyperthermic temperature [6].

Effect of TSL loaded with DOX on fibrosarcoma tumor in mice

The DOX loaded liposomes were administered to mice transplanted with fibrosarcoma tumor and the effect of drug delivered in various combinations of treatment was measured in terms of tumor growth ratio and percentage cure (Table 1). Tumor growth retardation in animals was small but significant when they are treated with heat or free DOX alone. However, combination of heat and free drug treatment showed substantial growth retardation of transplanted tumor. On the other hand, it was interesting to find that delivery of DOX encapsulated in TSL in combination with local heat treatment at 43°C for 30 min. produced profound effect on tumor regression indicating the efficient and enhanced action of DOX to tumors by this mode of delivery. A plausible explanation for observed effect may be that heat treatment destabilized liposomes resident in the vicinity of heated region of tumor resulting in therapeutically effective concentration of drug to tumor [6,7]. It, however, needs to be noted that one of the limiting factors in the success of thermosensitive liposomes can be their short lifetime in circulation. Therefore, investigators are directing their efforts towards preparation and use of long circulating thermosensitive liposomes for effective drug delivery in response to hyperthermia. Some progress has been made on research on this line in our laboratory and these results are under evaluation and communicated separately. It is hoped that liposomes based strategies may prove very useful in developing effective protocols for cancer therapy.

Table 1. Effect of liposomal DOX delivered intravenously to transplanted fibrosarcoma tumor in mice

Group	Treatment	TGR	% cure
1	Control	5.42 ± 0.24	-
2	Heat only	5.45 ± 0.46	4
3	Free drug	4.24 ± 0.26*	22
4	L-drug	4.46 ± 0.17*	18
5	F-drug+heat	3.75 ± 0.14	31
6	L-drug+heat	2.75 ± 0.23**	50

TGR = Tumor Growth Ratio
* Significantly different from absolute control with $p < 0.01$
**Significantly different from all groups with $p < 0.01$

ACKNOWLEDGEMENTS

We deeply thank Prof. P.C. Kesavan for his constant encouragement and support during this work. Dr. A.R. Gopal and Ms. Dipti Marathe are recipient of the Research Fellowship from Department of Atomic Energy and wish to acknowledge this support with their sincere thanks.

Abbreviations: DPPC: Dipalmitoyl phosphatidyl choline, DSPC: Distearoyl phosphatidyl choline, CF: 6-Carboxyfluorescein; DOX: Doxorubicin; TSL: Thermosensitive liposomes; TGR: Tumor growth ratio

REFERENCES

1. Gregoriadis, G. (1976). **New Eng. J. Med.** 295, 704.

2. Gregoriadis, G. (1991). **J. Antimicro. Chemother.** 28, supl.B, 39.

3. Yatvin, M.B., Weinstein, J.N., Dennis, W.H. and Blumentahl, R. (1978). **Science** 202, 1290.

4. Weinstein, J.N., Ralston, E., Lesreman, L.D., Klausner, R.D., Dragsten, P., Henkart P. and Blumentahl, R. (1984). In : Liposome Technology, (Gregoriadis, G. Ed.), CRC Press Inc., Florida,.USA, p.183.

5. Mayer, L.D. et al. (1989). **Cancer Res.** 49, 5922.

6. Gopal., A.R., (1996). Ph.D. Thesis, Mumbai University, Mumbai, India

7. Maruyama, K., Unezaki, S., Takahashi, N. and Iwatsuru, M. (1993). **Biochem. Biophys. Acta** 1149, 209-216.

10

NIOSOMES AS DRUG DELIVERY SYSTEMS

N. UDUPA

College of Pharmaceutical Sciences,
K.M.C.H. Manipal, Karnataka.

INTRODUCTION

Nonionic surfactant vesicles or niosomes which are similar to liposomes have been reported by Vanlerberghe et al. [1]. Niosomes can entrap both hydrophilic and lipophilic drugs, either in aqueous layer or in vesicular membrane which is lipoidal in nature. Niosomes are reported to attain and retain better stability than liposomes. They can prolong the circulation of the entrapped drugs. Because of the presence of nonionic surfactant they possess better intrinsic targeting potential and propensity towards to tumor, liver and brain. It may prove very useful for targeting the drugs for treating cancer, parasitic, viral and other microbial diseases more effectively. Non-phospholipid vesicular systems have been studied for many years and have largely involved investigation of dialkyl, dimethyl ammonium salts and other ionic amphiphiles. Most of amphiphiles are toxic and are unsuitable for use as drug carriers.

The handling and storage of the surfactants require no specific conditions. Niosomes behave *in vivo* like liposomes, prolonging the circulation of entrapped drug and altering its *in vivo* distribution and metabolic characteristics. Inclusion of cholesterol in the preparation of niosomes has been demonstrated to alter the properties of niosomes by markedly increasing the efflux of entrapped solute(s).

Nonionic surfactant based vesicles as vehicles for drug formulation have been found to reduce the systemic toxicity of many anticancer and antiinfective drugs. Secondly as carriers for enhanced delivery to specific cells niosomes may significantly improve the therapeutic index by restricting and localizing the drug effects to target cells. They are reportedly nontoxic and biodegradable.

In the preparation of various drug carriers like albumin microspheres, magnetic microspheres, carbohydrate spheres, cell containing multienzyme system and drugs, many surfactants like Tween 20, Tween 80, Pluronic F-68, Pluronic L-35 and other detergents have been proven to be pivotal and were found very useful in selective drug and enzyme targeting. Many nonionic surfactants like Tween and spans, cationic surfactants like cetrimide and sodium dodecyl sulfate are conventionally used with cholesterol to entrap drugs.

Azmin et al. [2] used nonionic hydrophilic surfactants like Tween-80 for making niosomes containing methotrexate and studied the pharmacokinetics of methotrexate after intravenous injection of niosomes to the mice. Chandraprakash et al. [3] made nonionic surfactant vesicles using lipophilic surfactants like Span-40, Span-60 and Span 80 and successfully entrapped methotrexate in to them. The tissue distribution of niosome entrapped methotrexate was found to be modified. These vesicles were also found to be osmotically responsive yet stable. Reports are available in literature pertaining to the use of niosomes as drug carriers for doxorubicin and sodium stilbogluconate in order to incorporate better targeting property [4-6].

Niosomes can be exploited to attain selective, however, differential drug distribution and release characteristics by judicious combination of surfactants. Liver can act as a depot for many drugs where niosomes containing drugs may be taken up by the liver where they are broken down by lysosomal lipase slowly to release the free drug and reenter the circulation. Niosomes can be used in the treatemtn of parasitic infection of liver, spleen and bone marrow.

The cardiotoxicity of adriamycin has been reported to be reduced by administering it contained in niosomes while their was no loss in therapeutic efficacy. Surfactants like Tween 80 also increased brain level of methotrexate. Similarly, analgesic effect and brain level of D-Kyotorphen was enhanced on incorporation of Tween 80 in niosomes. Nonionic surfactants like Triton X, Triton N, Brij and Tweens inhibited the motility of few microorganisms, thus they possess some intrinsic bacteriostatic effects.

NIOSOME PREPARATIONS INVESTIGATED BY MANIPAL GROUP

Preparation of surfactant vesicles using various surfactants was attempted and some anticancer drugs like methotrexate and vincristine sulfate and antiinflammatory drugs like diclofenac sodium were encapsulated in niosomes. An attempt was made to explore this approach for targeting anticancer and antiinflammatory drugs using surfactant vesicles. As encouraging results were observed, this technology may be promising in future for better administration of drug(s) to the target sites. The application of niosomes may be further extended to other toxic drugs to reduce their toxicity and to improve their therapeutic index.

Methotrexate was encapsulated in nonionic surfactant vesicles prepared using cholesterol, dicetyl phosphate and span 60 by reverse phase evaporation technique. Similarly, diclofenac sodium was encapsulated in niosomes prepared with Span 60, Tween 80 and poloxamer. Vincristine sulfate was encapsulated in niosomes based on span 40 and cholesterol (1:1). Significantly high, i.e. 90% entrapment could be achieved employing transmembrane pH gradient (inside acidic) drug active loading technique. The prepared niosomes were often characterized by studying their release profile, entrapment efficiency, distribution study, stability, etc.

ANTITUMOR ACTIVITY

Improved delivery of anticancer drugs to tumor tissues

Niosome encapsulated vincristine was found to enhance the antitumor activity against Ehrlich's ascites and sarcoma-180 models. The niosomal/free drug mean survival time values as high as 1.89 were achieved in Ehrlich's ascites infected animals. Multiple doses of niosomal vincristine and methotrexate increased the survival rate in mice. Tumor volume doubling time of S-180 tumors increased significantly in niosomal drug treated animals. An increase in doubling time reflects the supressed rate of proliferation of sarcoma. Subsequent to macrophage activation using encapsulated muramyldipeptide a more quantitative delivery of anticancer drugs to the tumor site could be achieved. Drug level at the tumor site was increased after macrophage activation.

Amelioration of vincristine and methotrexate toxicity

Toxicological effects of anticancer drugs after entrapping in niosomes were compared with those of free drug. The 50% lethal dose of 2.8 mg/Kg in BALB/c mice when observed for free vincristine increased to 4.8 mg/Kg with niosomal vincristine. A 30-day dose response survival studies in mice indicated that niosomal anticancer drugs were less toxic than free drugs.

Histopathological studies of skeletal muscle, spinal cord and aciatic nerve of niosomal vincristine treated rats confirmed the low level toxicity of the encapsulated vincristine. Unimpaired locomotor activity evidenced from rotorod performance and unaltered gait patterns of niosomal vincristine treated rats further confirmed the safety profile of niosomal vincristine. The separation of peripheral and bone marrow WBC counts upon niosomal anticancer drug treatment to mice, though marginally increased yet it was in significant.

Altered plasma kinetic and tissue disposition of anticancer drugs

Subsequent to intravenous administration, the niosome encapsulated anticancer drugs were cleared from the plasma much more slowly than free drugs. A markedly enhanced plasma concentration of drug was achieved in mice when it was administered in niosomes. Encapsulation of anticancer drugs also caused marked alteration in the tissue disposition of injected drugs. The tumor drug levels were enhanced significantly. This correlates well with the increased antitumor activity of niosomal anticancer drugs, the decreased blood levels in small intestine and skeletal muscle account for the reduced gastrointestinal and mycological toxicity of niosomal anticancer drugs.

From these investigations the following conclusions can be drawn:

Transmembrane pH gradient (inside acidic) drug loading process offers an efficient means for preparation of vesicular drug carriers for vincristine, with as high as 90% entrapment efficiency. Niosomal anticancer drugs have superior anticancer activity than free drugs. Enhanced drug retention in plasma and increased levels of anticancer drugs can be achieved by encapsulating them in niosomes. The decreased partitioning of niosomal vincristine to nonactive sites resulted in a significant decrease in the toxic side effects, myological and intestinal impairment of drugs. A more quantitative delivery of anticancer drugs to tumor site is possible after macrophage activation. The use of niosomes as anticancer drug carrier seems to be a certainly promising approach in cancer therapy of future.

Better antiinflammatory activity with niosomal diclofenac sodium

Intraperitonial, transdermal and oral administration of niosomal diclofenac sodium resulted in better antiinflammatory activity as compared to free drug administration. Thus niosomal drug delivery of antiinflammatory drugs may be a promising therapy for arthritis and other inflammatory conditions. Thus, there is lot of scope to encapsulate different drugs, specially toxic anticancer and antiinfective drugs in niosomes and to use niosomes as promising drug carriers to achieve better bioavailability, reduced toxicity and better therapeutic index.

FORMULATION AND EVALUATION OF METHOTREXATE LOADED NIOSOMES

Macrophages have been reported to effect a greater degree of phagocytic tumour cell kill following activation [7]. Muramyl dipeptide (MDP, N-acetyl muramyl 1-L-alanyl D-isoglutamine), is an activator of macrophages and does not exhibit toxicity and antigenicity. It is rapidly cleared from the body and of low *in vivo* efficacy in inhibiting tumour growth [8,9]. MDP carried by liposomes, neoglycoproteins or antibodies is selectively recognised and endocytosed by macrophages, improving the efficacy of their activation. The effectiveness of MDP incorporated in biodegradable gelatin microspheres (or as a MDP gelatin conjugate) in macrophage activation has been demonstrated both *in vivo* and *in vitro* [10]. Owing to their inherent and phagocytic activity macrophages are able to internalize liposomal as well as niosomal vesicles, as a result vesicular system are passively targeted to these cells.

Macrophages can be activated by their interaction with defined components of bacterial cell wall such as muramyl dipeptide and tuftsin, and immunoglobulin G associated tetrapeptide [11,12]. Macrophages are found in association with malignant tumours in a defined pattern suggesting that the most direct way to achieve macrophage mediated tumor regression is macrophage activation [13]. Since the vesicular drug carrier system like niosomes are rapidly bound and endocytosed by fixed and circulating phagocytic cells, thus provide convenient vehicle for the *in vivo* delivery of biologically active agents to phagocytic cells [14-16].

Liposome entrappped defense modulator muramyl dipeptide and its lipophilic derivatives, which are potent inducers of macrophage mediated antitumor activity were reported to have strong antimetastatic activity in experimental systems [17,18]. Vesicular drug carriers are transported by macrophages which are known to infiltrate tumor cells [19]. In the process it may be possible to take advantage of these activated macrophage system in delivering the antitumor agents, encapsulated within vesicles more quantitatively to tumor site.

In the present study, niosomes were prepared and loaded with methotrexate. Methotrexate loaded niosomes were evaluated for their shape, size, encapsulation, tissue disposition in mice bearing a transplanted S-180 tumour. The effect of macrophage activation on anticancer activity was also studied.

Preparation of methotrexate containing niosomes

Nonionic surfactant vesicles (Niosomes) encapsulated with methotrexate was prepared using Tweens and Spans. Niosomes were prepared by a method reported by Azmin et al. (1985) with slight modifications. Surfactant (Tween 80, 60, 40 or Span 60, 40, 20) (71.25mg), cholesterol (71.25 mg) and dicetyl phosphate (7.5 mg) were used as the lipid ingredients. These ingredients were dissolved in about 15 ml of diethyl ether in a round bottom flask. The solvent was evaporated under reduced pressure using a rotary evaporator. The rotating flask was positioned about 1.5 cm above a boiling water bath, thus a thin layer of the surfactants was deposited on the wall of the flask. Methotrexate (MTX) (5 ml solution; 10 mg/ml) was added to the flask slowly, while warming the flask at about 50°C with intermittant vortexing, until a good dispersion of the mixture was obtained. The MTX-entrapped niosomes were separated from the unentrapped MTX by dialysis as discussed by Hardy et al. [20]. Measurement of the niosome size was made using a microscope.

Preparation of 3H-MTX and 3H-MTX containing niosomes

Pure cold MTX (5 mg) (American Cyanamide Corporation) was added to 250Ci 3H-MTX (Amersham Corporation), made slightly alkaline and diluted to 5 ml with water. This solution was used to hydrate a thin film of lipids (Span 60, cholesterol and dicetyl phosphate:71.25 mg, 71.25 mg, 7 mg respectively) to from niosomes. After sonication the niosomal suspension was passed through a Sephadex G50 column to separate the entraped MTX from the free drug. The mean diameter of the niosomes was measured to be 4.5μm. Elution was carried out using normal saline. Normal suspension, which elutes first, was collected to a total volume of 15 ml, while 5 ml free MTX was collected as the second portion. One ml of the niosomal suspension collected was diluted to 9 ml with water and 1 ml of the resultant suspension was used to determine the percentage drug entrapment.

Entrapment studies

Niosomal entrapment of MTX was studied by liquid scintillate counter (LKB Wallace, Finland) where scintillate count of 1 ml sample of niosome and free MTX was made.

Table 1. Size distribution of formulated niosomes

Mean Size diameter (μm)	Number of niosomes in each range						% of niosome in each size range
	Span 60	Span 40	Span 20	Tween 80	Tween 60	Tween 40	
1.5	16	19	20	31	29	25	23.33
4.5	34	27	32	36	38	40	34.50
7.5	29	36	25	15	17	19	23.50
10.5	14	15	18	9	11	9	12.67
13.5	7	3	5	9	5	7	6.00

Large unilamellar niosomes were formed in the size range of 1.5 to 13.5 μm with a mean diameter being 4.5 μm (Table 1). The niosomes entrapped 25 to 50% of the MTX as shown in table 2.

Table 2. Encapsulation efficiency of formulated niosomes

Surfactant used	Amount of MTX dialysed (mg) in 300 minutes			Av. Conc. of MTX dialysed into saline ±SD (mg)	% coefficient of variation	% of MTX entrapped
Span 60	21.60	24.75	26.05	24.13 ± 2.29	9.48	51.70
Span 40	26.55	24.95	27.05	26.18 ± 1.10	4.20	47.60
Span 20	23.50	26.85	22.60	24.32 ± 2.24	9.21	51.40
Tween 80	41.35	35.50	34.55	37.13 ± 3.68	9.92	25.70
Tween 60	30.65	29.63	28.10	29.37 ± 1.28	4.34	41.30
Tween 40	26.25	27.05	25.95	26.42 ± 0.57	2.15	47.20

PHARMACOKINETICS

Mice implanted with Sarcoma 180 tumour cells were administered with 0.4 ml MTX niosomal suspension per animal (2.5 mg/kg). Seven mice implanted with S-180 were used for pharmacokinetic studies; the animals were divided into 3 groups which were given free MTX, niosomal MTX or niosomal MTX 2 days after macrophage activation. Blood samples were collected at 3.5, 7.5,15 and 30 min. and 1,2,4,6,8,12,24 and 72h and 1 ml of pooled blood sample was used for liquid scintillation counting. Three ml tissue solubilizer (BTS 460, Beckman, Finland) and 1 ml of 30% H_2O_2 were added to the blood sample and the mixture was allowed to stand for 6 h, after which 1 ml acetone and 5 ml liquid scintillant mixture was added. Acetone was added to make the toluene in the solubilizer miscible with water. Counting was performed by liquid scintillation. The results are as given in Table 3.

Table 3. Pharmacokinetic parameters of MTX in micre transplanted with S-180 tumours and treated with 3H-MTX-containing niosomes

Parameter	Free Drug	Niosomal MTX	MDP + Niosomal MTX
$(AUC)_0^\infty$ (µg/h/ml)	2.17	64.57	202.23
$(AUC)_0^\infty$ (µg/h/ml)	54.74	11464.16	22989.64
MRT (h)	25.275	177.53	113.68
K_{ss} (h)	0.0396	0.0056	0.0088
Vd_{ss} (ml)	1.11	0.287	0.059
Cly (ml/h)	0.0441	0.0016	0.0005

Results and discussion

The results of the pharmacokinetic studies as shown in Table 3 reveal that the concentration (area under the curve) of niosomal MTX increased three fold after macrophage activation with MDP-gelatin conjugate (64.6µg/h/ml vs 202.2 µg/h/ml) in mice implanted with S-180. The MTX -AUC of mice with S-180 after macrophage activation was twice of that obtained without macrophage activation. However, the mean residence time (MRT) of MTX decreased slightly after macrophage activation. The MTX elimination rate constant at steady state, K_{ss}, was slow in both cases. Volume of distribution (Vd_{ss}) decreased nearly by four folds after macrophage activation, i.e. from 0.2866 to 0.06 ml. Similarly, a three-fold decrease in the clearance rate (CLR) of MTX from 0.0016 to 0.0005 ml/h was recorded after macrophage activation. The improved bioavailability of MTX after macrophage activation was evidently due to the internalization of the MTX entrapped in niosomes (Table 3).

Improved MTX availability to tumours may be accounted for the improved tumour regression observed after macrophage activation with MDP-gelatin conjugates. Plasma MTX was higher in tumour bearing mice after administration of niosomal MTX as compared to free MTX. MTX concentration increased dramatically when administered in niosomes 2 days after macrophage activation. The treatment demonstrated improved tumour regression.

Plasma MTX was much higher when MTX in vesicular form was injected subsequent to macrophage activation than the drug was administered vesicular form with prior macrophage inactivation. Thus, macrophage activation using MDP-gelatin conjugate improved the efficacy of MTX entrapped in span 60 based niosomes.

Tissue distribution of niosome encapuslated methotrexate

Niosomes encapsulated with MTX were prepared as described earlier. The prepared formulations were studied for their tissue distribution was determined on mice bearing transplanted S-180 tumour. The effect of macrophage activation on tumour size was studied.

Determination of caliberation for MTX in different organs of mice transplanted with S-180 by HPLC with fluorescence detection

The method followed for the determination of methotrexate (MTX) in various organs of S-180 bearing mice was similar to that for the determination of MTX in plasma [21]. The mice was killed by survical dislocation and various organs like the Kidney, liver, spleen, lungs, brain and tumour were excised from the S-180 bearing mice two weeks after transplantation of the tumour. The tissues were weighed after drying the tissue on a coarse filter paper. One ml of water was added to every gram of the tissue and sonicated in an ice bath. The homogenate was vortexed for 5 minutes. Then, 0.3 ml of 10% acetic acid (containing known quantities of MTX for calculation of recovery) was added to precipitate proteins. Glutamic acid was used as an internal standard.

To each 0.5 ml of trichloroacetic acid extract, 0.5 ml of 5 M acetic acid sodium acetate buffer, pH 5.0 was added.   0.05 ml of 5% potasium permanganate aqueous solution was added to oxidize the contents. The samples were decolorised by adding 0.05 ml of a 3% v/v solution of hydrogen peroxide. The solutions were degassed using ultrasonic water bath for about 5 min. The resultant solutions were filtered through 0.5 μm nylon filters and 50 μl of the filtrate was injected through HPLC column, after suitable dilutions.

Plasma and tissue distribution of MTX following intravenous injection of commercially available MTX injection

Inbred male BALB/c mice, 6-8 weeks of age, weighing 18-20g transplanted with S-180 were used (10 mice per each group). The first group of mice was given intravenously, the commercially available MTX injection after one week of tumour transplantation at the dose of 5 ml MTX solution per Kg mice body weight (equivalent to 2.72 mg/kg). At predetermined intervals of 5,10,15,30 min. and 1,2,4,6,8,12,24 and 72 h blood was collected into clean heparin rinsed tubes, from the eye orbits of the animals, then, after cervical dislocation animals were autopsied and kidneys, lungs, spleen, liver, brain and tumour were excised and collected. At each predetermined time interval the blood and tissues were collected from three animals. The ratio of peak height for the MTX oxidation produced versus peak height of the internal standard oxidation product was used to determine MTX concentrations in plasma and tissues at various time intervals.

Plasma and tissue distribtuion of MTX following intravenous injection of niosomes suspened in 0.9% saline

The niosomes containing methotrexate were diluted with normal saline so as to get a concentration of 2.72 mg/5 ml. The second group of mice received intravenous injections of the niosomal suspension, at a dose of 5 ml niosomal MTX suspension/Kg body weight of the mice (equivalent to 2.72 mg MTX/Kg mice body weight). At predetermined intervals of 1,10,15 and 20 min. and 1,2,4,6,8,12,24 and 72 h blood was collected into heparin rinsed haemetocrit tubes, from the eye orbit of the mice. After cervical dislocation, the animals were autopsied and various organs along with the solid tumour were excised and the drug concentration in these tissues and plasma was estimated.

Plasma and tissue distribution of MTX following intravenous injection of niosomes suspended in 0.9% saline two days after macrophage activation with muramyl dipeptide-protein conjugate

MDP-protein conjugate was prepared with a water soluble carbodiimide (EDC1; 1-ethyl-3(3-dimethyl aminopropyl) carbodiimide HCL), according to the Schechan and Hess method [22]. EDC1 powder (30 mg) was added to phosphate buffer (2 ml, 0.05 m) at pH 4.7 containing 1.25 mg of MDP, and left for 1 h at 4°C to activate the gamma glutamyl carboxyl group of MDP. The phosphate saline buffer, pH 4.7 (2 ml, 0.05 m) containing 10 mg of gelatin was added to the activated MDP with agitation upto 40 h at 4°C. The *in vivo* activation of macrophages was carried out by intravenous injection of the MDP protein conjugate two days prior to the administration of niosomal MTX. The dose of MDP protein conjugate administered to mice was 1 µg MDP per mice.

The third group of mice received intravenous injections of the niosomal suspension at a dose of 5 ml of niosomal MTX suspension/Kg mice body weight (equivalent to 2.72 mg MTC/Kg mice body weight) two days after macrophage activation. Macrophage activation was carried out with the MDP gelatin conjugate 5 days after transplantation of S-180, by *in vivo* administration of MDP gelatin conjugate equivalent to 1 µg MDP/mice. At each pre-determined time intervals plasma, kidneys, liver, lungs, spleen, brain and tumour were collected from these mice.

Estimation of tumour volume on i.v. administration of free MTX niosomal MTX after macrophage activation

Inbred male BALB/c mice, 6-8 weeks of age weighing 18-20 g were selected and inoculated with S-180. The mice were then divided into three groups (ten mice in each group). One week after tumour implantation the first group of mice received free MTX intravenously, at a dose of 5 ml MTX solution/Kg mice body weight (equivalent to 2.72 mg MTX/Kg). The second group of mice received the same dose of MTX encapsulated in niosomes. The third group of mice also received the same dose of MTX encapsulated in niosomes, however in this group of mice macrophage activation was done two days prior to administration of drug (i.e., on the fifth day of tumour inoculation).

The mice were observed for one month after drug treatment for macroscopic signs of tumour and toxicity. The tumour dimensions were measured using vernier calipers. The tumour volumes thus measured were plotted against time and the test/control ratios (T/C ratios) of the tumour volumes were also compared.

Tissue content of MTX after administration in solution and in niosome encapsulated form, with and without macrophage activation.

It was observed that the liver plays an important role in the uptake of niosomal MTX as indicated by the higher tissue level of MTX compared to levels after free MTX administration (Table 4). The presence of MTX in the kidney at all time intervals was less when administered in the form of niosomes. The activation of macrophages further decreased the concentration of MTX in the kidney. The concentration of MTX in kidney when administered as niosomes was comparatively higher in the spleen as compared to solution treatment (administered).

No marked alteration in the lungs could be seen when the drug was given in the form of niosomes, however the concentration of the drug reaching the brain were significantly altered. Thus, uptake of MTX in liver and brain was higher after niosomal encapsulation similar to the investigation of Azmin et al. [2].

Significant differences in the disposition of MTX in tumour was observed when administered in the form of niosomes. The tumour concentration of MTX were higher after macrophage activation. Similar reports were made earlier by Gregoriadis et al. [14].

EFFECT OF NIOSOME ENCAPSULATION OF MTX AND MACROPHAGE ACTIVATION ON THE TUMOUR VOLUME

The maximum tumour volume reached in the group injected with MTX in solution was 35 nm^3 and the volume declined after 2 weeks of treatment (Table 5). The tumour volumes of treated niosomal MTX group decreased from the first day after the treatment. On the 20th day after niosome administration, the tumour volume was almost negligible, while on the 23-day the tumors regressed almost completely, without any signs of recurrence. In this group the T/C values were reduced to 0.05 on the 8th day after treatment, whereas with the administration of free MTX, the T/C values were not reduced to 0.5 even after one month of treatment. The free MTX was able to arrest the growth of the tumour, but did not induce much tumour remission. Niosomal MTX was able to produce almost total remission three weeks after treatment.

In the third group, where macrophage activation was effected before niosomal MTX administration, the tumour volume was reduced to a great extent on the 15th day of the treatment (Table 5).

Table 4 : Disposition of MTX in organs following I.V. administration (μg/g of organ homogenate)

Hours	1			4			8			12			24		
Organs	Free MTX	Nio MTX	Nio MTX + MDP	Free MTX	Nio MTX	Nio MTX + MDP	Free MTX	Nio MTX	Nio MTX + MDP	Free MTX	Nio MTX	Nio MTX + MDP	Free MTX	Nio MTX	Nio MTX + MDP
Liver	8.9	11.2	9.0	0.2	11.5	11.9	0.1	7.8	10.1	0.03	2.6	2.2	0.01	0.10	0.05
Kidney	24.3	6.3	5.4	8.6	4.0	3.0	6.8	3.8	2.2	4.03	2.50	1.80	1.60	1.70	0.80
Spleen	8.9	24.7	20.3	2.9	19.3	15.6	6.3	15.6	20.0	5.9	19.5	19.4	5.5	21.3	13.6
Lung	6.8	1.5	2.9	1.4	1.3	2.1	1.9	2.0	2.1	2.0	0.9	1.2	0.80	0.7	0.40
Brain	0.1	0.3	0.5	0.1	0.3	0.3	0.1	0.2	0.2	0.04	0.2	0.2	0.04	0.1	0.10
Tumour	17.2	20.4	27.2	18.3	29.2	47.3	21.2	36.5	61.2	21.9	50.4	80.6	22.6	80.3	100.3

The niosomal MTX with and without macrophage activation attained higher concentration in the brain. This may be due to the increase in total lipid concentration of the drug delivery system.

The steep rise in the tumor drug concentration clearly depicts the usefulness of niosomes as drug carriers for the delivery of MTX to solid tumour. The activation of macrophages enhances the delivery of the drug to the tumor interstitium in addition the activated macrophages also contribute to the antitumour activity.

Table 5. Effect of niosome encapsulation of MTX and macrophage activation on tumour volume

Days after tumour incubation	Tumour volume ratio (T/C)		
	Group I	Group II	Group III
7	0.797	0.859	1.021
9	0.759	0.739	0.836
10	-	-	0.735
11	0.723	0.626	0.668
12	-	-	0.602
13	0.718	0.554	0.540
14	-	-	0.478
15	0.722	0.503	0.417
16	-	-	0.360
17	0.722	0.450	0.296
18	-	-	0.233
19	0.728	0.380	0.188
20	-	-	0.136
21	0.737	0.324	0.056
23	0.733	0.261	-
25	0.721	0.119	-
27	0.702	0.042	-
29	0.688	-	-
31	0.661	-	-
33	0.583	-	-
35	0.569	-	-

The incorporation of antineoplastic agent in niosomes would markedly increase the delivery of the drug to the tumor, probably due to surfactant activity and better permeation of the drug through tumor. The activation of macrophage would elicit and negotiate a certain degree of tumor kill by its own merit.

The T/C values reached 50% within a week of treatment. This may be due to niosomal MTX being selectively delivered to the tumor interstitium by the activated macrophages, in addition to inherent antineoplastic activity of these macrophages.

CONCLUSION

Niosomal encapsulation and macrophage activation with muramyl dipeptide gelatin conjugate may be helpful for better targeted delivery of methotrexate to the tumor site because of surfactant activity and better permeation of drug and for better tumoricidal activity. Niosomal encapsulation of methotrexate also results in higher amount of methotrexate in liver, spleen and brain.

REFERENCES

1. Vanlerberghe, G., Handjani Vila, R.M., Berthelot, C., Serbg (1972). **Proc. 6th Internat. Congress Surface Activity**, Zurich, 139.

2. Azmin, M.N., Florence, A.T., Handjani Vila, R.M., Stuart, J.F.B., Vanlerberghe, G., Whittaker, J.S. (1985). **J. Pharm. Pharmacol.** 37, 237-242.

3. Chandraprakash, K.S., Udupa, N., Pillai, G.K., Uma Devi, P. (1993). **Drug Dev. Ind. Pharm.** 19(11), 1331-1342.

4. Rogerson, A., Cummings, J., Willmott, N., Florence, A.T. (1988). **J. Pharm. Pharmacol.** 40, 337-342.

5. Baillie, A.J., Florence, A.T., Hume, L.R., Muirhead, G.T., Rogerson, A. (1985). **J. Pharm. Pharmacol.** 38, 863-868.

6. Hunter, C.A., Dolan, T.F., Coombs, G.H., Baillie, A.J. (1988). **J. Pharm. Pharmacol.** 40, 161-165.

7. Adam, D.O. and Nathan, C.F. (1983). **Immunol. Today** 4, 166-167.

8. Adam, A., Petit, J.F., Lafrencier, P.,and Lederer, E. (1981). **Mol. Chem. Biochem.** 41, 27-47.

9. Candid, L.C., Carelli, L., Audibert, F. (1979). **J. Reticuloendothel. Soc.** 26, 631-641.

10. Tabata, Y., Ikada, Y. (1987). **J. Pharm. Pharmacol.** 42, 13-19.

11. Fogler, W.E., Fidler, I.J. (1985). **Cancer Res.** 45, 14-18.

12. Schlomo, D., Philip, G., Esther, T., Michael, F., Mati, F., Koichi, Y., Kenji, O., Harnaki, Y. (1986). **J. Med. Chem.** 29, 1961-1968.

13. Whiteworth, W.P., Charles, C.P., Joseph, E., Eugenie, S.K., Isaiah, J.F. (1970). **Cancer Metasta Rev.** 8, 319-351.

14. Gregoriadis, G., Neerunjun, D.E., Hunt, R. (1977). **Life Sci.**, 21, 357-370.

15. Schroit, A.J., Galligioni, E., Fidler, I.J. (1983). **J. Biol. Response Mod.** 2, 97-100.

16. Poste, G., Kirsh, R., Fogler, W., Fidler, I.J. (1984). In: Normal approach to cancer chemotherapy (Sunkara. ed.), Academic Press, New York, 166-221.

17. Fidler, I.J., Sone, S., Fogler, W.E., Barnes, Z. (1981). **Proc. Natl. Acad. Sci.**, USA, 78, 1680-1684.

18. Fidler, I.J., Barner, Z., Fogler, W.E., Kirsh, R., Bugleski, P., Poste, G. (1982). **Cancer Res.** 42, 496-501.

19. Gregoriadis, G. (1980) In: Liposomes in biological systems (Gregoriadis, G., Alison, M. ed.), John Willey and Sons Ltd., New York, 45-50.

20. Hardy, J.G., Kellaway, I.W., Rogers, J., Wilson, C.G. (1980). **J. Pharm. Pharmacol.** 32, 309-313.

21. Chandraprakash, K.S. Udupa, N., Uma Devi, P., Pillai, G.K. (1990). **Int. J. Pharm.** 61, R1-R3.

22. Shechan, J.C., Hess, G.P. (1955). **J. Am. Chem. Soc.** 77, 1067-1068.

11

LIGAND MEDIATED DRUG TARGETING: PRINCIPLE AND PERSPECTIVE

In Obliterative Magnoresponsive Chemotherapy of Tumour

S. P. VYAS

Department of Pharmaceutical Sciences,
Dr. Harisingh Gour Vishwavidyalaya,
Sagar 470 003.

INTRODUCTION

Most of the drugs introduced to clinical medicine exert their effects by interactive interference with cell and cell membrane related structure and functions through concentration dependent reversible interactions at specific receptor site. Obviously, to obtain a desirable therapeutic response, the correct amount of drug should be transported and delivered to the site of action with subsequent control of drug input rate. The distribution to other tissues therefore seems unnecessary, wasteful and a potential causes of toxicity. The developments over past decade indicate explicit progress in the area of controlled and targeted drug delivery. One ever sought after yet an attained goal in the clinical medicine has been the development of site or organ targeted drug delivery systems. The practical realisation of the concept shall be a great breakthrough in medical sciences. The precision, programmed site specificity of the system was poised as "magic bullet" by Paul Ehrlich. It not only should ensure of site specificity however, it should also mitigate toxicity of the drug (s) to non-target sites as a result of attenuated drug levels. The cell related biological regular events occurring in high order of specificity and precision offer basis for quantitative targeted drug delivery. There involves a number of essential bioligands for physiologic cell need and biosignalling. These operate through bio-ports referred to as receptors. The ligand receptor interactions are highly conserved and specific. Thus ligands or receptors could be exploited for targeted drug delivery, at the quantitative level in a well-defined manner. Let us discuss and define various facets and essentials of drug targeting.

TARGETING

Targeted drug delivery implies for effectively selective localization of a pharmacodynamic agent into the vicinity of pre identified (pre selected) target(s) in therapeutic concentration, with its minimum access to non-target normal cells.

In pharmacodynamic term time concentration profile of drug at target site is optimized whilst the drug burden to other non-target tissues that may manifest toxicity, is minimized, the drug delivery is referred to as site specific.

Rational of drug targeting

The rational for site specific targeted delivery may be appreciated as a set of desirable events including an exclusive drug delivery to pre-identified compartments with maximum potential intrinsic activity of drugs and concomitantly reduced drug access to irrelevant non-target cells. Invariably, every event stated leads to higher drug concentration at the site of action simultaneously results in to a lower concentration at non-target tissue circumventing toxic effects [1]. The high drug concentration at the target site is resultant of cellular uptake of the drug carrier system, then liberation of drug (Fig. 1).

Targeting is only significant if the target compartment is biologically distinguished from the other compartments, (where toxicity may occur), and also when the active drug could predominantly be delivered and accumulated in the immediate proximity of the target site [2].

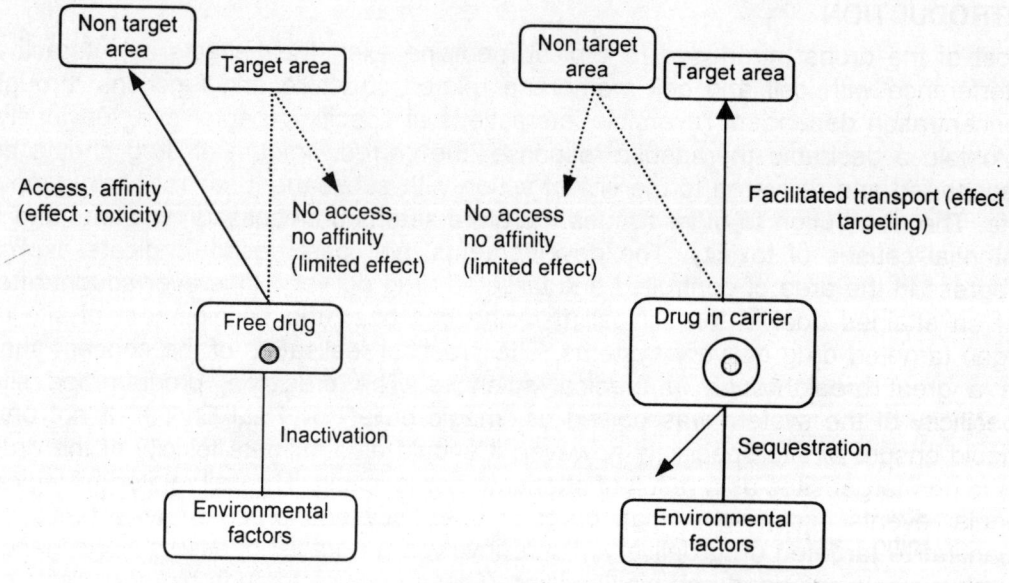

Fig. 1 : Principle of drug targeting [1]

Target

Target could be described as a cell or group of cells in minority (biologically a disease locus), identified to be in the need of treatment. Two distinctive cellular elements exist on the surface of the target cell(s) are to be critical considered in designing of carriers for targeting. They are:

1. Cell surface antigens
2. Cell surface receptors

Target organs / tissues

The appropriate targets for carrier mediate interactions are [3]:

(i) Cells *in vitro* for genome grafting or manipulation of DNA (genetic materials).

(ii) Accessible anatomical compartments, i.e. peritoneal cavity, cerebral ventricles, plural cavity, lungs, lymphatics, etc.

(iii) Macrophages and other phagocytic cells including Kupffer satellite cells, tissue macrophages and the blood macrophage or monocytes of MPS.

(iv) Nonphagocytic cells of RES including the liver endothelial cells, endocytic in nature.

(v) Lymphocytes and antigen presenting cells.

(vi) Tumor cells.

Carriers

Carrier is one of the most important entity essentially required for effective transportation of drug load(s). They **sequester**, **transport** and **retain** drug en route, while **elute** or deliver it into the **vicinity of target** extracellularly or intracellularly. Carriers can do so either through an ability, **inherent or acquired** (through structural modification), to interact selectively with biological targets. They however may be engineered to release the drug in the proximity of target cell lines, in need of optimal pharmacological action. Various carriers investigated and characterized include liposomes, niosomes, nanoparticles, microspheres, bio-conjugates, erythrocytes, neutrophils, supramolecules etc. They are at large colloidal in nature engineered for envisaged drug delivery.

Ligands

Ligands are indigenous or synthetic molecules or groups appended on to the surface of carrier. They selectively steer up the carrier to the prespecified tissues or organ (target) equipped with the ligand specific receptor units. Various ligands exploited for selective drug targeting include **antibodies, polypeptides, oligo-saccharides, viral proteins, endogenous hormones and fusogenic residues etc**. The ligands confer site recognition and specificity upon carrier/vector and help them to approach the respective target where they eventually deliver the drug.

Levels of targeting

Targeted drug delivery may be achieved by using carrier systems, where reliance is placed on exploiting both, their intrinsic pathway(s) that these carriers follow, and the bioprotection that they offer to drugs during transit through the body. The various approaches of vectoring the drug to the target site can be broadly classified as [4-8]:

1. Passive targeting
2. Active targeting
3. Inverse targeting
4. Physical targeting
5. Dual targeting

Passive targeting

The passive process which utilizes the natural course of (attributed to inherent characteristics) 'homing' of the carrier system, through which it finally identifies and eventually approaches the intended cell lines with in the body for its clearance. Size and surfacial charge play a critical role in passive carrier uptake.

Figure 2 shows the mechanical screening of colloidal carriers where particles larger than 10 μm are retained in lungs. Those smaller than 10 μm in size get sequestered in liver or spleen via opsonic endocytosis or phagocytosis. The smallest size less than 150 nm passes through fenestrate in liver endothelial and accumulated in sinusoidal spaces or may extravasate on tumor mass or via pinocytosis to some extent taken up in bone marrow.

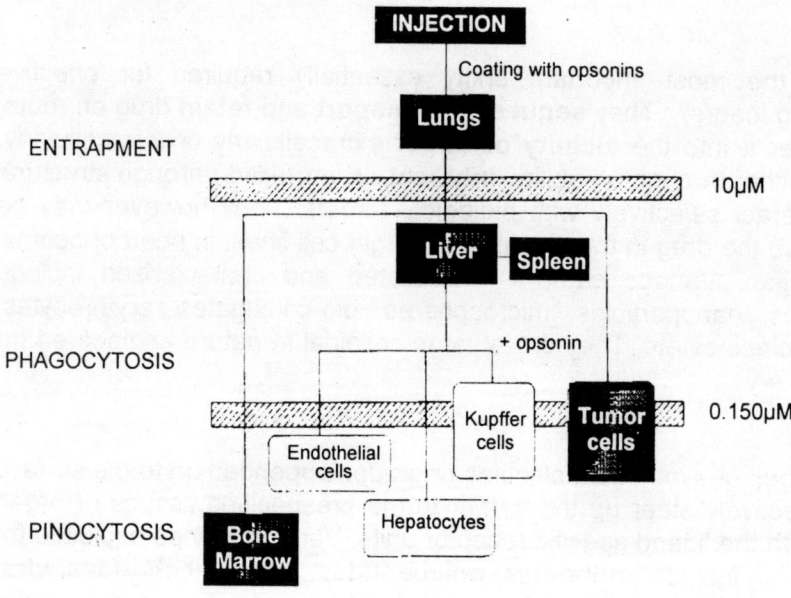

Fig. 2 : Schematic diagram of bio-fate of colloidal particles *in vivo*

Active targeting

The process of active targeting exploits modification or manipulation of drug carrier using some exogenous means, so that it can be identified and captured by particular cell lines. It is generally achieved by using specific uptake mechanisms, such as receptor dependent uptake of natural low-density lipoproteins (LDL) particles and synthetic lipid microemulsions from partially reconstituted LDL particles, coated with the apoproteins.

Active targeting is operative at three different levels and accordingly referred to as first order targeting (organ compartmentalization), second order targeting (cellular targeting) and third order targeting (intracellular targeting).

Inverse targeting

It is essentially based on successful attempts to circumvent and bypass passive biofate or uptake of colloidal carriers by reticuloendothelial system (RES). One strategy applied to achieve inverse targeting is to suppress the function of RES by a preinjection of a large amount of blank colloidal carriers or macromolecules like dextran sulphate [9].

Davis and Hansrani [10] reported that phospholipid microspheres emulsified with Polaxamer 338 showed the slowest RES uptake in mouse peritoneal macrophages *in vitro*. Illum et al. [5,11] reported that Poloxamine 908, is another hydrophilic nonionic surfactant, which diverts normal RES uptake of coated emulsion and coated nanoparticles (polystyrene microsphere) to inflammatory sites in rabbits. Recently, Lee et al. [12], suggested inverse targeting of drugs to the sites other than RES rich organs by coating the lipid micro-emulsion (LM) with polaxamer 308.

Bio-physical targeting

The selective drug delivery programmed and monitored at the external level (*ex-vivo*) with the help of physical means is referred to as physical targeting. In this mode of targeting, some characteristics of the environment are used either to direct the carrier to a particular location or to cause selective release of its contents. Examples are Magneto responsive, thermosenstive, external signal sensitive (pH, irradiation and electroimpulse) drug carrier composites or constructs.

Dual targeting

This classical approach of the drug targeting is based on the carrier molecules having its own intrinsic antiviral effect thus synergies the antiviral effect of the loaded active drug. Based on this approach, drug conjugates can be prepared with a improvised activity profile against the viral replication process [8]. A major advantage of strategy is that the virus replication process can be attacked at multiple points, excluding the possibilities of resistant viral strain development. Immunoconjugates anti-CD4, Abs-Ricin A complex is one of the representative example of this concept.

CELLULAR EVENTS IN TARGETING

Endocytosis

Endocytosis is a main cellular activity involved in the internalization of the colloidal and macromolecular carriers, summing the two processes of '**phagocytosis**' and '**pinocytosis**'. Endocytosis is defined as the internalization of plasma membrane with concomitant engulfment of extracellular material and extracellular fluid.

The process involves sequential steps:

- **Recognition** (mediated by coating of blood components, mainly opsonin and high density lipoproteins),
- **Adhesion** (attachment of the particle to the macrophage cells of the RES)
- **Digestion** (whereby the particles are transferred to phagosome, phago-lysosome and finally to digestive vacuoles).

Zippering: Multiple attachment of particle associated ligands with membrane receptors is an essential stimulus for phagocytic capture of particles.

Ligand mediated transcytosis

Ligand transcytosis suggests that exclusive localization of particulates does not occur necessarily within sinusoidal cells, but the particulate ligands may also end up in hepatocytes (in case, if hepatocyte is not capable to endocytose initially).

RECEPTOR

A large variety of receptor systems with important roles in controlling growth, differentiation, endocytosis, secretion, cell signaling and cell activation have been reported to be differentially expressed on macrophages and other cells (Fig. 3). However, some receptors are restricted to specific cell lines. The receptor-mediated endocytosis serves to selectively retrieve and assimilates various essential macromolecular bio-ligands from the extracellular environment. The process is dependent mainly on the existence of cell surface receptors.

Table 1. Cell specific receptors expressed by various cell types in the bio-environment

Cell types	Receptor(S)
Monocytes	Mannose 6-phosphate - t(n)GP, β-glucan, charge scavenger
Hepatocytes	Galactose -t(n)GP (high-density), HDL, LDL, EGF, IgA, transferrin
Enterocytes	Maternal IgG, dimeric IgG, transcobalmin II
Macrophages	Mannose-6-phosphatet (n)GP, galactose -t(n)GP, manGlcNAct (n)GP, fucosyl-glycoconjugates, AMPC
Kupffer cells	Mannose -t(n)GP, galactose-particles, polymeric negative charged proteins, complement factors, fucose, LDL, AMPC, fucosyl-glycoconjugates
T4 cells	Galactose -t(n)GP (low-density), interleukin, transferrin, CD4
Fibroblasts	Mannose-6-phosphate-t(n)GP, transferrin, transcobalminII, LDL, EGF, AMPC
Endothelial cells	
i. Liver	Monomeric negatively charged proteins, manGlcNAc--t(n)GP, Fc receptors
ii. Blood brain	Transferrin, insulin, cationic
iii. Lung, diaphragm and heart	Albumin
Mammary acinar cells	Growth factor
Renal tubular cells	Low molecular weight proteins (cationic)

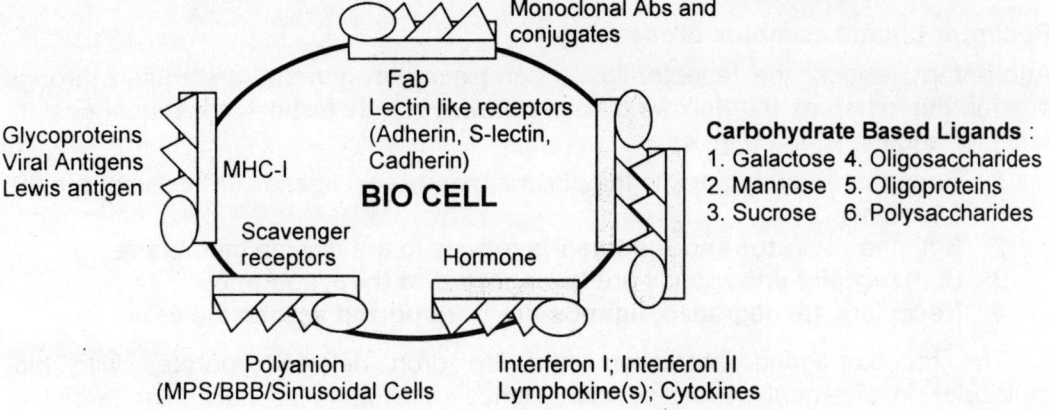

Fig. 3 : Distribution of receptors on bio-cell surface

Table 2. Cell specific receptors expressed by biocells with their preferred ligands

Receptors	Expression by various biocells	Ligands
1. Antibody and its conjugates		
Fc/C3b.receptors	Human/murine macrophages; peritoneal macrophages; Fc receptor bearing tumor cell lines	(a). Immunoglobulin IgG class (polyclonal or MoAb); Haptens; Fab' or F(ab)$_2$ immunological fragments
Complement receptor	Peritoneal macrophages	(b). IgM class
Surrogate receptors	Macrophage cell lines	(c). Palmitate derivatized IgG
2. Endogenous ligands		
Interferons (ganglioside expressing receptors); interleukin- I, II, IV,VI receptors	T-lymphocytes; hepatocytes; macrophages; tumor T-cell lines	(a). Endogenous cytokines & lymphokines
MHC class I & II	Resting & activated human T cell lines	(b). MHC classes
Insulin growth-factor (IGFII/Man 6P); Transferrin (Tf); r-T cell (rCD4) receptor; α_2 macroglobulin; gp120; complement receptors	Human monocytes; alveolar macrophages; proliferating cell lines; T4 cells; macrophages; monocytes; Kupffer cells	(c). Lectins & other protein receptor based ligands
3. Glyco-conjugates		
Galactose specific; 4GalNAc; asialoglycoprotein receptors	Kupffer cells; liver endothelial cells	(a). Glycosylated carrier
Scavenger receptors	Liver endothelia-monomeric Kupffer cells-polymeric	(b). Negative charged particles
Lectin receptors (galactose specific; ASGP; Mannosylated; mannose 6P fucosyl; and β-glucan) lympho-cyte homing receptors	Macrophage hepatic endothelium; macrophage leukocytes; lymphocytes, rat kupffer cells; proliferating cell lines	(c). Glyco-conjugates based on galactose; mannose; fucose; β-glucan; biantennary glycans & oligosaccharide with terminal reduciblegalactose residue; etc.

*Adopted & modified from [3,13,14].

Receptor Ligand complex processing

After internalization, the receptor-ligand complexes, in general, are routed through one or the other of the following four pathways with distinct consequences for receptor and the ligand (Fig. 4):

1. **Receptor recycle** back to the plasma membrane, ligands get delivered to the lysosomes.
2. Both the **receptor and the ligands** recycle to the plasma membrane,
3. Both receptor and ligands are **transported to the lysosomes**
4. Receptors are degraded, **ligands are transported across** the cells.

The receptor-ligand interaction mediated drug delivery operates with bio-molecules involvement. It is also some times referred to as molecular targeting. Immunological process exemplifies the targeted molecular bio-events. Judicious interplay and manipulation of activity course of these ligands could be utilized for targeted pharmacodynamic and immunological consequences. In order to signify receptor-ligand interaction mediated targeting

1. **Molecular targeting and immunology and**
2. **Tumor specific ADEPT / VEDEPT** strategies are discussed here.

MOLECULAR TARGETING AND IMMUNOLOGY

Immunoregulatory molecules

These include factors mediating help and suppression of antibody formation, viz., insulin like growth factors (IGF I & II), major histocompatibility complex classes (MHC class I & II), β-glucans and glycoprotein 120 (gp120).

1. IGF: Human monocytes and alveolar macrophages express insulin like growth factor II/Man 6P receptors. Human peripheral blood T-cells upon anti CD3 activation express receptor for IGFI, IGFII and insulin in a sequential manner [15].
2. MHC: Blood T-lymphocytes and monocytes/macrophages express Receptors for MHC molecules. MHC I molecule functions as transport module and internalized by coated pits. Class II MHC molecules carry a sulfated glycosamino-glycan (anionic polysaccharide) that is essential for antigen presentation [16].
3. β-glucans : Receptors for these particular immune activators are present on human monocytes and initiate phagocytosis of glucan, production of leukotrienes and release of lysosomal enzymes [17].
4. gp120 : MHC class II positive T-lymphocytes are capable of internalizing, processing and presenting this antigen. The HIV virus infected cells shed it abundantly [18].

Gp120 targeted CD4-HIV vaccine: A molecular targeting concept

Invasion of HIV in to target-cells involves two steps: binding virion to the receptors on target-cell follwed by fusion of the viral envelope with target cell plasma membrane. Two glycoprotein gp 120 and gp 121 play viral role in the infective events. Viral gp 120 binds to receptors on target cells. The major receptor expressed on target cell is

CD4. Since the CD4 receptors is exclusively expressed in abundance on T_H cell that is why HIV infection is said to be lymphotropic. Thus virus not only anchors to T_H cells via CD^+4 but also obstruct or arrests the participation of CD4 T_H cells in immunological communication thus corrupting / disabling the defense system.

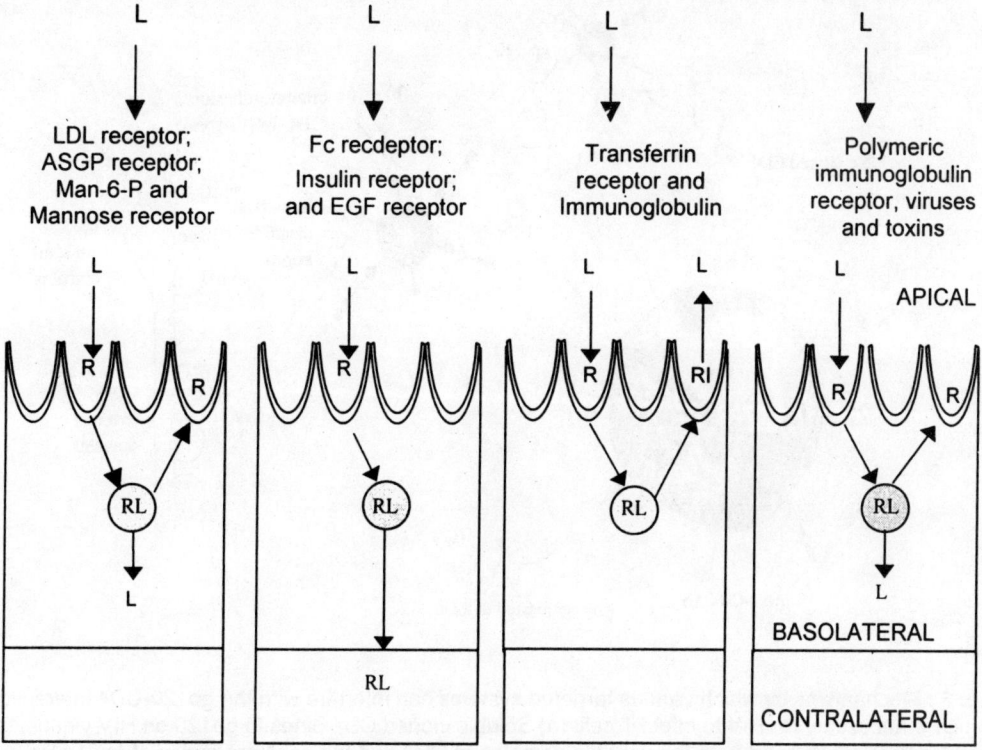

Fig. 4 : Pathways of receptor internalizing and recycling. Subsequent to entry into acidic endosomes, ligand and receptors are sorted and trafficked independently which may result into degradation, recycling or transcytosis of either molecule. L=Ligand, R=Receptor.

Gp120 of HIV has high affinity for CD4 and hence if more of soluble or circulatory CD4 are added, it may bind effectively to gp120 on HIV and thus could block viral binding to the host cells and can also inhibit syncytia formations. The major problem with soluble CD4 in humans is that CD4 has a half-life of only 30-120 minutes in serum and there is the necessity for regular injection. Copon and Ward [19] reported that the problem could be effectively overcome by linking CD4 gene to the constant-region gene of human IgG 1. The resulting CD4 immunoglobulin encoded by recombinant gene, is referred to as immunoadhesion molecule with high-affinity binding of gp120 of CD4, together with longer serum half life characteristics of IgG 1 (nearly 21 days) (Fig. 5).

MHC II targeting

The major histocompatability complex I and II can selectively be targeted with the help of their respective ligands (anti MHC antibodies) while the antigen (avidin, streptavidin) enroute may be deterred by encapsulating them into some carrier units like liposomes or nanoparticles. Encapsulated antigen following phagocytosis of ligand MHC I/II complex gets unmasked and processed by MHC I/II and subsequently presented to T cells for elicitation of cellular immunity. The concept is presented schematically in the figure 6 & 7.

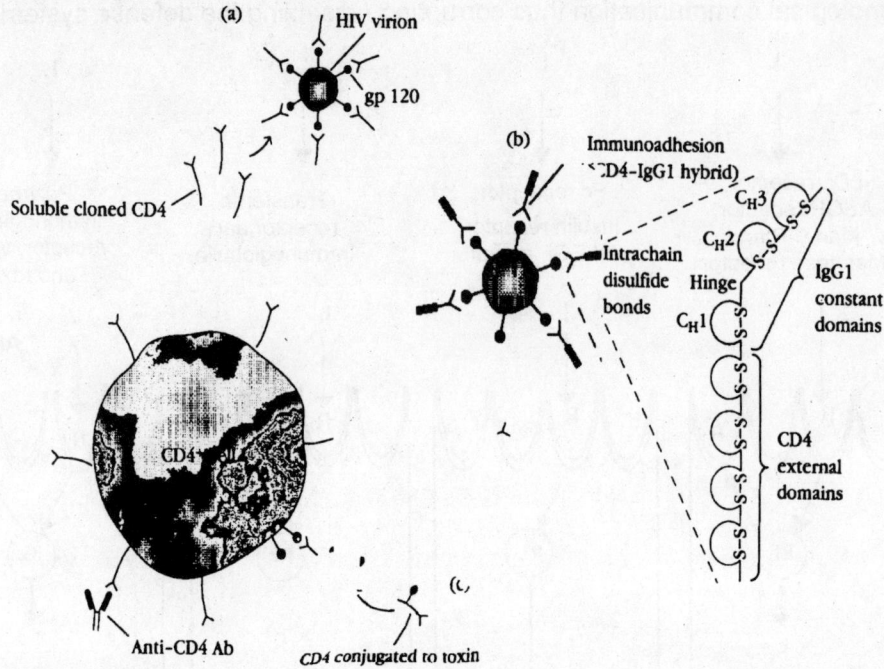

Fig. 5 : Mechanisms by which various targeted systems can interfere with the gp120-CD4 interaction, which is necessary for HIV to infect T cell. (a) Soluble cloned CD4 binds to gp120 on HIV virions. (b) Immunoadhesion: formed from the variable domains of CD4 and the constant region of IgG1 also binds to gp120 virions. (c) Immunotoxin: A bioconjugate prepared using CD4 and immunotoxin (i.e. ricin A) selictively binds to to viral gp120 expressed on HIV-infected cells, and subsequently leads to infected cell death.

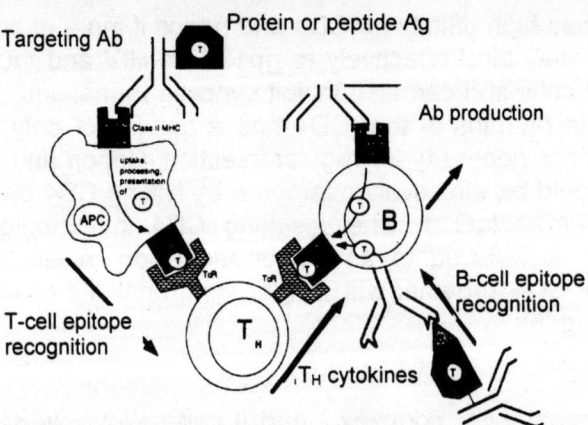

Fig. 6 : Schematic presentation of the proposed mechanism for the enhancement of immunogenicity by immunotargeting. T: T-helper cell epitope ; B : B-cell epitope; TcR : T cell receptor ; APC : antigen presenting cell; TH : T-helper cell

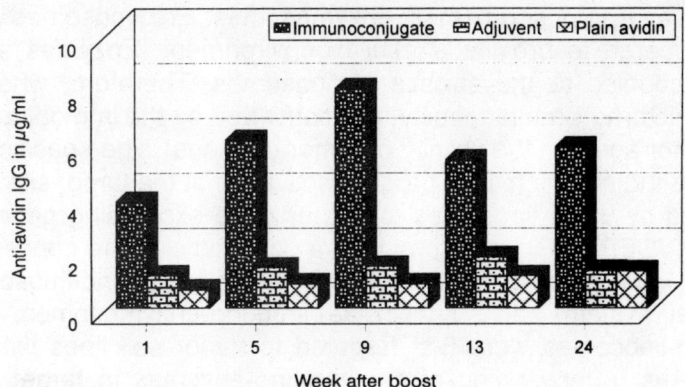

Fig. 7 : Shows significant immuno response when immuno conjugated avidin was used for BALB/C mice immunization. Approximately 8 times higher antibody titre was estimated using ELISA. The titre level remained consistently and comparatively high for more than 24 weeks. The strategy suggests for potentiation of immunization via MHC class II mole targeted antigen presentation.

Enzyme prodrug therapy based on antibody, virus or gene directed mechanisms (ADEPT/ VDEPT/GDEPT)

A novel strategy for the delivery of cytotoxic and antiviral agents to specific cell types is the prodrug activation by antibody-enzyme conjugates. Such antibody-coupled enzyme can be specifically delivered to the cell types that express antigenic determinant. Infact, the need for antibody internalization, which is one of the problems associated with immuno-conjugates, is addressed in this strategy known as ADEPT (antibody directed enzyme prodrug therapy) or VDEPT (virus directed enzyme prodrug therapy) or GDEPT (gene directed enzyme prodrug therapy). The formation of active derivatives in the close proximity of the target cells could lead to higher cellular and lower systemic concentration of the active drug. Vingerboeds and co-workers in 1993 [20] reported the coupling of the enzyme β-glucouronidase capable of activating the prodrug epirubicin-glucouronide, to epirubicin. It was found that pretreatment with enzymosomes (bearing no specific antitumor antibodies) or immunoliposomes (bearing no enzymes) was ineffective, but preincubation with immunozymes (enzymosomes) resulted in an enhanced antitumor activity of the prodrug.

The range of tumor antigen-targets and the prodrug chemistry make this enzyme/ prodrug/carrier seemingly a complex concept exploitable in cancer chemotherapy. There is a wide selection of antigen specific targets available, which provide the opportunities of targeting a range of tumors with MAb-enzyme conjugates (ADEPT) and a range of antigen markers are also available which might be used for selective expression of prodrug activating enzymes coded by genes in GDEPT. Sherwood [21] reported several enzyme-prodrug systems and proposed carboxy-peptidase G2 enzyme and a nitrogen mustard prodrug based enzymosomes for further clinical trials. Herpes simplex virus-thymidine kinase (HSV-tk) has been a leading candidate conceivably suitable for VDEPT based on large differential insensitivity to GCV (Gancyclovir) between cells expressing HSV-tk and parental cells.

An interesting strategy towards selective and specific chemo-therapeutics has been developed and proposed namely enzymosomes. Enzymosomes are liposomal constructs engineered to provide a *mini* bioenvironment. Enzymes are covalently immobilized or coupled to the surface of liposomes. Therefore, when a nontoxic prodrug is administered simultaneously, it is converted by the immobilized enzyme to a potent anti-tumor agent in the vicinity of tumor cell lines. The specificity of enzyme reaction provides the means to limit prodrug activation at the tumor site, through prior enzyme targeting by using liposomes, or via enzyme expressing gene delivery into the tumor cells (VDEPT). Figure 8 provides a schematic of the concept of targeted delivery of anticancer prodrug activating enzymes with immuno-liposomes (ADEPT based liposomal system), also known as immuno-enzymosomes. The enzyme bearing immuno-liposomes were first targeted to tumor cell lines with the help of appropriate MoAbs. After binding of the immuno-enzymes to target, a prodrug is administered, which is activated by cell bound immuno-enzymes in the close proximity of the tumor cells. Vingerboeds and co-workers [335] reported the coupling of the enzyme β-glucouronidase, capable of activating the prodrug epirubicin-glucouronide, to epirubicin. It was found that pretreatment with enzymosomes (bearing no specific anti-tumor antibodies) or immuno-liposomes (bearing no enzymes) were ineffective, but pre-incubation with immunozymes (enzymosomes) resulted into an enhanced antitumor activity of the prodrug.

It is the spectrum of activity provided by the choice of enzymes for ADEPT/VDEPT and the range of tumor antigen-targets that make these enzyme/prodrug/carrier seemingly a complex concept exploitable in cancer chemotherapy and gene therapy in the near future. There is a wide selection of antigen specific targets available, which provide opportunities of targeting a range of tumors with MAb-enzyme conjugates (ADEPT) and a range of antigen markers are also available which might be used for selective expression of prodrug activating enzymes coded by genes in GDEPT.

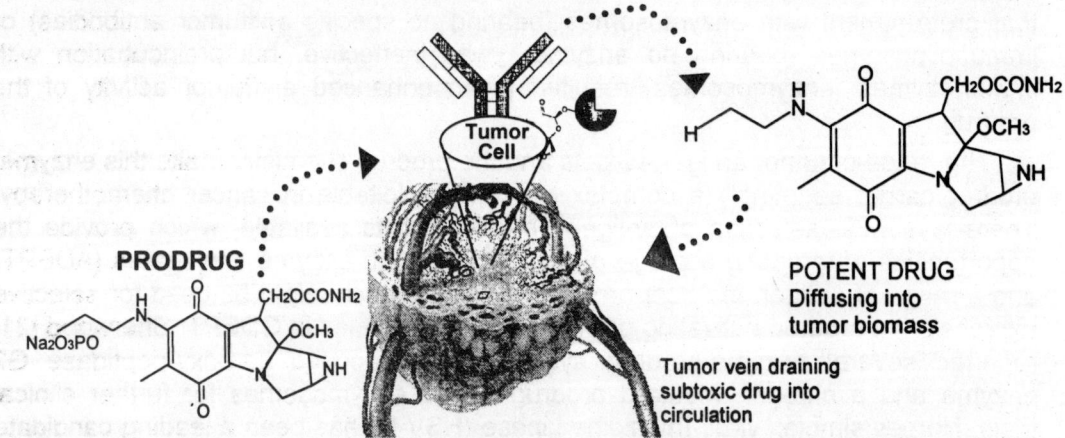

Fig. 8 : Schematic presentation of the concept of antibody directed enzyme pro-drug therapy (ADEPT) with immuno-liposomes (immuno-enzymosomes). The system first binds with the target cells, and then activate a pro-drug (simultaneously administered) in close proximity of the target cells.

Sherwood [21] reported several enzyme-prodrug systems and proposed carboxy-peptidase G2 enzyme and a nitrogen mustard prodrug based enzymosomes for further clinical trials. Herpes simplex virus-thymidine kinase (HSV-tk) has been a leading candidate conceivably suitable for VDEPT based on large differential insensitivity to GCV (Gancyclovir) between cells expressing HSV-tk and parental cells.

Table 3. The principle of ADEPT with the different prodrugs and enzyme systems reported in the literature

Prodrug	Enzyme	System
Benzoic acid mustards	Carboxypeptidase (CPG2)	CPG2-mAB conjugate
Phenol mustards	Carboxypeptidase (CPG2)	CPG2 and F(ab') fragments
Phenol mustards	Alkaline phosphatase (AP)	AP-mAB conjugate
Mitomycin derivatives	Alkaline phosphatase (AP)	AP-mAB conjugate
Phenol mustard	β-glucuronidase	MAb-β-glucuronidase conjugate
Psshenylenediamine mustard	β-Lactamase	MAb-β-Lactamase conjugate
Carboplatinum derivatives	β-Lactamase	MAb-β-Lactamase conjugate
Mitomycin C	β-Lactamase	MAb-β-Lactamase conjugate
Melphalan	Penicillin V/G amidase	Penicillin V/G amidase-mAb conjugate
Nitrogen mustards	Nitroreductase	Nitroreductase-mAb conjugate

Reddy and Low [22] has suggested the ADEPT approach that uses folic acid in place of monoclonal antibody in a recent review. In their studies, penicillin-V-amidase, a fungal enzyme known to hydrolyse the prodrug, doxorubicin-N-p-hydroxyphenoxyacetamide (DPO) to free doxorubicin, was conjugated to folic acid and tested for in vitro cytotoxicity. These workers suggested the use of this folate targeted enzyme pro-drug therapy *in vivo*, where factors such as tumor selectivity and immunogenic behavior can be more accurately assessed.

It is well documented that tumor mass or cells secret some tumor necrolizing factor, and angiogenesis factor which results in to creation of which results in to creation of small endothelial capillaries excessively high in volume. This meets out the need of rapidly growing tumor cells by profused blood and its containts supply. It is convincingly appreciated that selective blockade of blood supply with simultaneous release of chemotherapeutic agent could be a successful bio-physical therapy. In our laboratory we adopted the concept and prepared some polymer coated magnetic liposomes for embolization of blood supply at the target site vis a vis to modulate and manipulate drug delivery under the influence of oscillating / static magnetic field at external level. The work is discussed as follows.

POLY(PHTHALOYL-L-LYSINE) COATED MAGNETIC MLVS

Lipidic multilamellated vesicles containing drug and magnetite were prepared and lamellae of vesicles were coated using poly (phthaloyl L-lysine) by interfacial polycondensation technique.The prepared poly-plied multilamellar vesicles (MPP-MLVs), demonstrated passive embolization and controlled drug release. Measurement of magnetic responsiveness revealed that MPP-MLVs could be localized at preidentified target site with the help of an external magnetic field of appropriate strength. The localization in turn affects obliteration of vasculature leading to the pathological site. MPP-MLVs under magnetic field released the drug at significantly faster rate, indicating their potential in externally modulated drug pulsatilation. The prepared MPP-MLVs were studied for magnetic retention, size and shape, percent drug and magnetite loading, drug release with and without application of magnetic field, turbulence shock, and effect of magnetic field strength on drug release.

Site specific delivery of drug molecules often referred to as drug targeting is now gaining intense and continual attention of both academic and industry based research groups. Although the attempts have been marked by success to some extent, it is apparent that integrated and concerted multidisciplinary efforts yet required to be directed in order to develop some carrier systems stable physico-chemically in *in vitro* as well as in vivo with target oriented drug delivery potentials [23].It has been found and documented that systemic drug delivery is an undesirable way to treat local diseases like tumours, since it exposes normal body cells to cytotoxic effect of medicinal agent(s) generally associated with contraindicative manifestations. Localization of chemo-therapeutic agent at the pathological site would result in to manifold reduction in dose of administered agent vis a vis would generate an effective higher drug concentration [24]. The drug carrier systems suggested for drug targeting include, liposomes, niosomes, nanoparticles, nanocapsules, microemulsions, cellular carriers, drug macromolecule-conjugates, e.t.c. Microcapsules and microparticles have been studied and suggested for chemoembolization where vasculature obliteration was discussed as a consequence of particulate logging of blood vessels [25].

Carrier systems following administration in to the systemic circulation are mainly intercepted by cellular RES. Various approaches which could successfully be used to divert particles or drug carrier from RES predominant site have been reviewed and discussed [26]. These include, surface characteristics modification, i.e. coating of surface with bio-adhesive polymer [27], non-ionic surfactants [28], or cell or tissue specific antibodies [29]. Development of magnetic carrier system and its external navigation is one of the approach that allows Manoeuvring of carriers with the help of two dimensional magnetic field applied externally thus may be localized at pathological site, deterring its content from RES recognition and subsequent interception [30-36].

Liposomes have received considerable attention as carrier for delivery of chemotherapeutics especially to cancer cells. Being based on natural lipids they are biodegradable,nonimmunogenic and nontoxic. They can preferentially be localized in organs rich in RES.

Liposomes are spherical vesicles formed when phospholipids are confronted with aqueous media (Fig. 9). They consist of one or more concentric lipid bilayers surrounding aqueous phases. Liposomes are of particular interest since their structure bears great resemblance to of cellular membranes.

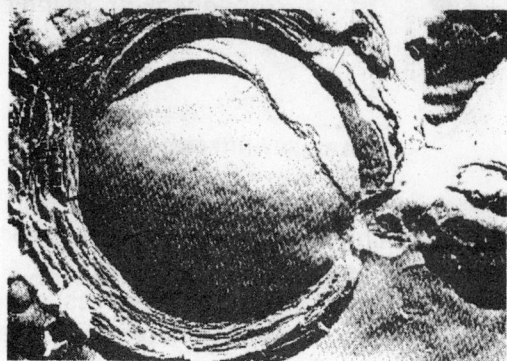

Fig. 9 : Freeze fractured SEM photomicrogarph liposomes

The event of selective and preferential localization has been considered to be of great advantages therapeutically. The vesicles are amenable to surface amelioration and target specific determinants may be attached/adsorbed as site sensing modules for navigation of the carriers. Targeting using ligand based vesicles needs great deal of bio-chemical knowledge to distinguish and to utilize the biochemical differences between normal and diseased cells in order to use them in site specific manner [31,37]. Yatwin et al suggested that local hyperthermia could successfully be utilized in preferential local drug release from liposomes [38]. In one of the approaches attempted, other than utilization of bio- chemical attributes for drug targeting was the development of magnetic microcapsules prepared by phase coacervation technique. The magnetic microcapsules demonstrated potential of active target localization at the site with the help of an external magnetic field [39].

Magnetic lipid or polymer based microspheres rely mainly on diffusional drug leakage from the carrier or on in vivo biodegradation of microsphere at a determined rate. Most of the patents discuss the intravenous administration of the magnetic microsphere or microcapsules so they circulate in capillary bed and subsequently retained there immobilized with the help of an external magnetic field until the therapeutic agent contained in the carrier system(s) is released [35,40,41].

The superdiamagnetic effect of magnetic field on one the component of liposomes vesicles was studied and the same was accounted for rapid/pulsed drug release of drug from liposomes under magnetic field. Lipid clustering which occurs at prephase transition temperature predisposes phospholipid domains to diamagnetic orientation in magnetic field and thereby facilitates drug release [42]. The preparation of magnetic liposomal vesicles and their characterization for possible use in chemotherapy of cancer has been discussed [43].

The liposomal vesicles however, are subjected to premature enzymatic attack or physical degradation and realizing the content Chang et al prepared and evaluated magnetic unilamellar liposomes based on polymerizable phospholipids [44].

The present study was aimed at preparation and characterization of polymer coated magnetic MLVs. The MLVs lamellae were coated using poly(phthaloyl-L-lysine) employing interfacial poly condensation technique (Fig. 10).

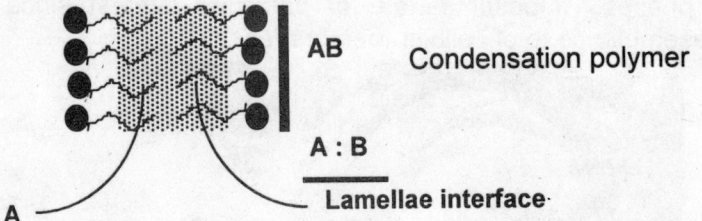

Fig. 10 : Schematic of interfacial condensation polymerisation at lipid water interfaces of liposomes

The magnetic lipid systems reported to suffer in vivo stability or under magnetic field release their contents rapidly, thus fail in generating a sustained release profile. Additionally, there are possibilities of loss of magnetic responsiveness as the diffusional permeability enhancement due to clustering of lipid component in magnetic field may allow release of magnetite as well. The developed system combines the characteristics of lipid vesicles and tere-phthalate polymer based microcapsule in magnetic field more consistent but facilitated release is expected, while during the course of size based embolization the contents would release slowly. Thus the developed MPP-MLVs system has potential of drug release modulation as well as of navigation to the target site under the effect of an external magnetic field.

MATERIAL AND METHODS

L-lysine, tere-phthaloyl dichloride, phosphatidyl choline (PC), cholesterol (CH), were used as supplied by Sigma chemical (U.K.) Methotrexate injection was obtained from Lederle Corporation. All other chemicals used were of AnalaR grade until unless mentioned and were obtained from Fluka Chem.,U.K.

EXPERIMENTAL

Preparation of MPP-MLVs: 100mg of phospholipid (PC), 50 mg of cholesterol, and 0.08 mMol of tere-phthaloyl chloride were dissolved in 2ml of chloroform in 50 ml round bottomed flask. The lipoidal solution was then dried down in to a thin film using a rotary evaporator. The solvent was removed completely leaving behind a thin film on the wall of round bottomed flask. The dried film was left rotating for 15 minutes to ensure complete removal of residual solvent. Subsequently, the film was left under the stream of nitrogen for 10 minutes. The completely dried lipid film was then hydrated using magnetite aqueous dispersion (5 ml) equivalent to 20 mg of magnetite and 1ml aqueous methotrexate solution containing 25 mg of methotrexate, at 45°C for an hour while the flask contents were layered with nitrogen to prevent possible oxidation of lipid due to atmospheric oxygen and were shaken gently to dislodge the lipids from wall of the flask. To the hydrated MLVs aqueous solution of L-lysine equivalent to 0.4 m Mol was added in order to affect interfacial polycondensation. The MLVs were shaken gently at 45°C for 3 hours. The unentrapped magnetite from MPP-MLV suspension was filtered off using millipore membrane filter (0.2 μm). The MPP-MLVs retained on filter were washed continuously using phosphate buffer saline (pH7.4) to remove free or unentrapped drug and magnetite particles. The MPP-MLVs was harvested by centrifugation at 5000 rpm for 20 minutes. The plain MLVs were prepared using the same method except in formulations, tere-phthaloyl chloride, l-lysine and magnetite were not used.

Table 4. Different formulation codes with their molar ratio

Components	MMV1	MMV2	MMV3	MPVs
DMPC	100	100	100	100
PA	----	----	10	10
Tere-phthaloyl chloride	0.08 M	0.08 M	0.08 M	----
PC	100 mg	50	50	50
Chol.	50 mg	75	80	50
Magnetite	100 mg	100	100	----
Drug	2.5 mg	25	20	20
L-lysine	0.4 M	0.4 M	0.4 M	----
Percent Drug	20	18	20.5%	10%
Magnetite	22.5	19.5	20.5%	----

Estimation of drug

Free/unentrapped drug was estimated in filtrate(s) collected of multiple washings by HPLC using BIO LAB system and employing method discussed by Azmin et al. [45]. A silica stainless steel reverse phase column (25 cm, length and 0.45 cm diameter),15% methanol in 0.5 m tris-phosphate buffer at a constant flow rate 1 ml .min-1 as mobile phase,and UV detector at wave length 303nm were used.

In order to estimate entrapped drug the MLVs prior to polymeric coating were lysed using 0.2% sodiumtaurocholate. The liberated drug on disruption of vesicles was estimated by HPLC.

Per cent drug entrapment

The drug estimated in filtrates (Df) after addition of that estimated entrapped was considered as total drug (Dt), then % drug entrapment was calculated using relation

$$\text{\% Drug Entrapment} = [Dt - Df / Dt] \times 100.$$

Estimation of magnetite

The magnetite concentration in filtrate was estimated using atomic absorption spectroscopy as suggested by Gallo et al . and difference of amount originally added for entrapment and that estimated in filtrates as free/unentrapped was considered as the amount entrapped and calculated as % entrapment based on initial weight.

Morphological characterization and size determination

The prepared magnetic liposomes and plain MLVs were observed microscopically for their shape. Average diameter of magnetic polyplied MLVs and plain PP-MLVs was determined by Malvern Master sizer.x SB.OD. The laser beam length was 14.3 nm. while the concentration of sample used was 0.012% w/w.

Magnetic responsiveness

Drug loaded magnetic polyplied MMVs evaluated for their magnetic responsiveness following the method discussed by Vyas and Malaiya [36]. MPP-MLVS suspension of known vesicles count per cubic ml was passed through a magnetic field of 8K Oe.The responsive MMVs were localized at the point of magnet application while those nonresponsive were passed through and collected in a beaker. The vesicles in suspension collected in beaker were counted and the difference from original count was considered as the number retained and used in the calculation of magnetic responsiveness.

Turbulence shock stability

The effect of turbulence shock on physical stability of the MPP-MLVs was studied by the method reported by Deloach et al. Plain MLVs and MPP-MLVs were passed through a 23 gauge needle at a flow rate of 10 ml per minute. After every pass an aliquot was withdrawn and after filtration through 0.2 μm millipore membrane, the filtrate was estimated for drug content.

Drug release profile

The MMVs and plain MLVs were studied for release profile of drug from them using dialysis sac method. Visking 8/32 dialysis tube (5cm) was filled with MPP-MLVsor MLVs suspension of known concentration and dialysed against phosphate saline buffer. *In vitro* release studies were conducted using a continuous flow appareatus as designed ans used by Ishii et al. A continuous flow rate pump to establish laminar flow at a rate ~ 0.36±2 Cm/s of 5% dextran 70 MLVs suspension through a cellulose tube 10 cm long and approximately 0.55±5 cm diameter. The cellulose dialysis tube was horizontally mounted passing through a bulk dialysing fluid, and magnetic fluid at some point. At this point magno responsive liposomes were retained releasing entrapped drug 5 FU at a rate in to dialysing fluid. The sample from dialysing fluid were withdrawn and estimated for drug content using a HPLC method. Free or plain 5 FU solution was treated similar way for release rate study. The drug release from magno responsive and plain MLVs was also characterized without the application of magnetic fluid. The content of beaker was mechanically stirred (250 rpm) continuously while the temperature was maintained at 37° C. The samples were withdrawn periodically with help of a hypodermic syringe fitted with a millipore membrane filter (0.2um).The volume withdrawn as samples was replaced by an equal volume of PBS (pH. 7.4). The release rate of drug was also determined by keeping the dialysis bag in magnetic field of various strength, i.e., 1.5, 2.0, 3.5, and 6 K Oe at different flow rates (Reno). The static magnetic fields were used by placing diamagnetic of known strength at a distance of 3 inches at either vertical sites of the dialysis tube.

RESULTS AND DISCUSSION

Multilamellar liposomes were prepared using phosphatidylcholine and cholesterol as principle vesicles components. The lipids solution in an organic solvent was taken in a round bottomed flask and the solvent was evaporated in a rotary flash evaporator leaving a thin film on the wall of the flask. The dried lipoidal film was hydrated using aqueous drug solution containing magnetite (20mg/5ml) dispersed in it, while in the case of plain liposomes hydration was accomplished using aqueous drug solution without magnetite.

The poly-terephthalamide plied multilamellar liposomes were prepared using the same procedure. However, tere-phthaloyl dichloride was added in to lipoidal solution as one of the component (0.08mM) while following hydration the MLVs were further incubated for 3 h with L-lucine (0.4mM) at 55. The addition of L lucine allowed formation of poythalamide wall on either sites of lipid domains (lipid/water interfaces). The vesicles were observed to be spherical, multilamellar and 3.5±5 μm in average diameter.

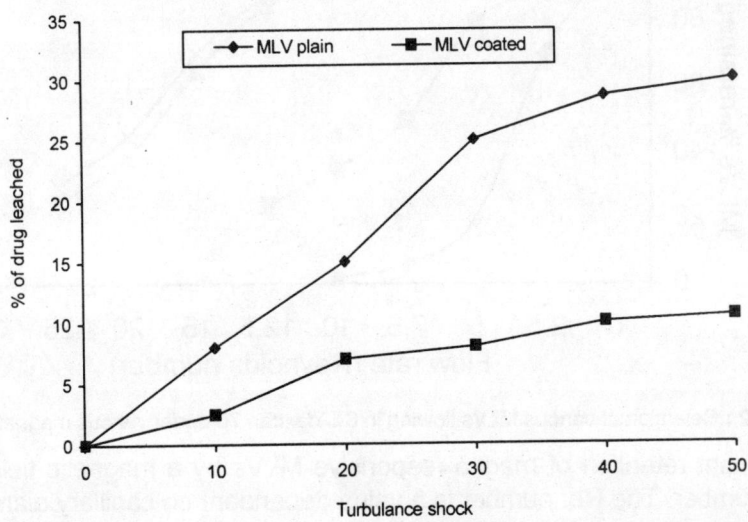

Fig. 11 : Effect of turbulance shock on stability of magno responsive liposomes

The vesicles as expected were found to be quite stable aginst physical stresses. Following 50 passes plain MLVs lost nearly 30% of the magnetite content as estimated by Atomic Absorption Spectroscopy. The polymer coated MLVs showed significant resistance to turbulance shock (Fig. 11). The percent magnetite leached out estimated to be nearly 10% after 50 passes. The values suggest significant stability improvization of MLVs following polymer coating.

The percent entrapment of methotrexate estimated in MLVs/MPP-MLVs was 18%w/w calculated on the basis of weight of methotrexate. Initially added for incorporation. The percent entrapment of magnetite in MLVs was determined to be 20% w/w of the actually added weight. The addition of magnetite at different concentration levels resulted in to products with varied magnetic responsiveness, maximum magnetic retention was recorded in the case of preparation containing 4-5% w/w of magnetite based on total liposomal component weight.

Magnetic responsiveness determined at flow rates corresponding to different Reynold's numbers in magnetic field of different strength revealed that a preparation exhibited the maximum magnetic responsiveness in a magnetic field of 6 K Oe. The percent magnetic responsiveness recorded for MPP-MLVs containing 7.5 mg of magnetite per 100 μ.mol of lipid(s) were 98.88, 90.00, 29.50 and 2.50 under magnetic fields of 1.5, 2.0, 3.5, and 6 K.Oe magnetic strength respectively.

Figure 12 shows the exhibited magnetic responsiveness by MPP-MLVs at flow rate that corresponds to Re no.10 in a magnetic field of 8 K Oe.

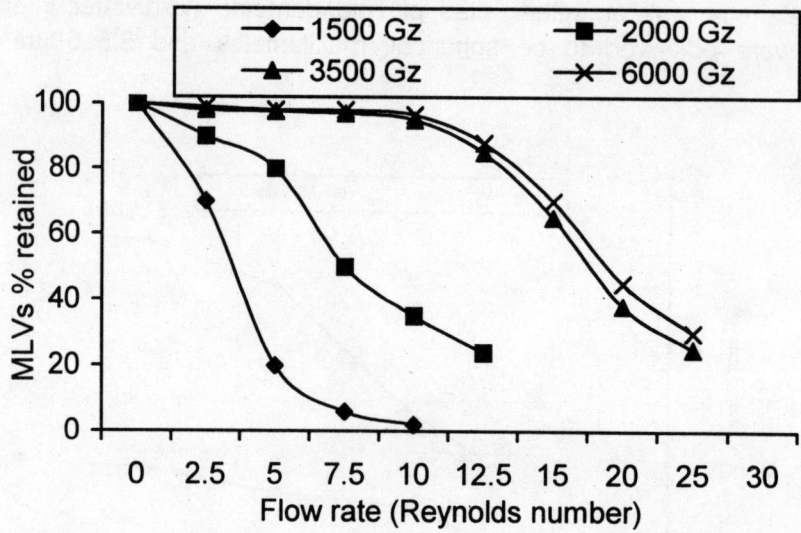

Fig. 12 : Retention of various MLVs flowing in 6% dextran 70 under various magnetic fields

The percent retention of magno responsive MLVs by a magnetic field at a varied Reynold's number. The Re. number is a value dependent on capillary diameter, density of dispersion and viscosity of medium. It is a dimensionless no. Figure 13 indicates that under a flow condition percent vesicle retention is dependent on magnetic field strength. It was also recorded that release of drug under magnetic effect was a time dependent event which increased significantly with time of magnet application. Furthermore, when magnet effect was combined with temperature a burst release at temperature near 41°C resulted (Fig. 14 & 15). This could be due to prominent clustering at near glass transition temperature resulting in to membrane defect and release of drug.

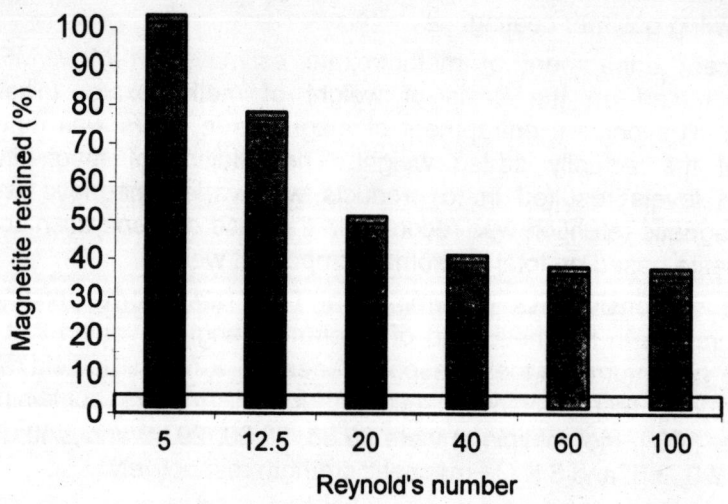

Fig. 13 : Magnetic retentivity of lipid vesicles at various Reynold's number

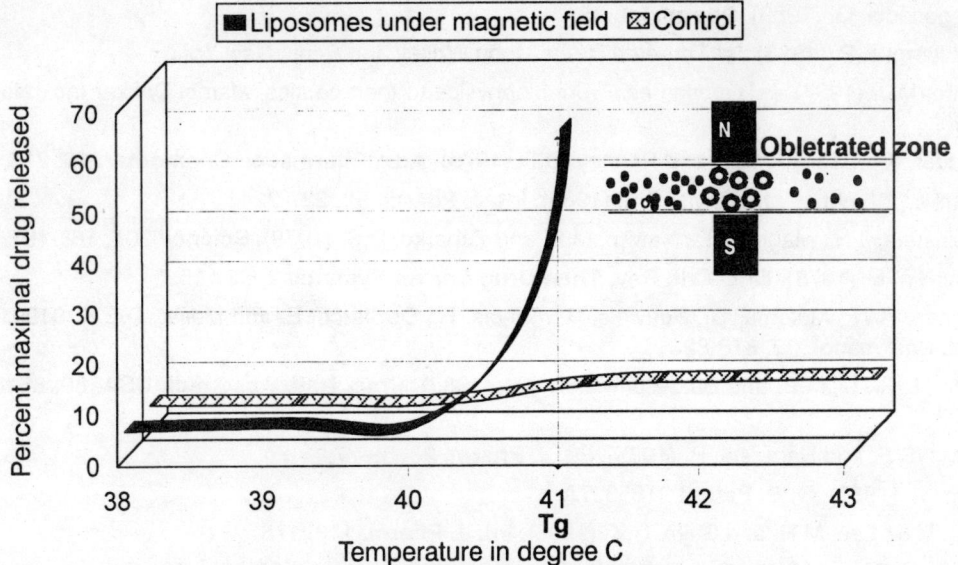

Fig. 14 : Effect of 7.5 T static magnetic field in liposome as a function of temperature

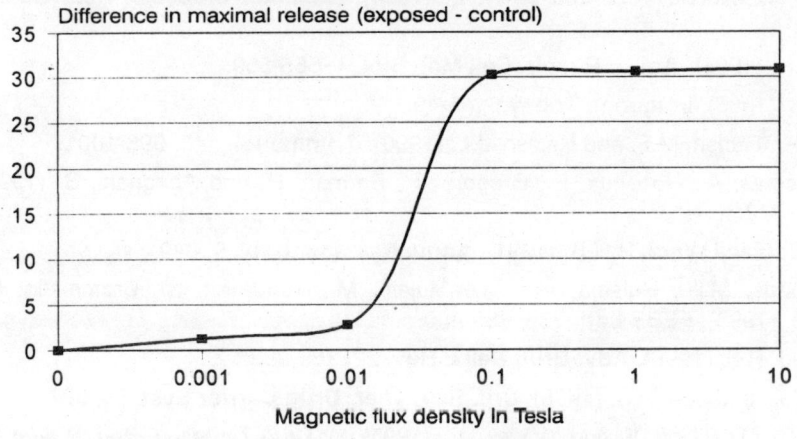

Fig. 15 : Magnetic field effect on liposome permeability at 41°C

It is therefore inferred from the study that lipid domains of MLVs can be coated with biodegradable poly tere-thalamide. The polymeric coats offer structural support to lipid membrane during clustering under magnetic field; however rapid drug release resulted. The relative agglomeration blocks flow in down stream thus embolization was negotiated with concomitant drug release. The strategy has high targeting potential and promises for chemoembolization.

REFERENCES

1. Gregoriadis, G. (1983). **Pharm. Int.** 33.

2. Goldberg, E.P. (1983). In: Targeted Drugs, John Whiley and Sons, New York.

3. Ostro, M.J. (1987). In: Liposomes: From biophysics to therapeutics, Marcel Dekker Inc., New York.

4. Widder, K.J., Senyei, A.E. and Ranney, D.F. (1979). **Adv. Pharmacol. Chemother.** 16, 216.

5. Illum, L., Wright, J. and Davis, S.S. (1989). **Int. J. Pharm.** 52, 221-224.

6. Weinstein, J.N., Magin, R.L., Yatwin, M.B. and Zaharko, D.S. (1979). **Science** 204, 188-191.

7. Torchilin, E. (1978). **CRC Crit. Rev. Ther. Drug Carrier Systems 2, 65-115.**

8. Jansen, R.W., Molema, G., Pouwels, R., Schols, R., DeClercq, E. and Meijer, D.E.K. 91991). **Mol. Pharmacol.** 39, 818-823.

9. Patel, K.R., Li, M.P. and Baldeschwieler, J.D. (1983). **Proc. Natl. Acad. Sci.** USA, 80, 6518-6522.

10. Davis, S.S. and Hansrani, P. (1985). **Int. J. Pharm.** 23, 69-77.

11. Illum, L. (1987). **G. B. Patent** 2185397A.

12. Lee, M.J., Lee, M.H. and Shim, C.K. (1995). **Int. J. Pharm.** 113, 175.

13. Molema, G. and Meijer, D.K.F. (1994). **Adv. Drug Deliv. Rev.** 14, 25-50.

14. Mosigny, M., Roche, A.C. and Bailly, P. (1984). **Biochim. Biopysic. Res. Commun.** 121, 579-584.

15. Rom, W.N. (1991). **Am. J. Respir. Cell Mol. Biol.** 4, 555-559.

16. Pernis, B. (1985). **Immunol. Today** 6, 45-49.

17. Czop, J.K., Gurish, M.F. and Kadish, J.L. (1990). **J. Immunol.** 145, 995-1001.

18. Lanzavecchia, A., Roosnex, E., Gregory, T., Berman, P. and Abrignani, S. (1998). **Nature** 334, 530-532.

19. Capon, D.J. and Ward, R.H.R. (1991). **Annu. Rev. Immunol.** 9, 649.

20. Vingerhoeds, M.H., Haisma, H.J., VanMujein, M., VandeRijt, S., Crommelin, D,J.A. and Storm, G. (1993). **FEBS Lett.** 336, 485-490.

21. Sherwood, R.F. (1996). **Adv. Drug Deliv. Rev.** 22, 269-288.

22. Reddy, J.A. and Loe, P.S. (1998). **Crit. Rev. Ther. Drug Carrier Syst.** 15, 587.

23. Burger, J.J., Tomilson, E. and McVie, J.G. (1985). In: Drug Targeting (Buri. P. and Gumma, A. Eds.), Elsevier Science Publishers, Amsterdam, New York, Oxford, pp.81-84

24. Ishii, F., Takamura, A. and Naro, S. (1984). **Chem.Pharm.Bull.** 32(2), 678-684.

25. Benoit, J.P. (1985). In: Drug Targeting (Buri, P. and Gumma, A. Eds.), Elsevier Science Publishers, Amsterdam, New York, Oxford. pp 95-117.

26. Illum, L. and David, S.S. (1985). In: Drug Targetting (Buri, P. and Gumma, A. Eds.), Elsevier Science Publishers, Amsterem, New York, Oxford, pp 65-80.

27. Goldberg, E.P., Iwlata, H., Terry, R.N., Longo, W.E., Levy, M., Lindheimer, T.A. and Cantrell, J.L. (1982). In: Affinity Chromatography and Related Techniques (Gribnau, T.C.J., Visser, J. and Nivard, R.J.F. Eds.), Elsevier, Amsterdam, pp.375-385.

28. Illum, L. and Davis, S.S. (1983). **J. Pharm. Sci.** 72, 1086.

29. Kaplan, M.R., Calef, E., Bercovici, T. and Gitler, C. (1983). **Biochim. Biophys. Acta** 728, 112.

30. Senyei, A., Widder. K.J. and Czerlinski, G. (1978) **J. Appl. Phys.** 49, 3578.

31. Widder, K.J., Senyei, A.E. and Scarpelli, D.G. (1978). **Proc. Soc.Exp. Biol. Med.** 58,141.

32. Driscoll, C.F., Morris, R.M., Senyei, A.E., Widder, K.J. and Heller, G.S. (1984). **Microvasc. Res.** 27, 353.

33. Gupta, P.K., Hung, C.T., Lam, F.C. and Perrier, D.G. (1988). **Int. J. Pharm.** 43,167.

34. Yarimoto. Y., Akimoto, M. and Yotsumoto, Y. (1982). **Chem. Pharm. Bull.** 30, 3024.

35. Ishii, F., Taktmura, A. and Ishigami, Y. (1990). **J. Dispersion Science and Technology.** 11(6), 581.

36. Malaiya, A. and Vyas, S.P. (1988). **J. Microencapsul.** 5(3), 243.

37. Jain, S.K. and Vyas, S.P. (1994). **J. Microencapsul.** 11,141.

38. Ishii, F., Takamura, A. and Noro, S. (1984). **Chem. Pharm. Bull.,** 32,678.

39. Yatvin, M.B., Weinstein, J.N., Dennis, W.H. and Blumenthal, R. (1978). **Science** 202, 1290.

40. Yoshida, H., Uesugi and Noro, S. (1980). **Yakagaku Zasshi** 100, 1203.

41. Yoshida, H., Uesugi and Noro, S. (1980). **Yakagaku Zasshi** 100, 1209.

42. Braganza, L.F., Blott, B.H., Coe, B.H. and Melville, D. (1984). **Biochim. Biophys. Acta.** 801, 66-75.

43. Liburdy, R.P. and Magin, R.L. (1985). **Radiat. Res.** 103, 266-275.

44. Chang, E.L. (1985). **US Patent** 67,579.

45. Azmin, M.N., Florence, A.T., Jandjani-Vila, R.M., Stuart, J.F.B., Vanlerberghe, G. and Whittaker, J.S. (1985). **J. Pharm. Pharmacol.** 37, 237.

12

DRUG DELIVERY CHALLENGES FOR BIOTECHNOLOGY BASED PRODUCTS

GOUR MUKHERJI

Ranbaxy Research Laboratories Udyog Vihar, Gurgaon

- Present status
- Industrial process affecting bio-tech drugs
- Oral drug delivery
- Nasal drug delivery
- Non-parenteral delivery
- Parenteral route

- Controlled drug delivery
- Various sites for protein and peptide delivery
- Targeting to specific tissues/organs
- Stability testing
- Suggested readings

PRESENT STATUS

The evolution of biotechnology and its role in commercial production of proteins and peptides with pharmaceutical applications has thrown considerable light on the challenges involved in their appropriate delivery. The first commercial production of re-combinant DNA technology based human insulin (Humulin, Lilly) in the year 1982 was the first of its kind. Subsequently, many other proteins and peptides of therapeutic value have emerged and have now become an integral part of our pharmaceutical industry.

The emergence of biotechnological products as therapeutics can be very well assessed by the fact that about 50 products comprised of 27 different molecules have been marketed in USA, Europe and Japan from 1982 to 1996. Over 1300 biotech companies in USA and 400 in Europe are conducting basic research in biotechnology. About 250 molecules are undergoing human clinical trials. Research investment in 1994 accounted to $ 7.7 billion by biotechnology companies. $ 14.9 billion were invested by traditional drug manufacturers, of which a significant percentage was devoted to biotechnology.

The delivery of these biotechnology based products is however not without any shortcomings. These biotechnology based products unlike conventional small drug molecules, are generally not therapeutically active when administered orally. An attempt is being made in this presentation to focus those areas, which demand for consideration in designing of an appropriate delivery system.

Some of the marketed biotechnology produced pharmaceuticals are presented in table 1.

INDUSTRIAL PROCESSES AFFECTING BIO-TECH DRUGS

A recent survey indicates that over 100 biotechnology based protein and peptide drugs, vaccines & monoclonal antibodies have been submitted for the approval with US-FDA.

Table 1. Marketed biotechnology produced pharmaceuticals

Product	Class
Aldesleukin	BRM
Antihemophilic Factor VIII(2)	Enzyme
Epoetin Alfa (6)	CSF
Filgrastim	CSF
Hepatitis B Vaccine (2)	Vaccine
Insulin (3)	Hormone
Interferon	BRM
Lenograstim	CSF
Liposomal Agents (5)	Liposome
Seprafilm	Surgical adjunct
Somatropin (5)	Hormone

(Values in parenthesis indicate number of products of the same molecule manufactured by different companies)

Inspite of the Goliath show of biotechnology products, they do have short comings in their process, storage, stability and formulation. This is because proteins are unstable due to hydrolytic, oxidative or thermal liability. Furthermore, there are chances of denaturation of the protein during process leading to unfolding of the protein and loss of tertiary structure.

Bio-tech products are susceptible to inactivation by various manufacturing processes. These include heating, freezing, thawing, dehydration, mechanical forces (shearing, shaking, atomization, compression) and radiation.

Physical instability of proteins and peptides

Physical instability of proteins may result in changes in the three-dimensional protein structure due to unfolding, changes in hydrogen bonding and changes in hydrophobic interactions. Globular proteins fold in such a way that the exposure of hydrophobic groups is reduced. On unfolding, they loose their globular structure and become highly susceptible to inactivation. The loss of the globular structure of proteins is referred to as denaturation.

Denaturation

Denaturation, by far, is the most extensively studied aspect of protein instability. It involves a change in the physical structure of protein rather than in its chemical composition. Denaturation can be reversible, or irreversible with reversible or irreversible functionality. Denaturation can be initiated by change in solution temperature, pH, organic solvent composition (e.g. alcohol). Some of the representative examples of denaturants are urea, salts, organic solvents, thiol reagents, guanidinum chloride, chelating agents and heavy metals.

Denaturation decreases the aqueous solubility of the protein and in addition, results in loss of biological activity, loss of crystallizing ability, alteration in reactivity of constituent groups, changes in molecular shape and susceptibility to enzymatic hydrolysis.

Aggregation and precipitation

Association of proteins to higher orders leads to aggregation, resulting in the formation of dimers, tetramers, hexamers and also macromolecular aggregates. This is an irreversible process and is primarily initiated by pH, solvent composition, ionic interaction strength, temperature and amount of denaturants. Denaturants are believed to bring about aggregation through the formation of partially unfolded intermediates, which have greater tendency to aggregate. Precipitation, which is the macroscopic equivalent of aggregation, usually occurs in conjugation with denaturation.

Surface adsorption

Surface adsorption of proteins is characterized by adhesion of proteins to surfaces. Loss of proteins and peptides by adsorption onto the walls of dosage form containers or delivery devices often referred to as "flocculation" or "frosting", is a common phenomena. The common adsorbing surfaces include polyethylene, paper, polychloride, plastic and glasswares.

A great deal of interest is presently shown in the delivery of bioactive proteins and peptides. The successful design of delivery systems for proteins and peptides depends on the understanding of their physico-chemical and biological characteristics.

ORAL DRUG DELIVERY

Among the various routes available for the delivery of therapeutic agents, the most popular route is the oral route. Oral route is the most preferred route since it is considered uncomplicated and safe. However, the oral route is not feasible for the delivery of peptides and proteins, as they have to undergo certain formulation challenges, such as:

1. degradation in the acidic environment of the stomach
2. enzymatic degradation in the small and large intestine
3. low mucosal bio-availability
4. rapid small intestinal transit
5. extensive first pass metabolism by the absorbing membrane and the liver

The oral bioavailability of most peptides and proteins accounts for less than 10% except for a few, for example thyrotropin releasing hormone, leupeptins and cyclosporine. Bioavailabilty of peptides and proteins can only be increased if they are capable of reaching the site of action in the biologically active form, which, however, needs to overcome certain barriers (Table 2).

Present research is largely focused on How to increase the effectiveness and safety of orally administered proteins and peptides? The strategies include the coating of proteins and peptides with polymer cross-linked with an azoaromatic group, complex emulsion systems, incorporation of enzyme inhibitor, etc.

NASAL DRUG DELIVERY

Anatomically, the pair of nasal cavities are separated by the nasal septum. The epithelium in the nasal cavity is covered by abundant microvilli, which provide a large surface area for absorption. The nasal mucosa is rich in vascular and lymphatic network. Nasal administration of a drug escapes first pass metabolism as the venous blood from the nose passes directly into the systemic circulation.

Table 2 . Factors that afffect protein and peptide absorption

Physiological	Physico-chemical
pH	Molecular size and shape
Digestive enzymes	Partition coefficient
Nature of the mucosal barrier	Aqueous-pH stability
Intestinal permeability and binding	Electrostatic charge
Carrier mediated transport	
Metabolism	
Dietary factors	

Generally, the intranasal route is considered appropriate for the intermittent delivery of peptides and proteins that are highly potent and have low molecular size. However, in achieving a systemic effect, this route stands next only to the parenteral route. The intranasal delivery of a peptide or protein is largely dependent on the size of the molecule. For example, metkephamid-a pentapeptide has 100% bioavailability whereas insulin with 51 amino acid residues has a bioavailability of less than 1%. In order to achieve considerable absorption by nasal route, permeation enhancers such as surfactants, bile salt derivatives, etc. are required.

A number of delivery systems have been studied for nasal delivery of peptide and proteins. Several mechanisms have been utilised to improve nasal bio-availability. These include pH modification, reverse micelle formation, alteration in membrane transport and enzyme inhibition. A representative example is the improvement in bioavailability by using glycocholate (as absorption enhancer) as displayed in table 3.

Table 3. Effect of glycocholate on bioavailability of some peptidal drugs

Molecule	# Amino acids	Bioavailability (%)	
		without	with
Glucagon	29	<1	70-90
Calcitonin	32	<1	15-20
Insulin	51	<1	10-30
Met-hGH	191	<1	7-8

COLONIC DRUG DELIVERY

The delivery of drugs and peptides by oral route to the colon has a wide and potential opportunity in the future. The enzymatic activities associated with the microflora of colon can be used as a tool for colon specific drug delivery. The large intestine has been appreciated as a promising site for the administration of poorly absorbable drug molecules for their improved bioavailability following oral administration. The colon is known to have somewhat less hostile environment with lesser diversity and intensity of enzymatic activities as compared to stomach and small intestine. In addition, the colon has a large retention time and appears to be highly responsive to agents that enhance the absorption of poorly absorbed drugs.

The absorption function of the colon has been mainly evaluated in connection with the transport of water, electrolytes and ammonia across the mucosa. However, there is no detailed study pertaining to the absorption of drug at this part of the gastrointestinal tract. Hence, the absorption mechanism is unclear. The principle route of absorption appears to be transcellular rather than paracellular.

Table 4. Advantages and limitations in colonic drug delivery

Advantages	Limitations
1. Relative lack of degradative enzymes as compared to stomach and small intestine	1. Significant protease enzyme activity
2. Low level of motility	2. Bioavailability influenced by fecal matter
3. Relative favorable pH as compared to stomach	3. Enteric formulations likely to release in the small intestine
4. High local concentration of absorption enhancers	4. Viscous contents affecting release rates; both drug dissolution and diffusion
5. GRAS absorption enhancer available	5. Diseases like diarrhoea influence colonic transit and absorption of drugs

A number of oral systems with a variety of approaches have been designed for drug release into the colon which include -

1. Prodrugs (e.g., Salicylazosulfapyridie)
2. Bioerosion of a polymeric coating which dissolves at a particular pH (e.g. Insulin coated with Eudragit LS)
3. Enzymatic degradation using the plethora of microorganism in the lower g.i.t.

NON-PARENTERAL DELIVERY

Some of the non-parenteral routes studied for their potentials in protein and peptide drug include transdermal, pulmonary, buccal, rectal and vaginal delivery.

Transdermal

The transdermal route offers a potential advantage over other routes like oral, nasal and ocular in that it has low proteolytic enzyme activity and thus forecasting a superior therapeutic and biological activity by a given peptide or protein. However, certain barriers like the lipophilic nature of the stratum corneum, the large molecular size and the hydrophilicity of proteins and peptides limit the penetration of these bioactive molecules across the skin. The delivery of peptides and proteins via the transdermal route by their simple application to the skin in a vehicle is very unlikely to produce any clinical effects. However, various approaches including the use of suitable penetration enhancers, iontophoresis and enzyme-responsive delivery systems show great promise in the future.

Various means by which the permeation of bioactives across the skin can be increased is being investigated across the globe. Once such approach is the use of penetration enhancers like dimethyl sulfoxide, azone and surfactants. Another approach involves the use of iontophoresis to delivery charged molecules into the body by an active diffusion mechanism. Delivery of insulin and Hyrotropin-releasing hormone in rats has been reported.

Recently, an enzyme-responsive transdermal delivery system for insulin delivery has been reported. Where in, the reservoir device loaded with insulin generates an electric pulse to open the skin pores, takes the blood samples, processes it using a glucose-oxidizing enzyme and accordingly adjusts the release and delivery of the appropriate quantity of insulin into the body. An other successful report involves the transdermal administration of leupiolide to normal human volunteers.

Pulmonary route

The respiratory tract consists of a nasopharyngeal region, a tracheo-bronchial region and lungs. Local delivery of conventional drugs including proteolytic and mucolytic agents, bronchodilators and sympathomimetic agents to the respiratory tract is accomplished via the airways because of their large surface area. Inspite of its advantages, this route hasn't received much attention. Only one product is available in the market. Zinc insulin crystals along with a propellant and a dispersant.

Buccal route

The buccal route has been successfully employed to deliver conventional small drug molecules to the oral mucosa for local, as well as systemic therapy. Buccal mucosa offers a much larger surface area for the placement of protein and peptide delivery systems such as buccal tablets, gels, patches, etc. Among the various non-conventional route of administration, this route offers potential advantages for its accessibility in administration. Nevertheless, the buccal route is effective for only small peptides.

Rectal and vaginal route

The mucous membrane of the rectum and vagina offers potential for absorption of soluble drugs. Conventionally, tablets, gels and suppositories, were used for administration through these sites. The vaginal route is not commonly used for systemic delivery of drugs. The vaginal epithelium consists of stratified squamous cells, which act as a barrier to absorption of drugs. The vaginal route has not been fully exploited for its potential in the delivery of bioactives. The rectum is about 15-20 cm in length and is non-motile in the resting state. The rectal route has the following advantages:

1. Avoidance of hepatic first-pass metabolism,
2. Devoid of GI irritation,
3. Large dose of drug can be administered
4. Targeting to lymphatic system can be achieved

PARENTERAL ROUTE

Parenteral route is the most effective route for the administration of bioactives, since, better therapeutic profile is achieved following administration by this route. However, the biological half-life for proteins and peptides administered by this route is very short. This leads to the repeated administration of bioactives in cases as desired. Furthermore, the potent activity of bioactives requires minimal administration at a given particular time, which might lead to quantitation and assessment of the stability, and other problems related to the formulation. In addition, administration of protein and peptides poses certain challenges during formulation which are -

1. Sensitivity to heat, radiation and chemical (gaseous) treatment
2. Presence of pyrogens / endotoxins
3. Sensitivity to pH, ionic strength, temperature and stabilizers
4. Degradation on freezing
5. Storage between 2°C and 8°C
6. Injection of diluent for reconstitution aimed at the side of the vial to present foaming and destruction of the protein
7. Reconstituted product not to be stored

The various components involved in formulation of parenteral products are:

1. **Solubility enhancers** :- e.g. lysine or arginine, sodium dodecyl sulphate
2. **Anti-adsorption/anti-aggregation agents** :- These are used to reduce adsorption of active proteins to interface. e.g. albumin, phospholipids and surfactants and optimum pH.
3. **Buffer components** :-These are included in the formulation for solubilization and stabilization.
4. **Preservatives and anti-oxidants** :- e.g. ascorbic acids, sodium formaldehyde sulfocylate, Phenyl mercuric nitrate.
5. **Osmotic agents** :- e.g, dextran, sucrose, sodium chloride

Process

1. Aseptic technique
2. Filtration sterilization (0.2 / 0.22 membrane filters) before vial filling
3. Freeze drying

Table 5. Some of the potential contaminants in recombinant protein products

Origin	Contaminant
Host related	viruses, bacteria; host derived proteins & DNA; glycosylation variants ; N- and C- terminal variants; endotoxins (from gram negative bacteria)
Product related	amino acid substitution and deletion; denatured protein; conformational isomers; dimers & aggregates; disulfide pairing variants; deamidated species; protein fragment
Process related	growth medium; components; purification reagents; metals; column materials

CONTROLLED DRUG DELIVERY

Chemical approach

Proteins and peptides are highly susceptible to hydrolysis and proteolytic degradation. This can be prevented by certain chemical modification of the protein and peptides at molecular level. The chemical modification includes carbonyl reduction, N-terminal to C-terminal cyclization and dehydro-aminoacide substitution. One promising approach to minimize proteolytic degradation is derivatization of the protein molecule into a inactive prodrug. These prodrugs acts as transient molecules and on reaching the delivery site transform into their biologically active form. However, the approach is successful only with those prodrugs, which are capable of releasing the parent compound.

Large numbers of prodrugs are of bioreversible type. Bioreversible derivatization involves functional groups such as the carboxy, hydroxyl, thiol, amino and amido groups present in amino acids and peptides. The most common approach in prodrug formation is the esterification of carboxyl, hydroxy and thiol functional groups. Esterification is widely used since the availability of enzymes for hydroloysis of these ester prodrugs are plenty.

Osmotic pumps

Drug delivery systems based on the principle of osmosis presents a strong means for controlled drug delivery. Osmotic devices have been used as implantable systems and in simple oral tablet formulations. Osmotic pumps offer many advantages over other controlled drug delivery systems.

Alza is a leading pharmaceutical concern, which developed the elementary osmotic pumps under the trade name OROS, for oral controlled release. Today a number of osmotic pumps are available. To cite a few, they are Procardia XL (Nifedipine), Acutrim (Phenyl propanolamine), Minipress XL (Prazosin), Volmax (Salbutamol), etc.

Recently, a new concept of OSMAT has come into existence. This novel system exploits the properties of hydrophilic polymers to hydrate and swell in an aqueous environment, thereby providing an intrinsic semi-permeable gel barrier across which osmotically triggered drug release could occur. Delivery of antigens by mini-osmotic pump has been recently proposed.

Approaches for controlled drug delivery are:
1) Chemical
   - polyoxyethylene glycol attachment to proteins changes circulation half-life
   - chemical modification of proteins
2) Open loop system
   - mechanical pumps for continuous infusion
   -"ALZET" and "DUROS" osmotically driven systems (ALZA's s.c. implantable minipump)
3) Closed loop systems
   - Biosensor- pump combinations
4) Protein delivery by self regulating systems
   - competition between glycosylated insulin and glucose for concanavalin A binding sites
5) Protein delivery by microencapsulated secretary cells
6) Implantation of Langerhans cells in diabetics to restore insulin production in a typical bio-feedback fashion

SITE SPECIFIC DELIVERY

Site-specific drug delivery can be defined as delivery of drugs to a specific site. Various routes of administration have been investigated to deliver proteins viz-a-viz oral, mucosal, pulmonary and transcutaneous. However, administration via these routes often requires delivery vehicles and/or permeability enhancers, which assist in the transfer across the delivery site. The deliveries of proteins and peptides have also been achieved to specific sites of action such as organs, tissues, cells and molecular targets. As in the case of route of administration, targeting to specific site too requires the aid of a delivery vehicle that relies on the specific properties of the protein or peptide to be delivered. Few examples of site-specific drug delivery are listed in table 6.

Table 6. Some examples of site-specific drug delivery

Site targeted	Comments
Route of administration	
Transdermal	Assisted by iontophoresis or ultrasound
Pulmonary	Liquid and dry-powder aerosol delivery
Mucous membranes	Aerosol-mucin charge interactions
Oral/intestinal	Small particles, protei-carrier complexes
Systemic circulation	
Injection	Prolong or sustain circulation
Specific tissues or organs	
Tumors	Neovascularization markers are targeted
Lungs	Aerosol, liposomal delivery
Brain	Target the transferrin receptor
Intestines	Protect against proteolysis and acid hydrolysis
Eyes	Mucin charge interactions
Uterine horns	Form biodegradable gel in situ
Bones	Hydroxyapatite binds bone-promoting growth factor
Skin	Methylcellulose gels
Cellular/intracellular	
Macrophages	Small particles are phagocytosed
Tumor cells	Fusogenic liposomes to deliver intracellular toxins
Molecular targets	
Tumor antigens	Antibody-enzyme conjugates activate prodrugs
Fibrin/site of clot formation	Fusion proteins combine targeting with toxin
Carbohydrate receptors	Mannose and galactose used to target receptors

The success in delivering proteins and peptides noninvasively has been modest. The challenges posed by proteins and peptides for successful delivery are well discussed earlier. In order to achieve a successful delivery, permeation enhancers have frequently been used to enhance membrane permeation and transport of unmodified proteins and peptides.

VARIOUS SITES THROUGH WHICH PROTEIN AND PEPTIDES CAN BE DELIVERED

Intestine via oral delivery

Oral delivery is the most convenient and accepted route for drug delivery. However, in the case of peptides and protein drug molecules very little success has been gained. The problems encountered in oral delivery have been discussed earlier.

The absorption of peptides and proteins following oral delivery is very little. Hence, they have to be formulated suitably so that the same can be absorbed across various passage routes across the intestinal lining especially through the Peyer's patches. Peyer's patches have been identified as a potential site for the uptake and transport of drugs, as they act as a key component in the lymphatic system of the intestines. Delivery of protein and peptide incorporated in poly(lactide-co-glycolide) (PLGA) nanoparticles in the size range of $\cong 100$ nm have been studied. Similarly, polyanhydride microspheres, which exhibited strong bioadhesive properties to the mucous lining of the intestines, have been reported. Further, it has been demonstrated that co-administration hGH with α-amino acids could significantly enhance the bioavailability of hGH. This enhanced bioavailability could be due to the complex formed between hGH and the α-amino acid which might have been responsible for passage across the epithelial lining. However, the exact mechanism is not clear.

Through mucous membrane

The high vascularity and accessibility of the mucous membranes have made this tissue a potential route for protein and peptide delivery. Mucous membranes of buccal, nasal, vaginal and rectal have been frequently investigated. Among these, nasal route has been investigated at large. Delivery through this route has been mostly attempted using aerosol. Large aerosol particles ($>10\mu m$) or drops which are capable of delivering the protein or peptidal drug through the nasal mucosa. However, in order to achieve success through this route, co-administration of permeation enhancers and protease inhibitors are recommended. Extensive and productive research in this field has led to the availability of certain marketed products which includes, buserelin, demopressin, oxytocin and calcitonin.

Vaginal delivery of calcitonin following encapsulation into esterified hyaluronic acid (Hyaff™) microspheres have been reported. Here, the microspheres adhere to the mucosal tissue by charge interactions, allowing slow degradation of microspheres and thus releasing the calcitonin slowly. Further, these microspheres protect the calcitonin from proteolytic digestion while adhering to the mucosal tissue.

Skin

Investigation for delivery of proteins and peptides through transdermal route has been studied extensively. However, the success via this route is remained limited. Few reports indicating the successful delivery of peptides and proteins are; antiflammin1, insulin, interferon γ and erythropoeitin, which were delivered with the aid of electrical charge and low-frequency ultrasound.

Lungs

Among the noninvasive routes for the delivery of proteins and peptides, the pulmonary route has been the most encouraging. This route has been proved to be attractive for the systemic delivery of peptide and protein pharmaceuticals. Delivery through this route involves the use of dry or liquid particles which are inhaled with the help of dry-powder dispersers or liquid aerosol generators or nebulizers. However, the delivery is largely size dependent. Particles of $<10\mu m$ in diameter are trapped in the nasal passages, throat, larynx and bronchial walls while those less than $5\mu m$ can penetrate deeply into the alveoli of the lungs, wherein the alveoli provide a large surface area ($80\text{-}140 \ m^2$) for rapid transfer into the pulmonary circulation. Despite several challenges in pulmonary delivery, several proteins and peptides are currently under investigation i.e., insulin, LHRH, hGH, G-CSF.

TARGETING TO SPECIFIC TISSUES/ORGANS

Tissues possess certain specific physical/chemical characteristics, which have been exploited for delivery of proteins and peptides to specific sites. Specific characteristics include elevated blood flow, selective membrane permeability overall net charge, pH conditions, receptors present on these tissues, etc.

Lungs

In addition to delivery of drugs through the lungs for systemic availability, targeting of drugs to the lungs for pulmonary disorders can be achieved. Patients suffering from cystic fibrosis have been treated with DNase, which cleaves DNA released from leukocytes that have been accumulated in the fluid of the lungs and thus helps in expelling this fluid from the lung and improves the condition of the patient. Other proteins studied in this area include cyclosporin, interferon and α-1 antitrypsin. Liposomes have been used in targeting proteins to the lungs. Targeting superoxide dismutase (SOD) entrapped in liposomes to the pulmonary epithelium has been reported. Thus, preventing tissue damage to lungs where in long-term therapy is required. Targeting of liposomes to pulmonary epithelial cells were achieved by using a surfactant protein A (SP-A). The pulmonary epithelial cells present in the lungs, express a high affinity SP-A receptor.

Intestines

Chemotherapeutic agents generally targeted to rapidly dividing cells for example, epithelial cell lining the small intestine. A recent study has shown that calcium-alginate microbeads trapped with TGF-β_1, when exposed to low pH conditions, caused the beads to shrink and prevent the release of TGF-β_1, thus, protecting the TGF-β_1 from harmful effects of lower pH. However, subsequent passage of the microbeads into the small intestine, the pH increase, leading to rapid release of TGF-β_1. The study has revealed that alginate entrapped TGF-β_1 could be delivered to the intestinal epithelial cells and inhibit cell proliferation.

Brain

Delivery of peptides and proteins to the brain is limited due to the presence of blood-brain barrier. The direct injection of protein or peptide drugs into the brain is not desirable because of the poor diffusion of these molecules in parenchymal brain tissue. However, presence of specific receptor-mediated pathway in the blood-brain barrier has paved way for site-specific delivery of proteins and peptides. Transferrin receptors are abundantly present on the vascular endothelium of brain capillaries and these receptors are internalized by the endothelial cells. This allows the blood-brain barrier to be bypassed by using transferrin or transferrin-receptor antibodies as carrier of proteins such as antibodies and neuropeptides.

Tumors

The need for large supply of blood and the demand for highly vascularized tissues to maintain the rapid growth of tumor have been considerably exploited. New-blood-vessel formation provides a general target by which drugs may be directed to rapidly developing tumors. The use of antibodies against tumor derived vascular endothelial cells have been explored to target these rapidly developing blood vessels. The subsequent injection of anti-TEC antibodies has been shown to suppress tumor growth significantly.

Uterine horns

Biodegradable hydrogels entrapped proteins have been studied to prevent post-surgical adhesions. Tissue plasminogen activator (tPA) or urokinase plasminogen activator (uPA) containing biodegradable hydrogels proved to inhibit post-surgical adhesions significantly.

1. Increase in the rate of elimination of free drug tend to increase the need for targeted drug delivery
2. Higher input of drug-carrier conjugate to maintain the therapeutic effect
3. For maximizing the targeting effect, the release of drug from the carrier should be restricted to the response compartment
4. Drugs with high total clearance are good candidates for targeted delivery
5. Response sites with a relatively small blood flow require carrier mediated transport

Liposomes

The biomedical and biotechnological potentials of the intravenously administered liposomes as drug- and gene delivery systems appear to be a success. The knowledge of the interaction of these bilayered vesicles with the bio-environment has paved the way for the advances in the rational design of vesicle constructs vis-à-vis sophisticated advances in formulation technology. With the versatility of the liposomal systems in biomedical application of the varied types, the future holds promise for more liposome-based biotechnological products in the market in the next decennia. The delivery system has achieved tremendous success in not only targeting to reticuloendothelial system (RES)-originated ailments (passive targeting) but also in RES-avoidance (inverse targeting), long circulatoery (Stealth) and ligand mediated targeting (active targeting) approaches. The table 1 outlines some of the bio-medical applications of the liposomes that are investigated in the literature. The prolonged circulation of liposomes in the circulatory system, which is essentially for targeting to sites other than RES-rich organs. This has been achieved in majority for the small vesicles (less than 50 nm) extravasate through fenestrae). However, the challenges demand for engineering an approach in order to accommodate large proteins and macromolecules in the aqueous or lipid domains as in the case of haemosomes (blood surrogate) and proteoliposomes. Larger and long circulatory vesicles could also accommodate sufficient quantities of cytokines (for immunomodulation) and genetic materials (for gene therapy). Liposomes have realized some of their potential for immunomodulation application with IRIV (Immuno-potentiating reconstituted influenza virosomes) and oral vaccines, but there is still a lot to do before their use can be optimized for the clinical trials.

Gene therapy, immunomodulation, anti-microbial and cancer therapy may attain a novel dimension.

Table 7. Potential bio-medical applications of liposomes with predicted or investigated studies

Liposome associated drug/gene/macromolecule	Route	Application	Desired attributes
Plasmid DNA, Antisense oligonucleotides	IV, IA, IM, IT, topical and oral	Gene and antisense therapy	High yield DNA incorporation, Fusogenic (cationic, virosome, pH sensitive), targeted
Haemoglobin (Hb), synthetic oxygen transporters	IV	Blood surrogates	High yield Hb entrapment, stability, long circulating
Endogenous cytokines (IL, IFN, TNF, GM-CSF) Exogenous products (lipo-polysaccharide, lipid A trehalose, muramyl-dipeptide)	IV, IM, SC, IT	Immuno-modulation	High yield incorporation, stability, controlled clearance rates, targeted
Antigens and allergen extracts	IM, SC, oral	Desensitization	High yield allergen entrapment, stability
Anticancer and antimicrobial drugs	IT	Site specific lung therapeutics	Stability as aerosols, localized targeting within the respiratory tract

STABILITY TESTING OF BIOTECHNOLOGICAL PRODUCTS

The evaluation of stability of biotechnological products may necessitate complex analytical methodologies, including bio-assays.

Selection of batches is done on the following lines.

- Drug substance (bulk material) - 3 batches
- Critical intermediates - generation of data
- Drug product (final container product) - 3 batches

Storage conditions

- Temperature - real time stability at proposed product storage temperature
- Humidity - stability data to be generated for products in humidity non-protecting containers

- Accelerated and stress conditions - Careful selection of conditions for useful support data
- Light - on a case by case basis
- Container / closure
- Stability after reconstitution of freeze dried products

Testing frequency

- Shelf life of 1 year or less proposed: real time stability for first 3 months and 3 months intervals thereafter
- Shelf life greater than 1 year: every 3 months during first year, every 6 months during second year and annually thereafter, should be studied and supportive stability profile and data should be generated.

Regulatory filing

- 6 months data for proposed storage greater than 6 months
- Case-by-case data for proposed storage less than 6 months

In regulatory requirements the proposed conditions for storage and stability behavior with supportive data are demanded. Similarly, in case of less than 6 months storage it is desirable that the product case individually be dealt and related data should be generated.

REFERENCES

1. Mize, N.K. et al. (1997) **Exp. Dermatol.** 6, 181-185.
2. Mitragotri, S., Blankschtein, D. and Langer, R. (1995). **Science** 269, 850-853.
3. Nivern, R.W. (1995). **Crit. Rev. Ther. Drug Carrier Syst.** 12, 151-231.
4. Adjei, A.L. and Gupta, P.K. (1997) Lung Biology in Health and Disease: Inhalation Delivery of Therapeutic Peptides and Proteins (Vol 107), Marcel Dekker, New York.
5. Byron, P.R. (1986). **J. Pharm. Sci.** 75, 433-438.
6. Sayani, A.P. and Chien, Y.W. (1996). **Crit. Rev. Ther. Drug Carier Syst.** 13, 85-184.
7. Bonuci, E., Ballanti, P., Ramires, P.A. Richardson, J.L. and Benedetti, L.M. (1995). **Calcif. Tissue Int.** 56, 274-279.
8. Wang, W. (1996). **J. Drug Target.** 4, 195-232.
9. Fix, J.A. (1996). **Pharm. Res.** 13, 1760-1764.
10. Desai, M.P. (1996). **Pharm. Res.** 13, 1838-1845.
11. Mathiowitz, E. et al. (1997) **Nature** 386, 410-414.
12. Delgodo, C., Francis, G.W. and Fisher, D. (1992). **Crit. Rev. Ther. Drug Carrier Syst.** 9, 249-304.
13. Pettit, D.K. et al. (1997). **J. Biol. Chem.** 272, 2312-2578

14. Sedlik, C., Perraut, R., Bonnemains, B. and Leclerc, C. (1996). **Immunobiology** 195, 105-118.

15. Nakaoka, R., Tabata, Y. and Ikada, Y. (1995) **Vaccine** 13, 653-661.

16. Nakanishi, M., Uchida, T., Sugawa, H., Ishiura, M. and Okada, Y. (1985). **Exp. Cell Res.** 159, 399-409.

17. Hirabayashhi, H., Nishikawa, M., Takakura, Y. and Hashida, M. (1996). **Pharm. Res.** 13, 880-884.

18. Pardridge, W.M. (1995). **Adv. Drug Deliv. Rev.** 15, 109-146.

19. Ohizumi, I. et al. (1997). **Biochem. Biophys. Res. Commun.** 236, 493-496

20. Mizuguchi, H., Nakanishi, M., Nakanishi, T., Nakagawa, T. and Mayumi, T. (1996). **Br. J. Cancer** 73, 472-476.

13

NEW DRUG DELIVERY SYSTEMS - RESEARCH AND TECHNOLOGY IN INDIA

AMARJIT SINGH

Vice-president,
Panacea Biotec Ltd., New Delhi

INTRODUCTION

Till recently and over the past quite a few years the number of products introduced by pharmaceutical companies in India has been only a few. The ones introduced are mainly based on simple delayed release formulations using trivial technologies. Although in the developed countries New Drug Delivery (NDD) technology development has been very significant and several advanced New Drug Delivery Systems (NDDS) have been introduced in the market. As is evident from the comparison between the World and the Indian Market figures.

The objective of the new drug delivery systems/devices is to promote the therapeutic efficacy of the drug and to minimize its toxic effects by augmenting the amount and persistence of drug in the vicinity of the target cell, while reducing the drug exposure of non-target cells. This is a system, which include altering and controlling the absorption, blood levels, metabolism, organ distribution and cellular uptake. Controlled drug delivery approaches can result in sustained, relatively constant, effective drug levels in the body, with an avoidance of undesirable saw tooth kinetics.

The current global market for NDDS products is estimated at about $ 20-22 billion, which is around seven percent of the total global pharmaceutical market. This segment is anticipated to grow at the rate of 16 percent per annum. About 50 percent of the total global NDDS sales are realized from oral controlled release products.

In the field of Novel Drug Delivery the estimate of Indian market is a part of 8% of total which it shares with many. On figurative basis it comes to be negligible to nil. Further, to drill up more to find out distinctive locus of contribution, an attempt has been made to redefine world market estimate in terms of region and segmental shares. The product categories including liposomes, monoclonal antibodies, nasal drug delivery systems, implants, transdermal systems and variable release preparations have been considered and percent of world market contribution was calculated. It was found that again India shares a negligible fraction with rest of the world estimates in terms of market wealth. While calculating taking Indian market in ablation, amazingly, the market estimate for New Drug Delivery comes to be 1.3% of total market estimate. The status ignites for a quest for cause responsible for situation hitherto. It could be realized that buying capacity of Indian is a big stigma, which presses them, compromised to an economic therapy rather preferring a convenient one.

The population proportion which even could afford for convenient therapy do not get the products for constraints which pharmaceutical units face at the floor. They include availability of basic materials, their cost composition and reproducibility characteristics. It has been realized that most of the raw materials used in development of new drug delivery systems are not easily available. In case they are imported, the cost factor increases exponentially giving a distinctive and incremental rise in product price.

Table 1. NDDS - Region wise Market (World) 1996
(All figures in US$ Million as on 1990)

S.No.	Category	Region				
		World	USA	Western Europe	Japan	Rest
1.	Total world Markets (growth % p.s.)	7065	2750	2050	1708	557
2.	% share	100	39	29	24	8

Table 2. Region wise, segment wise market estimates (World) 1996
(All figures in US $ Million as on 1990)

S.No.	Category	World	USA	Western Europe	Japan	Rest
1	Liposomes	860	356	268	184	52
2	Monoclonal antibodies	1150	495	287	276	92
3	Nasal Drug Delivery Systems	450	78	207	133	32
4	Implants	50	26	1306	705	209
5	Transdermal Systems	1160	495	302	277	86
6	Variable release products	3305	1263	938	820	284
	Total	6975	2713	2015.6	1697.5	549.9

The selection and production of a product is largely dependent on market demand. As discussed the New Drug Delivery Systems have limited target population hence they are not priority preparations for pharmaceutical manufacturers.

Furthermore, to set up a plant besides, raw material, sophisticated ancillaries and equipments their cost and availability impose another obstacles. The ancillaries include sophisticated coating equipments, polymer film coating rolls and pan, moulds, osmo drillers, electronic chips, precise vestibules and bio-sensors bio-chips, etc. The systems involve physico-chemical, biological and biomedical variables and principles in their design therefore to check upon their functionality, batch to batch variability, stability and other related parameters expertise are the utmost need. In Indian scenario, there exists a gap between academia (the source of expertise) and industries hence New Drug Delivery Systems can not conceivably be adopted. The inception of concept and its formations in to practical reality involves avoidance of patent impediment; due to poor availability of literature on patents it becomes difficult to deal with such requirements. It is needless to mention that finally to test bioequivalence or clinical efficacy as per FDA requirements only a few institutions competent. This imposes another barrier to New Drug Delivery Systems for clinical use. A fundament question arises in regard to the relevance of clinical evaluation. It is obvious that in cases where a good correlation exists between plasma level(s) and clinical response, the plasma concentration may be relies upon. However, where therapeutic effects are induced or where irreversible toxicity occurs or where functional tolerance is one of the possibility or where peak, trough levels differences are large or where some other reason for no relation between plasma levels and clinical effects, it is imperative or will probably be necessary to carry out clinical studies for FDA approval. Thus need of such laboratories, in the development of NDDS could be realized and focus of attention may therefore be placed on them equivocally [1].

Table 3. Market Estimates for Controlled Delivery Systems (India)
(Values Rs. in Crores) [2].

S.No.	Item	1990	1996
1	Total indigenous drug market	3300	7700
2	Market for new delivery systems	15 (0.45%)	100 (1.3%)
3	**Individual systems**		
	Liposomes	- -	15
	Mab	- -	17.5
	Nasal systems	- -	4
	Implants	- -	0.5
	TDS	- -	11.5
	VR products	14.3	50

There are several factors responsible for this gap between the Indian and the global market, e.g.,

1. The market needs in India have traditionally been economic therapies and not convenience therapies
2. Lack of availability of advanced polymers and raw materials
3. Lack of ancillary specialized equipment's e.g. precise coating machines,
4. Gap between academic research and industrial product development
5. Poor access to research and patent literature

6. Inadequate facilities to demonstrate bio-equivalence/clinical efficacy due to lack of international standards.

However, the scene is changing very fast and recently a number of pharmaceutical manufactures have chosen NDD as a thrust area of research. The buying power in Indian market is increasing so convenience therapies are being seen as potential products. Industry-academia relationships are being established, many performance excipient, polymer and other raw materials manufactures have opened Indian outlets, large number of scientists are visiting international meetings, exhibitions, etc. and the establishment of internet, e-mail and access to international databases on Pharmaceutical and Medical Research and Patents has made to easy for the scientists to be up-dated on issues.

The continual research all over the globe made liposomes a clinically acceptable strategy for leishmaniasis. Likewise many more liposomal products with added values and therapeutic characters are likely to come in world market. An assortment of such products under various phases of clinical trials is presented in table 2. Liposomes as accessory artificial cells in manipulating immune response have proven great potential. Being the liposomal vaccines safe and effective in performance re going to be clinical reality of future.

Our company's efforts on above line exemplifying how NDD research can be converted into a business opportunity. Our company introduced a Transdermal Gel of Nimesulide for the first time and a Microemulsion based delivery system for cyclosporine. The company grew consistently in turnover from 43.63 Cr. (1994-95) to 60.50 Cr. (1995-96) to 91.9 Cr. (1996-97) and R&D expenditure from about 1 Cr. (1994-95) to 6.97 Cr. (1996-97).

Several other NDD systems are at an advanced level of development in our laboratories, their development, clinical trials, patenting issues and marketing have been planned to support a consistent growth in business of the company and make it strong force not only in Indian but even global market environment even after 2005 when IPR and patent issues are in force.

The different types of NDDS are [4]

- Transdermal Drug Delivery Systems
- Transmucosal Drug Delivery Systems (Buccal Strips)
- Implantable Drug Delivery Systems
- Nasal Drug Delivery Systems
- Oral Controlled Release Drug Delivery Systems (Osmotic pumps, ion exchange)
- Liposomes & other targeted drug delivery systems (Nanoparticles, Niosomes, etc.)

In order to overcome patient compliance barrier the variable release products, which mainly include osmotic pumps, are significant members of NDDS.

In conclusion there are many areas where R & D work has to be carried out and there is a lot of potential for development work.

Table 4. Liposome based products developed or under development [3].

System*	Drug	Target disease	Status	Product
Liposomes *(Intravenous)	Nystatin	Systemic fungal Infections	Phase II	Aronex, USA
Liposomes *(Intravenous)	All-trans retinoic acid	Leukemia	Phase II	Aronex, USA
Liposomes *(Intravenous)	Anamycin	Kaposi's sarcoma Refractory breast cancer	Phase II/III Phase I/II	Aronex, USA
Novasome *(Intramuscular)	Newcastle disease virus	Newcastle disease (Chicken)	Licensed by USDA	Vineland, USA
Novasome *(Intramuscular)	Avion retrovirus	Vaccination of breeder chickens	USDA	Vineland, USA
Liposomes (AmBisome) *(Intravenous)	Amphotericin B	Systemic fungal infections, Visceral leishmaniasis	Approved in 18 countries including Europe & USA	NeXstar, USA
Liposomes (DaunoXome) *(Intravenous)	Daunosome	Advanced Kaposi's sarcoma Breast and other solid tumors	Approved by FDA in UK and Sweden Phase II	NeXstar, USA
Liposomes (VincaXome) *(Intravenous)	Vincristine	Solid tumors	Under preclinical development	NeXstar, USA
Liposomes (MiKasome) *(Intravenous)	Amikacin	Serious bacterial infections	Phase II	NeXstar, USA
Novasome (Eschewrichia coli 0157:H7) *(Oral)	E coli 0157:H7 (killed)	E coli 0157 infections	Phase I	Novavax, USA
Novasome (Shigella flexneri 2A vaccine) * (Oral)	Shigella flexneri 2A	Shigella flexneri 2a infections	Phase I	Novavax, USA
Liposomes (Doxil) *(Intravenous)	Doxorubicin	Kaposi's sarcoma Refractory tumors	Approved by FDA Phase II	SEQUUS, USA
Liposomes (Amphocil) *(Intravenous)	Amphotericin B	Systemic fungal infections	Approved in UK, Russia, Finland, Ireland & Europe	SEQUUS, USA
Liposomes (D99) *(Intravenous)	Doxorubicin	Metastatic breast cancer	Phase III	The Liposome Company, USA

(Contd.)

Liposomes (ABLC) *(Intravenous)	Amphotericin B	Systemic fungal infections	Approved in UK	The Liposome Co., USA
Liposomes (D53) *(Intravenous)	Prostaglandin E_1	Systemic inflammatory diseases (ARDC, AMI, SEPSIS/SIRS)	Phase II	The Liposome Co., USA
IRIV liposomes (Epaxal-Berna vaccine) *(Intramascular)	Inactivated hepatitis A virions	Hepatitis A	Approved in Switzerland	Swiss Serum & Vaccine Institute, Switz.
IRIV liposomes (Trivalent influenza vaccine) *(Intramascular)	Haemagglutinin /neuraminidase from approved influenza strains	Influenza	Phase III	Swiss Serum & Vaccine Institute, Switz.
IRIV liposomes (HAV/HB-IRIV combined vaccine) *(Intramascular)	Genetically engineered hepatitis B antigens (HAV)	Hepatitis A and B	Phase I	Swiss Serum & Vaccine Institute, Switz.
IRIV liposomes (Diphtheria/ tetanus/hepatits A combined vaccine) *(Intramascular)	Diphtheria and tetanus toxoids; inactivated HAV virions	Diphtheria, tetanus and hepatitis A	Phase I	Swiss Serum & Vaccine Institute, Switz.
IRIV liposomes (Hepatitis A & B/ Diphtheria/ tetanus/hepatits A combined vaccine) *(Intramascular)	Inactivated HAV virions; Diphtheria and tetanus toxoids	Hepatitis A and B, diphtheria, tetanus and influenza	Phase I	Swiss Serum & Vaccine Institute, Switz.

Abbreviations: Novasome = Non-phospholipid pausilamellar vesicles; IRIV = immunopotentiating reconstituted influenza virosomes

Gradation of NDD systems

1. Criteria
2. Market potential/product performance reliability
3. Ease of technology development and up-scaling
4. Development time
5. Cost of R & D, scale-up, machinery
6. Availability of clinical trials/Bioequivalence studies facilities

PHARMACEUTICAL RESEARCH IN INDIA

Since independence, Indian pharmaceutical industries have grown significantly. It had followed a typical growth pattern starting with trading activities, moved on to repackaging and marketing, further shifted to manufacture and distribution and further on the manufacture of bulk drugs primarily to meet captive and domestic requirements and finally moving in to the exports of both bulk drugs and formulation to the developed countries [5].

In India, so far, not much effort has been directed in the area of NDDS. The sole and significant example that can be cited here, is the recent licensing arrangement between Ranbaxy and Bayer AG for the development of a once-a-day dosage form of ciprofloxacin.

With the opening up of the economy and enforcement of GATT (General Agreement on Trade and Tariff) agreement, Indian pharmaceutical industry would face the challenge of increasing focus on international pharmaceutical companies in the sub-continent. In this context, many of the Indian pharmaceutical companies are gearing themselves up for being truly international generic companies especially for the advanced countries practicing stringent regulatory guidelines. Some of these Indian companies have also initiated research in the area of new drug discovery and delivery in order to come true India based research companies. It include Ranbaxy, Torrent, Zydus-Cdila, SPARC, Wockhardt, Dr. Reddy's Laboratories, Orchid, Panacea Biotec etc. However, they are faced with the dilemma of huge R&D investment and long gestation period before they hit the successful drug condidate.

NDD systems of potential market value in India

1. Variable release products (Osmotic pumps, Liquid SR products for children)
2. Liposomes (Anticancer, Antifungal drugs)
3. Microemulsions
4. Nasal Delivery Systems (Peptide drugs)
5. Transdermal systems
6. Transmucosal systems (Buccal, Oesophagal delivery systems)
7. Implants (Microsphere based CR vaccines, hormones, etc.)

Similarly, for the treatment of dreaded diseases, which provide no choice for therapy option, the liposomal preparations have great potential. Adding to promising systems is microemulsion, which claims for improvised therapeutic indices of drug substances, which are otherwise poorly available on oral administration. Nasal drug delivery particular of peptidal drug(s), which for well identified reasons, can not be administered through conventional oral route, presents therapeutical promises. The systems not only offer patient compliance but also produce better clinical pharmacodynamic effects. Likewise, systems, which ensure for localized as well as better systemic availability of drug, are mucoadhesives for buccal applications. They may be effective drug delivery tool in safe and effective delivery of proteinaceous drugs. Implants which ensure for protracted and effective therapeutic performances especially for drugs like anti tuberculosis agent, anti fertility agents or vaccine could be the most preferred posteriority of NDDS [6].

The areas in which research is being carried are as :

1. Basic research at cellular and molecular level
2. Formulation development work
3. Polymer synthesis and standardisation to suit individual needs

Account of status in regard to NDDS dealing with raw material requirement, their availability, formulations which are under developmental stages, machinery required and their availability vis a via technological knowledge in terms of technical knowledge are given in table 5.

Table 5. Technology status with respect to above types of NDDS in India is summed up as follows:

Drug Delivery System	Raw Materials	Formulation	Machinery	Mfg. Technology
Transdermal drug delivery systems	Polymers, backing membranes, plasticizers, release control membrane (imported)	Several labs working on different drugs	Indigenous machines not available	Dormant because of resources constraints
Liposomes	Phospholipids - imported	Lab. Scale techniques available	Lab. Scale available comm. scale to be imported	Not established (one product tech. transferred - Amphotericin B)
Implants	Some polymers available, others to be imported	Simple systems available. Programmable under development	Not available	Not available
Aerosols	MDI actuators still being imported	Well-established. Although restricted to some companies	Available	Available
Nasal delivery systems	NA	NA	NA	NA
Microspheres, Microcapsules	Some polymers available rest imported	Formulation know-how exists	Established to limited extent	Not well established
Osmotic pumps	Some polymers available, rest imported	Formulation technology available	Not available	Not well established
Mab	Mabs available only on lab scale	Little attention on formulation. Only basic research. Lack of coordination	Not available	Not well established

In India there are packets of excellence where commendable work is in progress. The spectrum of work they are specialized in, institutions and places of their laboratories are given table 6.

Table 6. The following are major labs where the R & D work is under progress [7]

Central Drug Research Institute, Lucknow	Liposomes of antitubercular drugs. Transdermal tapes, implants, oral systems
Indian Institute of Chemical Biology, Calcutta	Plant glycosides for DDS. NDD for leishmaniasis treatment
Dept. of Biochem. Univ. of Delhi	Liposomes, Recombinant toxins
Cancer Research Institute,	Liposomes of anticancer drugs
Dept. of Pharm. Sciences, Univ. of Saugar	Liposomes, osmotic pumps, virosomes, niosomes and nanoparticles.
Institute of Microbial Technology, Chandigarh	Macromolecular congrugates
Central Leather Research Institute, Chennai	Transdermal, Microencapsulation
Bombay College of Pharmacy, Mumbai	Transdermals, Spheronisation, Hydrogels
University Department of Chemical Technology, Mumbai	Polymers, Transdermal, Microencapsulation, ion-exchange, bioadhesive polymers
All India Institute of Medical Sciences, New Delhi	Implants, Liposomes
University Institute of Pharm. Sci., Panjab University	Matrix tablets
National Chemical Laboratory, Pune	Microencapsulation, polymers
Shri Chitra Tirunal Medical Res. Inst., Trivandrum	Microspheres
National Institute of Immunology, New Delhi	Controlled release vaccines
CU Shah College of Pharmacy, Mumbai	Rectal Delivery
Bhabha Atomic Research Centre, Mumbai	Radiation cured polymers systems
College of Pharmacy, Manipal	Niosomes in Cancer Chemotherapy
KMK College of Pharmacy, Mumbai	Oral and Transdermal systems
B.V. Patel PERD Centre, Ahmedabad	Oral, Ophthalmic and implants

Now that we are aware of the needs of R & D of NDDS in India, for commercialisation of the laboratory level research, it is recommended that industry-academic interaction be formalised. The successful development of NDDS will be dependent on successful teaming up of multidiscipline scientists.

REFERENCES

1. Jones, T.M. (1989). Improved drug delivery: A perspective from industry. In: Novel drug delivery and its therapeutic application. (Presscott, I.F. and Nimmo, W.S. Eds.), John Wiley and Sons, Chichester, pp.23-31.

2. Technology in New Drug Delivery Systems. A status report prepared under the National Register of Foreign Collaborations, October 1992, Department of Science & Technology, New Delhi.

3. **Trends in Biotechnology** (1995). 13, 527.

4. Skelly, J.P. (1989). Drug regulation and novel drug delivery systems. In: Novel drug delivery and its therapeutic application. (Presscott, I.F. and Nimmo, W.S. Eds.), John Whiley and Sons, Chichester, pp.341-351.

5. Singh, P. (1994). **Eastern Pharm.** 17-22.

6. Breimer, D.D. (1989). Drug delivery and therapeutics in the future. In: Novel drug delivery and its therapeutic application. (Presscott, I.F. and Nimmo, W.S. Eds.), John Whiley and Sons, Chichester, pp.353-355.

7. Singh, A. (1998). New drug delivery systems: Research and technology in India. In: Programs and proceedings of first symposium on advances in technology and business potential of new drug delivery systems. Mumbai, pp.130-135.

14

USE OF LIPOSOMAL CHELATING AGENTS IN THE AMELIORATION OF HEAVY METAL INTOXICATION

JAI RAJ BEHARI
Industrial Toxicology Research Centre
P.Box 80, Mahatma Gandhi Marg Lucknow 226 001

- Introduction
- Experimental

- Results and Discussion
- References

INTRODUCTION

Cadmium is recognised as a toxic metal due to its increasing environmental or occupational exposure to humans [1]. As a result of chronic exposure to cadmium renal tubular dysfunction's have been reported in animals as well as in human [2]. After its entry into the body cadmium is transported initially bound to albumin and other proteins and reaches liver, where cadmium gets released from this protein. The released cadmium induces the synthesis of metallothionein in liver. Most of cadmium is subsequently sequestered by this protein [3]. A small portion of metallothionein bound cadmium is released into plasma and gets transported through glomerular membrane brush border of the proximal tubules and reaches lyposomes where metallothionein is split from cadmium which becomes the toxic principle in the cell [4]. Capacity of synthesising metallothionein by renal cells determines the fate of kidney damage/nephrotoxicity of cadmium. Administration of chelating agents is so far the most effective management of heavy metal poisoning. The treatment with chelating agents is effective in cadmium intoxication specially if given soon after exposure [5]. The same chelators are not effective in cases of often prevalent chronic exposure to cadmium. The chelating agents being hydrophilic in nature get excreted rapidly and large doses are required to be administered. This results in their toxicity and imbalances of trace metals in the body since they also bind with chelating agents and get excreted from the body. Further treatment of cadmium poisoning is limited due to the inability of chelating agents to reach and mobilize cadmium from its intracellular storage sites as hydrophilic chelating agents are excreted rapidly [6].

Liposomal encapsulation of a variety of drugs has been shown to be an attractive method for the delivery of drugs to the intracellular sites. Liposomes protect these drugs from inactivation or premature loss before they reach the target organ, thereby enhances their efficacy [7]. Earlier work on tissue distribution of free and liposomal EDTA has already demonstrated higher uptake and prolonged retention of this chelating agent in the tissues [8].

Among chelating agents used diethylene-triamine-pentaacetic acid (DTPA), triethylene-tetramine hexaacetic acid (TTHA), meso-2,3-dimercaptopropanesulfonate (DMPS) and N-benzyl-D-glucamine dithiocarbamate (NBGDTC) have exhibited an increased potential for mobilization of cadmium from the body of exposed animals [9-12].

Experiments were carried out using chelating agents encapsulated in liposomes to examine their potential in mobilizing cadmium from the body of exposed animals. Role of different size of vesicles and lipid composition was examined and their potential as carrier for different chelating agents was evaluated in terms of cadmium mobilization.

EXPERIMENTAL

DTPA containing liposomes were prepared by the method based on induction of fusion of preformed vesicles by means of dehydration and controlled rehydration [13]. DTPA retention by DRV liposomes on incubation with mouse plasma was examined. Although liposomal formulations were used immediately after their preparation, it was found that 93-95% of the entrapped DTPA in liposomal preparations remained associated with vesicles upto 30 days storage. After incubation with plasma at 37°C for 1 hr. more than 90% of the chelator was retained by the carrier and the retention was reduced to 80% after 3 hr. of incubation. DTPA, free or liposome encapsulated, was administered intravenously to mice (control as well as those preexposed to cadmium, 0.01 mmol/kg, two injections given i.p. at an interval of 48 hrs. in vivo). Kinetics of DTPA (radiolabelled) was examined by withdrawing blood from tail vein daily for 3 days. Cadmium exposed animals treated with DTPA were sacrificed for their tissue mobilization of cadmium and compared with respective controls. Tissue levels of cadmium were assayed after acid digestion and atomic absorption spectrophotometry. Uptake of liposomal DTPA by tissue after i.v. injection as adjudged by the DTPA radioactivity data showed that 24h. After injection the level of DTPA in liver of normal mice was 15% of injected dose, while the corresponding value in cadmium loaded mice was 63%. It thus seems that DTPA injected into cadmium loaded mice binds to metal and its excretion is thereby delayed. Similar pattern of retention of DTPA was also observed upto 24 h in liver and spleen. In comparison the levels of DTPA in the liver and spleen of mice treated with the free chelator were practically nil in both normal or cadmium exposed animals at 24 h. On the other hand small amount of DTPA in kidney of both groups had more of chelator in free form. The pattern upto 72 h showed a higher retention of chelator in all the organs examined when given in the liposome encapsulated form [13].

Cadmium chelation by DTPA was examined by measuring cadmium levels in tissue and its excretion in urine and feces. Both liposomal DTPA and free DTPA removed cadmium from liver, lung and spleen of cadmium exposed animals. The liposomal DTAA however, showed slightly better efficacy. In the blood a different pattern of action was observed throughout the period of 72 h following chelator injection where as the levels of cadmium were generally lower in animals given liposomal DTPA than those administered free DTPA. Excretion of cadmium in urine and feces was significantly higher in liposomal DTPA treated animals (compared to free DTPA treatment). From these results it could be suggested that the treatment of cadmium poisoning with liposomal DTPA would present the kidney with lower concentration of cadmium for clearance thereby reducing the nephrotoxicity of the metal due to longer retention of cadmium in the body organs by virtue of its strong binding with metallothionein. Our experiments with dehydration rehydration vesicles having larger size might also be limiting the chelator entry into the cells thereby restricting the availability of chelator, which is also hydrophilic [13].

Effect of liposome encapsulated meso-2,3-dimercaptosuccininc acid (DMSA) was further examined on biochemical and trace metal alteration in cadmium exposed rats. DMSA was encapsulated in egg phosphatidyl choline and cholesterol (1:1) dehydration rehydration vesicles prepared as already described. Male albino rats preexposed to cadmium (0.2 mg/kg intraperitoneally daily for 3 days) followed by treatment with DMSA (30 µmole/kg intravenously) were examined for the activity of r-Glutamyltranspeptidase (rGT) in kidney and alkaline phosphatase in serum and urine. Cadmium, copper and zinc concentrations were determined in organs. r-GT a renal brush border enzyme and marker of kidney damage was inhibited. Serum alkaline phosphatase was lowered and its levels in urine increased by cadmium treatment. DMSA treatment after exposure to cadmium was able to restore the level of r-GT in kidney. Liposomal DMSA restored the levels of kidney/serum and checked the enzyme elimination via urine more efficiently. There was also better restoration of trace metal levels (Cu and Zn) in the organs (liver, kidney and spleen) by treatment with liposomal DMSA compared to free DMSA. The results on mobilization of cadmium from the body organs were however not so encouraging which may be attributed to the larger size of the vesicles [14].

In order to potentiate the efficacy of DMSA by attempting its targeted delivery in the biological system for mobilization of stored cadmium deposits. DMSA was encapsulated in small unilameller vesicles and then administered to mice pre-exposed to cadmium. Liposomes composed of egg PC and cholesterol were prepared by making thin film hydrated with DMSA solution followed by sonication procedure using a probe sonicator for 3 min x 1 min. rest for 10 cycle and gel filtration of the material on sephadex G-75 column. Small unilameller vesicles so produced entrapped 8-9% DMSA which was administered to mice which had earlier received 0.5 mg/ Cd/kg along with 109-CdCl$_2$. Distribution of radioactive cadmium as examined in body organs, including liver, kidney, testis, spleen as well as in the low and high molecular weight protein fractions of liver. Results showed that injections of DMSA led to mobilization of cadmium from the liver with liposome en-capsulated DMSA exhibiting significantly enhanced efficacy compared to the free material. Elimination pattern form protein fractions was also of similar order. Cadmium was removed from both high as well as low molecular weight protein frac-tions by free DMSA, while DMSA encapsulated in liposomes was more efficient in cadmium mobilization from the low molecular weight protein fraction. Injection of DMSA (Free) led to a 20 fold increase while liposomal DMSA resulted in 32 fold inc-rease in urinary cadmium excretion monitored over a period of 7 days. A delayed and less effective response by free DMSA compared to enhanced fecal elimination of cadmium throughout the period of treatment was observed by liposomal DMSA [15].

The intracellular delivery of chelating agents becomes an important factor in the treatment of cadmium poisoning. The enhanced elimination of cadmium via the feces was observed as a result of treatment with liposome encapsulated delivery of DMSA.

Influence of size of liposomes and the role of liposomal lipid composition was examined in potentiating the efficacy of triethylene-tetramine-hexaacetic acid (TTHA) against cadmium intoxication. TTHA was encapsulated in small unilameller vesicles (SUVs) or dehydration rehydration vesicles (DRVs) and its effect was examined in amelioration of cadmium toxicity. Mice were administered cadmium (0.2 mg/kg body wt.) as $CdCl_2$ intraperitoneally daily for 5 days. After a period of four weeks rest, they were given two intravenous injections of TTHA as free material or encapsulated in liposomes (0.16 mmole/kg) at a gap of 48 hours. Urinary and fecal elimination of cadmium and its distribution in the liver, kidney and spleen was monitored after TTHA treatment. The results of the present investigation reveal that administration of SUV-TTHA was most effective in mobilizing cadmium from liver, kidney and spleen of cadmium exposed animals followed by DRV-TTHA and free TTHA (Table 1). Enhancement in excretion of cadmium through urine and its elimination via feces was also observed by all the three treatments. Relatively highest cumulative excretion of cadmium by SUV-TTHA treatment was in correlation with the pattern of cadmium mobilization from the body organs [16].

Table 1. Effect of TTHA encapsulated in liposomes (DRV or SUV) on the mobilization of cadmium from the body organs of preexposed mice

Treatment	Liver	Kidney	Spleen
Cd-Sal	20.4±0.81	17.85±0.41	3.87±0.20
Cd-TTHA	14.07±0.67*	15.18±0.72*	2.60±0.51
Cd-TTHA via DRV	12.81±0.56*	14.21±0.92*	2.33±0.19
Cd-TTHA via SUV	9.19±0.51*+	12.92±0.59*	1.76±0.26*

Cadmium content expressed as ug/g fresh tissue.
Each value represents mean ±SE of six animals.
*p<0.05 when compared to cadmium saline.
±p<0.05 when compared to cadmium TTHA..pa.

The higher efficacy of SUV-TTHA may be due to the fact that the higher curvature of smaller liposomes gives rise to a lower surface pressure than that of larger liposomes making them more stable and available for circulation in blood for longer duration [17]. Further studies were conducted involving modulation in composition of liposomes. In this study mice were injected with cadmium as cadmium (II) chloride (0.5 mg/kg b.wt.) intraperitoneally daily for five days. Four weeks after the last injection of cadmium they were administered three injections of TTHA encapsulated in liposomes composed of either phosphatidyl choline: cholesterol (TTHA-PC-Lip) or sphingomyelin:cholesterol (TTHA-SM-Lip) in 1:1 molar ratio at a gap of 48 h. Urinary and fecal elimination of cadmium and its distribution in liver, kidney and spleen were examined.

The mobilization of cadmium by TTHA as free drug, TTHA-PC-Lip or TTHA-SM-Lip from Liver, kidney and spleen of cadmium loaded mice is shown in Table 2 Free TTHA treatment significantly removed cadmium from liver and kidney compared to saline treated group. Treatment with TTHA-PC-Lip or TTHA-SM-Lip mobilized higher amount of cadmium from liver and mobilized cadmium from spleen also but these treatments were not so effective in removing cadmium from kidneys. The efficacy for mobilization of cadmium from liver and spleen was maximum by TTHA-SM-Lip treatment. Distribution of cadmium in hepatic and renal metallothionein was also examined in different treatment groups. The results indicated that the reduction in cadmium content in metallothionein was in the order TTHA-SM-Lip>TTHA-PC-Lip> free TTHA>N-Saline treatment. Significant enhancement in the cumulative excr-etion of cadmium via feces was observed by TTHA-SM-Lip (2.48 fold) compared to saline treatment over a period of eight days. TTHA-PC-Lip (1.9 fold) or free TTHA (1.4 fold) were less effective. in removing cadmium from feces. Cumulative excretion of cadmium from urine exhibited similar pattern. The enhanced removal of cadmium through urine and feces indicates increased availability of TTHA to intracellular cadmium. The Cadmium-TTHA complex formed may get removed both through urine as well as through bile/feces since TTHA is delivered via liposomes [18].

Table 2. Effect of TTHA encapsulated in liposomes on the mobilization of cadmium (μg/g) in the body organs of cadmium exposed mice

Treatment	Liver	Kidney	Spleen
n-Saline	ND	ND	ND
Cd-Saline	21.56±0.94	18.43±0.89	3.81±0.37
Cd-TTHA	18.56±1.00[a]	2.06±0.95[b]	3.56±0.58
Cd-TTHA via DRV	16.84±0.83[b]	14.39±1.18[a]	2.31±0.16[a,d]
Cd-TTHA via SUV	14.16±0.59[c,e]	14.88±0.76	1.33±0.08[e]

The value are expressed as mean ±SE of 5 animals
a) $p<0.05$; b)$p<0.01$; c)$p<0.001$ compare to cd-saline; d)$p>0.05$; e) $p<0.001$ compared to Cd-TTHA

Lipid composition of liposomes plays an important role in their delivery to the target sites. Enhanced removal of cadmium from liver and spleen by TTHA-SM-Lip clearly exhibits that it increases the availability of the chelator at the site of cadmium accumulation. It is also known that cadmium gets accumulated in hepatic parenchymal cells [19]. The enhanced delivery of liposomes having sphingomyelin in their composition to parenchymal cells in liver has also been demonstrated [20]. This could be responsible for enhancing the efficacy of TTHA in removing cadmium from liver and spleen when administered as TTHA-SM-Lip. These results are consistent with enhanced mobilization of cadmium from MT and its enhanced elimination via feces. The removal of cadmium from kidney shows that TTHA is reaching kidney more in hydrophilic form since free TTHA mobilized more cadmium compared to liposome encapsulated forms. These results suggest that modulation of liposomes composition could be helpful in the delivery of the chelating drug to the target sites.

In order to target liposomes to the parenchymal cells, the storage site of cadmium, attempt was further made to prepare targetable liposomes and deliver DMSA through these carriers. Evidence exists that ß galactoside residues or mannoside residues present on the surface of liposomes can bring about selective uptake of liposomes by parenchymal cells or non parenchymal cells respectively [21]. It was attempted to deliver DMSA to these cadmium storage sites for mobilization of cadmium in a target specific manner using galactosylated liposomes as carriers. DMSA encapsulating liposomes composed of egg PC, chlestrol and phosphatidylethanolamine (7:2:1) were prepared by sonication procedure to obtain small unilamellar vesicles. After separation of unencapsulated material liposomes were incubated at 20°C for 20 min with 15 mM concentration of glutaraldehyde and 20 mg p-amino-phenyl-ß-D galactoside. The suspension was then dialysed against phosphate buffered saline (PBS) to separate the uncoupled product [22].

Mice exposed to cadmium were administered two injections (intravenous at a gap of 48 hrs.) of 15 mmoles/kg of DMSA either in free form or encapsulated in plain liposomes (PC-Chol-PE) or in galactosylated liposomes along with appropriate controls. Urine and feces of animals were collected in metabolic cages and the animals were later sacrificed for collection of body organs, viz. liver, kidney and spleen. Liver from two animals in each group was utilized for preparation of hepatocytes after liver perfusion [23]. Analysis of cadmium and trace metals, viz. zinc and copper was carried out by atomic absorption spectrophotometry.

RESULTS AND DISCUSSION

Results showed that the mobilization of cadmium from the body organs was in the order gal-lip-DMSA>Lip-DMSA>DMSA. The urinary excretion was enhanced by treatment with DMSA in either from and exhibited the same order. Cadmium was removed from kidney only by gal-lip-DMSA treatment (Table 3)

Table 3. Mobilization of cadmium from the body organs and hepatocytes of mice exposed to cadmium followed by administration n-saline DMSA in free form, DMSA encapsualted in liposomes or DMSA encapsulated in galactosylated liposomes

Treatment	Liver	Kidney	Spleen	Hepatocytes
CD-saline	24.67±1.20	19.07±1.50	3.26±0.25	0.87±0.60
Cd-DMSA	21.50±0.86	14.37±0.54	1.77±0.18	0.57±0.07
Cd-Lip-DMSA	19.37±0.87	14.05±0.82	1.36±0.10	0.43±0.10
Cd-Gal-Lip-DMSA	17.41±0.67	8.33±0.95	0.74±0.20	0.34±0.03

Values are expressed as µg/g tissue or hepatocytes derived from 1g liver. Each value represents mean ± SE of 6 animals. Comparison was made by one way analysis of variance (ANOVA) and $p < 0.05$ was taken as significant.

Almost similar pattern was observed in the elimination of cadmium via feces. Mobilization pattern of cadmium from hepatocytes although followed similar order the results were not significant when comparison was made between the liposomal DMSA and gal-lip-DMSA group. It could be due to overall low content of cadmium in hepatocytes used for the analysis from the liver of each animal.

The results of these studies reveal that interaction of liposomal DMSA with cadmium improved the mobilization/removal of cadmium from the body organs especially liver and spleen. Only galactosylated liposome encapsulated DMSA lowered the level of cadmium from the kidneys of cadmium exposed animals. It may be due to removal of the metal from liver in such a fashion that its retention in kidneys is prevented as well as there is mobilization from this organ when DMSA is given through this carrier. The removal of cadmium from the body is also expected to be relatively safe through slow and sustained release of the metal chelator complex, when chelator is administered through targetable liposomes.

REFERENCES

1. Nriagu, J. O. (1981) Cadmium in the environment, Vol-II, Wiley Intersciences, New York.

2. Friberg, L., Piscater, M., Nordberg, G. F., Kjellstrom, T. (1974). Cadmium in the Environment, CRC Press, Cleval and Ohio.

3. Nordberg, M. and Nordberg, G. F. (1987). **Experimentia** (Suppl) 52, 669-675.

4. Nordberg, G. F., Jin, T. and Nordberg, M. (1994) **Environ. Health Prespect.** 102, 192-194.

5. Cantilena, L. R. Jr. and Klaassen, C. D. (1982). **Toxicol. Appl. Pharmacol.** 63, 173-180.

6. Stather, J. W., Smith, H., Bailey, M. R., Birchall, A., Bulman, R. A. and Crawley, F.E.H. (1983). **Health Phys.** 44, 45-52.

7. Rahman, Y. E. (1988). Use of liposomes in metal poisoning and metal storage disease, In: Liposomes as drug carriers: Recent trends and progress, (Gregoriadis, G. Ed), Wiley, Chichester, pp 485-495.

8. Rahman, Y. E., Rosenthal, M. W., Cerny, E. A. and Morette, E. S. (1974). **J. Lab. Clin. Med.** 83, 640-647.

9. Basinger, M. A. and Jones, M. M. (1988). **J. Toxicol. Envirn. Health.** 23, 77-89.

10. Kojima, S., Ono, H., Kiyozumi, M., Honda, T. and Takadata, A. (1989). **Toxicol. Appl. Pharmacol.** 98, 39-48.

11. Jones, M. M., Singh, P. K., Gala, G. R., Atkins, L. M., Smith, A. B. (1988). **Toxicol. Appl. Pharmacol.** 95, 507-514.

12. Jones, S. G., Holscher, M. A., Singh, P. K. and Jones, M. M. (1990). **Toxicology** 61, 73-83.

13. Behari, J. R. and Gregoriadis, G. (1992). **Int. J. Pharm.** 79, 213-221.

14. Behari, J. R., Srivastava, S., Gupta, S. and Srivastava, R. C. (1991). **Bull. Environ. Contam. Toxicol.** 47, 827- 833.

15. Srivastava, S., Gupta, S., Behari, J. R. and Srivastava, R. C. (1991). **Tox. Lett.** 59, 121-131.

16. Behari, J. R., Gupta, S., Srivastava, S. and Srivastava, R. C. (1993). **Industrial Health** 31, 29-33.

17. Lin, D. and Huang, L (1989). **Biochemistry** 20, 7700-7707.

18. Gupta, S., Srivastava, S., Behari, J. R. and Srivastava, R. C. (1995). **Industrial Health** 33, 83-88.

19. Cain, K. and Skilleter, D. M. (1980). **Biochem. J.** 188, 285-288.

20. Chow, D. D., Essien, H. E., Padki, M. M. and Hwang, K. J. (1989). **J.Pharmacol. Exp. Ther.** 248, 506-512.

21. Ghosh, P., Das, P. K., Bachhawat, B. K. (1982). **Arch. Biochem. Biophys.** 213, 266-270.

22. Weissig, V., Lasch, L. and Gregoriadis, G. (1989). **Biochem. Biophys. Acta** 1003, 54-57.

23. Berry, M. N. and Friend, D. S. (1969). **J. Cell. Biol.** 43, 506-520.

15

PHARMACODYNAMIC AND PHARMACOKINETIC EVALUATION OF LIPOSOMES OF INDOMETHACIN

P.V. DIWAN, P. SRINATH, V. RAVIKANTH and S.P. VYAS[1]

Pharmacology Division,
Indian Institute of Chemical Technology, Hyderabad - 500 007 (AP).

[1]Department of Pharmaceutical Sciences,
Dr. H. S. Gour Vishwavidyalaya, Sagar - 470 003 (MP).

- Introduction
- Cytopathology of rheumatoid synovial lining cells
- Preparation of liposomes
- Tissue distribution profiles of free and liposomal indomethacine

- Results and discussion
- Conclusion
- References

INTRODUCTION

Liposomes have been investigated over the past few decades as a system for the delivery or targeting of drugs to specific sites in the body. These are phospholipids based vesicles consisting of concentric aqueous and lipid layers alternating with each other. Because of their structural versatility in terms of size, composition, surface charge, bilayer fluidity and ability to incorporate almost any drug regardless of solubility or to carry their surface cell specific ligands, liposomes have the potential to be tailored in a variety of ways to ensure the production of formulations that are optimal for clinical use. This includes controlled retention of entrapped drugs in the presence of biological fluids, prolonged vesicle residence in the circulation and enhanced vesicle uptake by target cells. Accumulated *in vivo* evidence particularly in areas such as cancer chemotherapy, antimicrobial therapy, vaccines, diagnostic imaging and the treatment of ophthalmic disorders has indicated clearly that some liposome entrapped drugs and vaccines exhibit superior pharmacological properties to those observed with conventional formulations [1].

Rheumatoid arthritis (RA) is a chronic disease of immune etiology that is dominated by its erosive and destructive effects on articular structure. The pathogenesis of the disease involves both humoral and cellular immune responses resulting in tissue destruction and inflammation. The pathological features of the lesions which are considered characteristic of the advanced stages of the disease include villous hypertrophy, proliferation of synovial connective tissue (pannus), subintimal infiltration with mononuclear cells and irreversible destruction of joint tissues. The proliferation of synovial tissue is associated with the presence of inflammatory cells and organized in an invasive front that progressively destroys cartilage and sub-chondral bone. Although these changes are characteristic of well-developed rheumatoid disease, since their disorders tends to be insidious in onset and biopsies are generally not performed during the initial phases of the disease, the sequence of the events leading to these lesions is often difficult to elucidate.

CYTOPATHOLOGY OF RHEUMATOID SYNOVIAL LINING CELLS [2]

Most commonly, normal synovial cells are disposed as a single cell layer. Electron microscopic studies of normal synovial lining cells in man have revealed that they are comprised of two major types, namely macrophage - like phagocytic cells containing numerous vacuoles with vesicles and little endoplasmic reticulum (Type A cells), and fibroblast-like cells revealing a well developed endoplasmic reticulum (Type B cells). The Type A cells exhibit monocytic differentiation antigens, receptors for Fc fragments of immunoglobulin and the C3 components of complement and HLA Class II antigens as well as containing lysosomal enzymes. Cells with this phenotype have been shown to account for about 30 - 50% of eluted from the synovium of RA patients. In addition to these phagocyte cells another cell type has been identified which expresses HLA Class II antigens but lacks Fc receptors, and macrophage/monocyte differentiation antigens on its surface (Type B). These cells constitute about 10% of synovial lining cells found in the sub-synovial tissue of RA patients and are most likely to be of fibroblast origin.

In rheumatoid joints the most striking histological feature is a proliferating multilayered synovium revealing distinct cytomorphological changes. Ultra structural examination of human rheumatoid joints have demonstrated that the initial erosion of articular cartilage is associated with an abundance of proliferating cells characterized by abundant cytoplasm and large, pale, multiple, prominent nuclei. In the last stage of the disease the characteristic lesions are those of an inflammatory vascularized pannus. Infiltration of synovial membrane, particularly with lymphocytes and cells of the monocyte, macrophage lineage, characterize the inflammatory lesions in the joints of patients with chronic rheumatoid arthritis. At this stage, destruction of joint tissue occurs in areas contiguous with inflammatory cell mass as well as in regions adjacent to bone marrow distant from the inflammation. In the inflamed synovium the production of collagenase in mesenchymal derived cells appear to the responsible for the degradation of collagen and distortion of the architecture and the function of the joints. Despite the fact that the inflammatory stage of rheumatoid synovitis is characterized by an intact network of interacting cytokines, soluble mediators that are released by many cell types that are capable of influencing cellular function in an autocrine/panacrine fashion, it remains unclear which cell type or soluble mediator is most important in maintaining the inflammation in rheumatoid arthritis.

In most models of rheumatoid synovitis it is argued that the T cells orchestrate the local inflammatory response. In response to an orthotropic agent such as virus or bacterial cell wall fragment, T cell activation is initiated, the antigen specific T cells preferentially multiply in the synovium or recruit and/or influence other cells through the collaboration of lymphokines. Although this process may be true for initiation of rheumatoid arthritis, in the chronic stage of the disease it would appear that the dominant cell type involved in maintaining the inflammatory response is the mononuclear cell. Several lines of direct evidence exist to support this contention viz. (a) the T cells present in synovial tissue are small and express low numbers of cell activation markers. (b) Their cytokine products are present only in very small concentration in synovial tissue and fluid. (c) There is no evidence that there is clonal expansion of a T cell population in the joint tissue. In contrast, the macrophage-like cells are highly activated, an observation based on their morphology, and enhanced surface Ia expression and the presence of significant quantities of macrophage derived cytokines in synovial cells and fluid. The cytokine profile in the rheumatoid synovium suggests that inflammation may be sustained by factors produced by the macrophages and fibroblasts in the synovial membrane.

Inflammation is a primary, immune or non-immune response of the body through which it repairs tissue damage and defends itself against infections. The function of inflammation is to deliver plasma and cellular components to extravascular tissue. The initiating event may be infection, irradiation, (auto) immune reaction, sprains, bruise or allergy. This is followed by increased vasodilatation and vasopermeability (hypereheia and edema); infiltration of neutrophils (pns) and mononuclear cells and fibrosis or cleaning after the damage is repaired. The involvement of phagocytic cells as well as increased vasopermeability offer excellent opportunities for the use of colloidal drug delivery systems such as liposomes, lipid microspheres, niosomes etc. It was recognized that sites of inflammation show local proliferation of phagocytic cells and these phagocytic cells such as polymorphs and activated lymphocytes wriggle out from blood vessels into the edema. This leads to the logical conclusion that liposomes, which can be rapidly cleared from the circulation by the same cells, should enhance the delivery of the encapsulated drug into the sites of inflammation or infection. To increase the uptake by circulating monocytes, liposomal surface may be tailored conveniently to impart negative charge.

Arthritis is a painful disease, which is affecting almost 1% of the population, especially older people. It causes painful swelling, immobility and possibly a loss of function of mainly peripheral synovial joints. Nonsteroidal anti-inflammatory drugs normally suppress the production of arachidonate metabolites, which are initiators and maintain inflammation. Indomethacin belongs to this category and is a popularly used NSAID for the treatment of arthritis.

It is an established fact that, vascular permeability increases at the diseased sites, as is evident in case of tumors and inflammation. Inflammatory mediators such as leukotrienes, bradykinins are involved in increasing the vascular permeability processes. These mediators open the gaps between the adjacent endothelial cells at the level of post capillary venule. This pathophysiological condition may be exploited for effective target delivery of nonsteroidal antiinflammatory drugs to the sites of inflammation in arthritic subjects. A schematic representation of accumulation of liposomes in inflammatory region [3] is given in Fig.1.

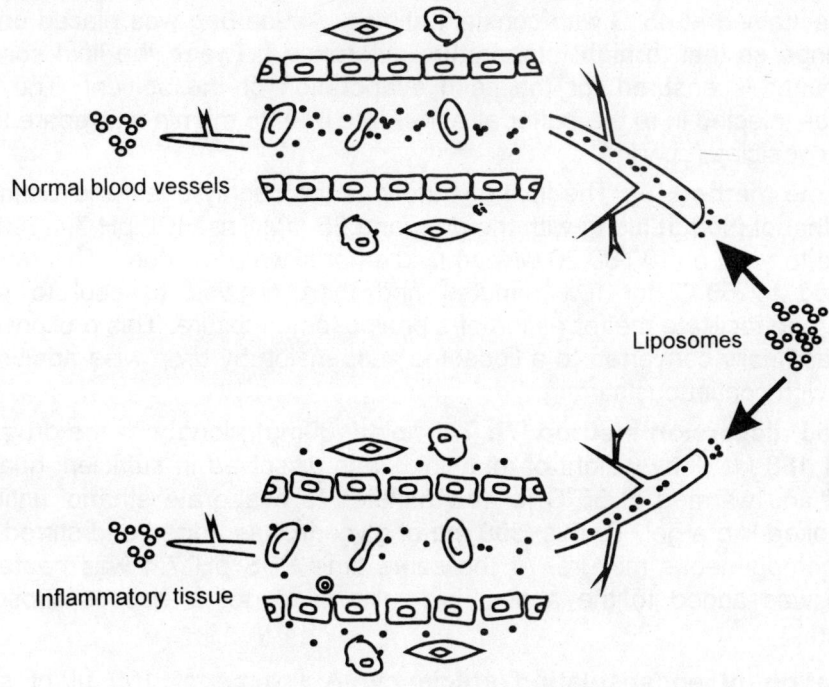

Normal blood vessels

Liposomes

Inflammatory tissue

Fig. 1 : Distribution and accumulation of liposomes in the vascular lesions

In the present work, we aimed at developing an optimal liposomal formulation of indomethacin, taking into consideration the influence of lipid composition and size of the liposomal preparation. Pharmacodynamic and pharmacokinetic evaluations were done in male wistar rats to assess the in vivo performance of this drug carrier system.

PREPARATION OF LIPOSOMES

Various methods such as thin film hydration; ether infusion, proliposome method and high-speed dispersion method were used for the preparation of liposomes with varied lipid compositions. The liposomes were characterized based on size, encapsulation efficiency, lamellarity and in vitro drug release profile. A brief description of various methods of preparation of liposomes is presented below.

Thin film hydration method: Multi lamellar vesicles (MLV) were prepared by conventional method described by Shaw et al. [4]. Specified quantity of lipid(s) and the drugs were dissolved in chloroform in a round-bottom flask. The solvent was evaporated under reduced pressure to get a thin film. The flask was stored overnight under vacuum to remove traces of the solvent. The lipid film was hydrated with phosphate buffered saline pH 7.4, just above the transition temperature of the lipid mixture.

Ether infusion method [5]: Lipid mixture and the drug were dissolved in diethyl ether at a concentration of 2mg/ml keeping on ice after complete drying. A sage syringe (pump) coupled to a crimped 19-gauze needle with polypropylene tubing was employed for infusion process. The other end of the tube was dipped in PBS pH 7.4, maintained at 45°C with constant stirring. An ice bag was placed on top of the syringe so that, a high temperature difference between the lipid solution and the buffer is ensured for the flash evaporation of the solvent. The lipid solution was injected in to the buffer at a flow rate of 0.25 ml/min to prepare large unilamellar vesicles (LUV).

Proliposome method [6]: The lipid mixture was thoroughly dried and dissolved in warm ethanol (80mg) along with the drug and 25 mM Tris-HCl, pH 7.4(200mg) was added to yield a (100:80:20 w/w/w) lipid:ethanol:water mixture. This mixture was heated to 60°C for few minutes and then allowed to cool to room temperature to facilitate the formation of a proliposome mixture. This proliposome mixture was finally converted to a liposome suspension by drop wise addition of the buffer with continuous stirring.

High speed dispersion method [7]: The lipid (100mg) along with the drug and poloxamer 188 (10% by weight of total lipid) was dissolved in sufficient quantity of ethanol and warmed at 50°C for few minutes to evaporate ethanol until the product looked like a gel. To this, 300 mg of glycerin was added and stirred well to get a homogeneous mixture. At the same time PBS pH 7.4 was heated to 50°C and was added to the above lipid mixture to get a viscous liposomal suspension.

Determination of encapsulation efficiency: A volume of 100 μl of stock liposomal dispersion was taken in a standard flask and 50 μl of 10% w/v Triton X-100 was added, vortexed thoroughly and allowed to incubate at room temperature for 4 h, for complete release of the drug from the liposomes. Volume of the solution was made up to 100 ml and the absorbance was noted at 320 nm using double beam spectrophotometer (Shimadzu, Japan).

Determination of lipid content: Determination of lipid content gives an idea about efficiency of the method of preparation of liposomes. A volume of 100 μl of the liposomal dispersion was taken and the total phosphorous was measured as per the method described by Rouser et al. [8].

Electron microscopic study: A small volume of stock solution of vesicles in PBS was fixed with Osmium oxide at a final concentration of 0.5% for 30 minutes on ice. Then the samples were negative stained on formvar coated copper grids with 0.5% uranyl acetate and examined under the microscope.

***In vitro* release of indomethacin from liposomes:** A volume of 1 ml of liposome preparation was taken in a dialysis tube and both the ends were tied. The dialysis bag was suspended in 40 ml of PBS pH 7.4 maintained at 25 ± 2°C and the solution was stirred at 200 rpm. Periodically 1 ml samples were drawn and absorbance was noted at 320 nm using a double beam spectrophotometer (Shimadzu, Japan). The volume of the buffer was maintained at 40 ml through out the experiment.

Pharmacodynamic evaluation: Indomethacin encapsulated liposomes were evaluated for anti-inflammatory activity by two experimental models. They are briefly described as follows.

Carrageenan induced rat paw edema model: The carrageenan paw edema was induced as described by Winter et al [9]. Male Wistar rats each weighing 150 ± 10 gm was divided in to five groups containing five rats per group. Each group of rats was given one formulation as follows. Empty liposomes were given to the first group (1ml/kg). Second group was given with free indomethacin (3 mg/kg). After 1 hr, the right hind paw was injected intraplanterly with 0.1 ml of 1% carrageenan solution. The edema volume was measured periodically up to 5 h using a plethysmometer (Ugo Basile, Italy) and percent inhibition of edema volume was calculated using the following equation.

$$\% \text{ inhibition of edema} = \frac{(V_{control} - V_{treated})}{V_{control}}$$

Where, $V_{control}$ = Mean edema volume of rats in control group.

$V_{treated}$ = edema volume of each test rat.

Adjuvant arthritis model [10]: Male wistar rats weighing 200 ± 20 gm were given a single intradermal injection of 0.25 ml of Freund's adjuvant in to the subplanter area of the right hindpaw. Rats were divided into three groups containing five rats in each group and the test preparations were administered intraperitonially once a day for 15 consecutive days, beginning one day before the injection of the adjuvant. At regular intervals paw volume of both the paws was measured by plethysmometer.

Statistical analysis of the above data was performed by ANOVA. P value <0.01 was considered significant.

TISSUE DISTRIBUTION PROFILES OF FREE AND LIPOSOMAL INDOMETHACIN

Plasmakinetics and tissue distribution studies were carried out in male wistar rats weighing 200 ± 10 gm. Rats were divided into 5 groups containing 5 rats. First group was given free indomethacin (12 mg/kg) and remaining groups were given liposomal formulations with various lipid compositions at the same dose intravenously. Following the treatment, blood samples were collected from retro-orbital puncture and rats were immediately sacrificed and various tissues such as liver, kidney, spleen, paw, heart, lung, and brain were removed, weighed and stored at -20°C until further analysis. To each organ, required amount of methanol was added and homogenized for few minutes and the homogenate was centrifuged at 4000 rpm, the supernatant was collected and assayed for indomethacin by HPLC method as described by Taro et al. [11] with slight modifications. The method may briefly be described as follows: To 50 µl of serum, 50 µl of standard samples of indomethacin in methanol were added at various concentrations of 0.1, 0.2, 0.4, 0.6, 0.8, 1.0 and 2.0 µg/ml and vortexed for few seconds. A volume of 50 µl of acetonitrile was added to the above to precipitate proteins. To this, 100 μl of 1 μg/ml solution of naproxen in methanol was added and vortexed for 30 sec. and kept on ice for 10 minutes. The samples were centrifuged for 20 min. The supernatant was injected to the HPLC system (Shimadzu LC-10A, Japan) equipped with UV spectrometer. Acetonitrile: water: acetic acid (80:20:1) was used as mobile phase at a flow rate of 0.6 ml/min and wavelength was fixed at 254 nm. Calibration curve was found to be linear between 40 ng/ml and 2 μg/ml with the following regression equation:rsp=0.00087 (amt) - 0.00597. Using PK analyst software program did pharmacokinetic analysis. Statistical significance of the data was analyzed by using ANOVA ($p < 0.05$).

RESULTS AND DISCUSSION

Table 1 shows the effect of lipid composition and charge on encapsulation efficiency of indomethacin in multilamellar vesicles (MLV). Except ether infusion method, all the other three methods produced multilamellar vesicles. Based on encapsulation efficiency, thin film hydration method was found to be better method for encapsulation of indomethacin in phosphatidyl choline liposomes. It was observed that inclusion of positively charged lipid (stearylamine) increased the encapsulation efficiency of the drug. However inclusion of phosphatidyl glycerol, a negatively charged phospholipid didn't significantly alter the encapsulation of indomethacin compared to neutral liposomes (PC:CH-1:1).

Table 1. Effect of lipid composition on encapsulation of indomethacin in Egg phosphatidylcholine based liposomes using various methods of preparation

Lipid composition	Encapsulation efficiency			
	Thin film hydration method	Proliposome method	Ether infusion method	High speed dispersion method
PC	13.65 ± 2.51 (3.33)	11.64 ± 3.56 (3.47)	11.62 ± 3.42 (3.47)	14.35 ± 4.73 (2.85)
PC:CH (1:1)	14.31 ± 1.72 (3.67)	13.23 ± 4.27 (4.10)	13.75 ± 5.30 (3.03)	14.21 ± 2.31 (2.56)
PC:CH:SA (1:0.5:0.1)	31.8 ± 6.20 (2.96)	2.97 ± 3.90 (4.22)	26.12 ± 7.36 (3.17)	18.96 ± 3.48 (2.74)
PC:CH:PE (1:0.5:0.16)	26.7 ± 7.01 (3.01)	18.42 ± 2.86 (3.79)	18.4 ± 8.91 (3.5)	13.67 ± 4.56 (2.65)
PC:CH:PG (1:0.5:0.2)	24.6 ± 3.61 (3.75)	14.1 ± 2.01 (4.06)	16.5 ± 4.21 (3.11)	14.10 ± 2.78 (3.11)

Each experiment was repeated in triplicate.
Total lipid content in each experiment was kept at 5.8 mg/ml
Average lipid content in each preparation is expressed as mg/ml in parantheses

It may be assumed that, as indomethacin is an acidic drug, its encapsulation was better when a basic lipid such as stearylamine is used because of the electrostatic interaction of the drug with the bilayers. Determination of lipid content of a liposomal formulation reflects the efficiency of method for the preparation of liposomes. It was observed from the lipid content data from the above table that, proliposomal method was an efficient method for the preparation of multilamellar vesicles.

MLVs were sonicated by using a Branson ultrasonifier at 100% duty cycle for 7 min and were further extruded through 0.05 µ polycarbonate membrane to get small unilamellar vesicles (SUVs). This also removes titanium particles if any present in the dispersion.

Table 1 also shows the effect of lipid composition and charge on encapsulation of indomethacin in large unilamellar vesicles (LUV) prepared by ether infusion method. This method resulted in heterogeneous size population of liposomes as observed by transmission electron microscopy.

Based on encapsulation efficiency, LUVs were observed to be not better candidates for encapsulation of indomethacin in liposomes compared to MLVs with various lipid compositions tried. As indomethacin is a lipophilic drug it will be incorporated in to the lipid layers. In the LUVs, inspite of bigger size, the volume of the lipid compartment will be lower than the aqueous compartment. Therefore, encapsulation efficiency was not improved. Incorporation of cholesterol did not affect the encapsulation efficiency both in MLVs and LUVs but as cholesterol was found to impart the rigidity to bilayers and increase the stability it was used in all the preparations. As in case of MLVs, inclusion of stearylamine improved the encapsulation of the drug significantly (about 26%).

There is a limitation of size for the use of colloidal drug carriers for the effective localization at the inflammatory sites. It has been reported that, particles of size range <100 nm will be efficiently deposited at the inflammatory sites. Though for hydrophobic drugs MLVs are suitable drug carriers, because of size limitation, MLVs were further sonicated and used for in-vivo studies.

In vitro release studies are often performed to predict how a delivery system might work in ideal situations, which might give some indication of its performance. Figure 2 shows comparative drug release study performed from MLVs, SUVs and LUVs prepared with same lipid composition (PC:CH:SA-1:0.5:0.1). About 18% of the encapsulated drug were released from MLVs at 6 h whereas; LUVs released around 32% and about 50% of the encapsulated drug from SUVs. From figure 2 it is evident that, the percent drug release from MLVs was much lower compared to unilamellar vesicles. It may be accounted for the number of aqueous barriers to be crossed in order to be released outside. The high cumulative percent drug release from SUVs may be due to the high area to volume ratio of these vesicles compared to LUVs and MLVs.

It is evident from Fig. 3 that, there is a significant difference in percent inhibition of edema volume between the free and encapsulated indomethacin at a dose of 3 mg/kg. To understand the advantage in using sub-micron size range of particles, SUVs (50nm) and LUVs (100nm) were used for the animal experiments. At 3h, percent inhibition of edema was ~ 55% with SUVs and ~ 50% with LUVs whereas with free indomethacin it was only 40% at the same dose. It may be assumed that liposomes were localized at the inflammatory site thereby anti-inflammatory activity was more than the free drug.

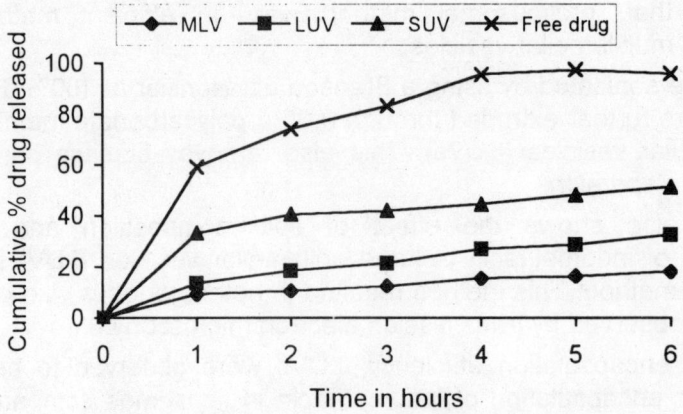

Fig. 2: Effect of lamellarity and size on drug release profile from phosphatidylcholine based liposomes. The lipid composition was PC:CH (1:1)

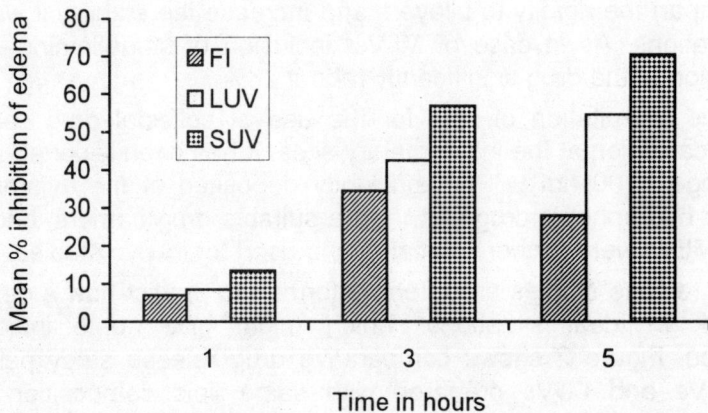

Fig. 3 : Inhibitory effect of free indomethacin and lipo-indomethacin on carrageenan induced paw edema in rats (Dose : 3 mg/Kg)

In case of Freund's adjuvant arthritis model (Table 2), peak swelling of the paw was observed on 2nd day with free indomethacin whereas, it was 5th day with liposomal indomethacin and neither the free drug nor encapsulated indomethacin could prevent the inflammation. Ulcer indices were determined on 18th day by the method described by Robert et al. [12]. It was found that, ulcer index with encapsulated indomethacin was 1/3rd that of free indomethacin (Fig. 4). It may be concluded that, encapsulated indomethacin showed higher efficacy than the free drug in inhibiting the inflammation both in acute and chronic inflammatory models.

Table 2. Effect of free and encapsulated indomethacin on edema volume, induced using Freund's adjuvant. Test preparations were given by i.p. equivalent to a dose of 3 mg/Kg of indomethacin

Treatment	Average edema volume (ml)-days after inoculation with adjuvant								
	1	2	3	5	7	9	11	13	15
Empty liposomes	1.10 ± 0.22	1.67 ± 0.13	1.13 ± 0.15	1.54 ±0.32	1.64 ± 0.17	1.61 ± 0.19	1.65 ± 0.18	1.54 ± 0.21	1.57 ± 0.26
Free Indomethacin	1.34 ± 0.20	1.32 ± 0.25	0.89 ± 0.12	1.22 ±0.20	1.28 ± 0.13	1.31 ± 0.43	1.27 ± 0.11	1.19 ± 0.45	1.17 ± 0.31
Liposomal Indomethacin	0.96 ± 0.10	1.26 ± 0.15	0.77 ± 0.06	1.31 ± 0.17	1.14 ± 0.36	1.09 ± 0.73	1.10 ± 0.91	0.91 ± 0.11	0.90 ± 0.28

Number of animals - 5 ($p<0.01$)

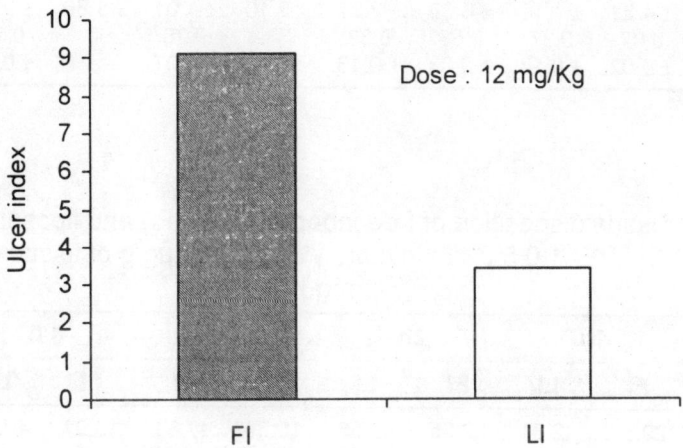

Fig. 4 : Ulcerogenicity of free and encapsulated indomethacin administered intravenously in male Wistar rats. Ulcer index was measured 6 h after the drug administration

A comparative pharmacokinetic study was performed between free indomethacin and liposomal indomethacin by measuring the drug levels in various tissues upto 24 h after the administration of the formulations. The organ concentration of indomethacin with free and lipo-indomethacin preparations are shown in Tables 3 to 6.

Table 3. Tissue disposition of free indomethacin (FI) and liposomal indomethacin (LI) (PC:CH-1:1) in male Wistar rats (μg/g of tissue ± S.D.) Dose 12 mg.Kg (i.v)

Organ	1h		2h		4h		8 h		24 h	
	FI	LI	FI	LI	FI	LI	FI	LI	FI	LI
Liver	29.84	39.16	22.35	47.43	16.54	49.86	19.01	41.03	7.14	30.18
	± 3.56	± 5.21	± 4.25	± 0.86	± 2.18	± 2.15	± 4.02	± 2.26	± 2.26	± 3.12
Kidney	26.31	12.96	24.18	15.28	22.15	11.56	19.69	8.31	18.01	5.69
	± 4.28	± 2.63	± 5.10	± 3.75	± 2.68	± 2.40	± 1.87	± 2.12	± 2.55	± 0.95
Spleen	6.41	9.89	5.21	12.13	4.54	15.95	4.10	11.26	2.16	8.15
	± 1.02	± 0.78	± 1.91	± 3.18	± 0.99	± 4.38	± 0.86	± 2.91	± 0.54	± 2.01
Lung	8.86	16.03	8.49	21.85	7.28	26.16	5.49	14.10	2.56	7.11
	± 0.69	± 4.12	± 0.97	± 3.78	± 0.76	± 4.25	± 1.28	± 3.15	± 0.63	± 2.04
Brain	1.21	0.50	1.56	0.48	1.42	0.36	0.99	0.31	0.78	0.26
	± 0.37	± 0.13	± 0.13	± 0.20	± 0.21	± 0.11	± 0.33	± 0.12	± 0.16	± 0.10
Heart	12.48	5.38	9.62	6.98	6.18	3.76	4.13	2.11	1.81	1.01
	± 4.21	± 1.10	± 3.89	± 2.23	± 2.10	± 1.01	± 1.86	± 0.54	± 0.56	± 0.26
Paw	0.07	0.37	0.06	0.32	-	0.28	-	0.24	-	0.15
	± 0.02	± 0.14	± 0.03	± 0.13		± 0.07		± 0.10		± 0.06

Table 4. Tissue disposition of free indomethacin (FI) and liposomal indomethacin (LI) (PC:CH:PE- 1:0.5:0.16) in male Wistar rats (μg/g of tissue ± S.D.) Dose 12 mg.Kg (i.v)

Organ	1h		2h		4h		8 h		24 h	
	FI	LI	FI	LI	FI	LI	FI	LI	FI	LI
Liver	29.84	42.31	22.35	49.55	16.54	47.81	19.01	40.65	7.14	32.11
	± 3.56	± 2.15	± 4.25	± 1.26	± 2.18	± 4.53	± 4.02	± 2.16	± 2.26	± 4.18
Kidney	26.31	11.75	24.18	10.24	22.15	8.13	19.69	7.29	18.01	4.51
	± 4.28	± 1.11	± 5.10	± 1.65	± 2.68	± 2.42	± 1.87	± 1.01	± 2.55	± 1.15
Spleen	6.41	9.01	5.21	15.10	4.54	13.18	4.10	11.40	2.16	9.28
	± 1.02	± 0.90	± 1.91	± 4.36	± 0.99	± 1.86	± 0.86	± 2.11	± 0.54	± 1.36
Lung	8.86	15.78	8.49	22.98	7.28	19.07	5.49	15.67	2.56	9.18
	± 0.69	± 2.15	± 0.97	± 1.01	± 0.76	± 4.01	± 1.28	± 4.26	± 0.63	± 2.22
Brain	1.21	0.51	1.56	0.46	1.42	0.39	0.99	0.28	0.78	0.24
	± 0.37	± 0.20	± 0.13	± 0.11	± 0.21	± 0.10	± 0.33	± 0.13	± 0.16	± 0.10
Heart	12.48	6.44	9.62	5.16	6.18	4.28	4.13	3.01	1.81	2.76
	± 4.21	± 2.22	± 3.89	± 0.99	± 2.10	± 1.21	± 1.86	± 0.69	± 0.56	± 0.93
Paw	0.07	0.39	0.06	0.35	-	0.31	-	0.26	-	0.21
	± 0.02	± 0.18	± 0.03	± 0.14		± 0.12		± 0.13		± 0.08

Table 5. Tissue disposition of free indomethacin (FI) and liposomal indomethacin (LI) (PC:CH:PG- 1:0.5:0.20) in male Wistar rats (µg/g of tissue ± S.D.) Dose 12 mg.Kg (i.v)

Organ	1h		2h		4h		8 h		24 h	
	FI	LI	FI	LI	FI	LI	FI	LI	FI	LI
Liver	29.84 ± 3.56	48.90 ± 2.29	22.35 ± 4.25	51.29 ± 1.18	16.54 ± 2.18	55.61 ± 3.12	19.01 ± 4.02	49.21 ± 1.20	7.14 ± 2.26	39.76 ± 2.15
Kidney	26.31 ± 4.28	14.71 ± 3.18	24.18 ± 5.10	16.12 ± 3.75	22.15 ± 2.68	13.37 ± 2.15	19.69 ± 1.87	11.73 ± 1.01	18.01 ± 2.55	8.16 ± 2.61
Spleen	6.41 ± 1.02	13.21 ± 2.61	5.21 ± 1.91	19.28 ± 2.10	4.54 ± 0.99	16.89 ± 0.46	4.10 ± 0.86	15.03 ± 0.95	2.16 ± 0.54	12.45 ± 1.67
Lung	8.86 ± 0.69	21.37 ± 4.65	8.49 ± 0.97	27.16 ± 2.86	7.28 ± 0.76	25.60 ± 1.98	5.49 ± 1.28	19.31 ± 3.15	2.56 ± 0.63	11.45 ± 2.56
Brain	1.21 ± 0.37	0.30 ± 0.11	1.56 ± 0.13	0.24 ± 0.09	1.42 ± 0.21	0.22 ± 0.10	0.99 ± 0.33	0.18 ± 0.06	0.78 ± 0.16	0.12 ± 0.02
Heart	12.48 ± 4.21	4.81 ± 1.23	9.62 ± 3.89	4.58 ± 1.42	6.18 ± 2.10	3.65 ± 0.96	4.13 ± 1.86	2.81 ± 0.73	1.81 ± 0.56	1.10 ± 0.38
Paw	0.07 ± 0.02	0.40 ± 0.11	0.06 ± 0.03	0.36 ± 0.15	-	0.32 ± 0.10	-	0.28 ± 0.13	-	0.26 ± 0.09

Table 6. Tissue disposition of free indomethacin (FI) and liposomal indomethacin (LI) (PC:CH:SA- 1:0.5:0.1) in male Wistar rats (µg/g of tissue ± S.D.) Dose 12 mg.Kg (i.v)

Organ	1h		2h		4h		8 h		24 h	
	FI	LI	FI	LI	FI	LI	FI	LI	FI	LI
Liver	29.84 ± 3.56	44.15 ± 1.62	22.35 ± 4.25	47.17 ± 2.67	16.54 ± 2.18	48.70 ± 2.62	19.01 ± 4.02	42.36 ± 2.90	7.14 ± 2.26	35.18 ± 3.15
Kidney	26.31 ± 4.28	15.76 ± 2.17	24.18 ± 5.10	13.18 ± 1.16	22.15 ± 2.68	12.01 ± 3.11	19.69 ± 1.87	9.65 ± 0.98	18.01 ± 2.55	6.23 ± 1.21
Spleen	6.41 ± 1.02	11.61 ± 0.99	5.21 ± 1.91	14.98 ± 2.51	4.54 ± 0.99	13.01 ± 1.11	4.10 ± 0.86	12.59 ± 3.20	2.16 ± 0.54	11.01 ± 3.16
Lung	8.86 ± 0.69	18.19 ± 2.66	8.49 ± 0.97	23.55 ± 4.25	7.28 ± 0.76	21.01 ± 3.19	5.49 ± 1.28	16.31 ± 3.15	2.56 ± 0.63	9.47 ± 2.29
Brain	1.21 ± 0.37	0.33 ± 0.12	1.56 ± 0.13	0.26 ± 0.09	1.42 ± 0.21	0.21 ± 0.06	0.99 ± 0.33	0.16 ± 0.09	0.78 ± 0.16	0.13 ± 0.04
Heart	12.48 ± 4.21	5.44 ± 1.79	9.62 ± 3.89	4.20 ± 0.86	6.18 ± 2.10	4.01 ± 0.95	4.13 ± 1.86	3.33 ± 1.25	1.81 ± 0.56	2.58 ± 1.20
Paw	0.07 ± 0.02	0.20 ± 0.09	0.06 ± 0.03	0.17 ± 0.08	-	0.15 ± 0.07	-	0.12 ± 0.04	-	0.11 ± 0.03

C_{max} (29.8 µg/g of the tissue) in liver was achieved after 1 h of administration of free indomethacin, which further gradually decreased to about 7 µg/g of the tissue after 24 h. Significantly high amounts of drug accumulations in liver could be the possible reason for the hepatotoxicity of this drug during the therapy. Thus the incorporation of indomethacin in liposomes had enhanced the total amount of drug accumulation in liver. The drug level was always greater than that of free indomethacin at any point during the study period. Peak drug level in liver with liposomal formulation was achieved within 4 h and declined gradually and high drug levels were detected even after 24 h. Of the four lipid compositions tried, localization in liver was highest with PC:CH:PG (1:0.5:0.2) molar composition.

T_{max} of indomethacin in spleen was found to be 1h and the drug concentration continuously decreased upto 24 h in the free drug administered group. However, with encapsulated indomethacin, T_{max} was observed to be equivalent or slightly more than 2 h. The total amount of drug accumulated in spleen was greater with encapsulated form than with the free form with all the lipid compositions tried. Liver and spleen are considered to be RES-rich organs and the high accumulation of drug with encapsulated form may be explained and by the possible uptake of this system by macrophages concentrated in these organs.

Detectable concentrations of the drug in the inflammatory tissue were found only upto 2 h when free indomethacin was administered to arthritic rats. However, detectable levels of the drug were found even upto 24 h when encapsulated drug was administered as various liposomal formulations. Drug levels with liposomal formulations were much higher than the free indomethacin at all the intervals of the study and the rate of fall of the drug level with liposomal preparation was also seen to be slow. Liposomes comprising of PC:CH:PG (1:0.5:0.2) showed highest localization in the inflammatory tissue compared to all other liposomal formulations prepared and the C_{max} in the paw was achieved 1 h after administration of the liposomes. High accumulation of negatively charged liposomes in inflammatory tissue may be accounted for by the rapid uptake of negatively charged vesicles by the circulating monocytes and further extra-vascularization of these monocytes at the inflammatory site.

Drug level in the brain with free indomethacin was higher than with the encapsulated form. This could be the reason for higher frequency of CNS disturbances observed in patients with long term therapy with indomethacin.

After 24 h, concentration of indomethacin was 2 to 6 folds higher with free drug over the encapsulated drug of the various liposomal systems studied. PC:CH:PE (1:0.5:1.6) and PC:CH (1:1) showed almost identical level of drug localization in brain and the concentrations were higher than the other two formulations.

With free indomethacin, the highest drug concentration was observed in kidney followed by the liver. At all time intervals of the study period, indomethacin concentration was about 1.5 to 2 times higher than the liposomal formulations. Almost a similar drug profile was observed in the heart. However the drug levels were more than 2 fold higher with free drug compared to the encapsulated formulations.

With all the liposomal formulations studied more drug was localized in lung compared to free drug formulation. Localization of the drug in lung was more with negatively charged liposomes than with positive or neutral liposomes. This is in confirmation with earlier report on the fate of empty liposomes in vivo. The possible reason for high accumulation of the drug in lungs with liposomal formulations may be due to the physical trapping of the vesicles in the highly perfused vasculature of the lung.

From the above biodisposition data, it is evident that the favorite sites of accumulation of encapsulated indomethacin are liver, spleen, confirming its in vivo fate similar to that of any other colloidal drug delivery system.

The relatively high localization of free drug in kidney and brain could be the possible reason behind the toxicity of indomethacin during the long-term therapy. But interestingly localization of encapsulated indomethacin in these organs was significantly lower than that of the free drug formulations.

Table 7. Pharmacokinetic parameters of free indomethacin (FI) and liposomal indomethacin (LI) after i.v. administration to male Wistar rats (dose 12 mg/Kg)

Parameter	FI	LI-1 PC:CH(1:1)	LI-2 PC:CH:PE (1:0.5:0.16)	LI-3 PC:CH:SA (1:0.5:0.1)	LI-4 PC:CH:PG (1:0.5:0.2)
AUC_{0-t}	478.26 ± 47.2	386.78 ± 38.1	397.26 ± 36.6	363.95 ± 27.25	300.75 ± 20.65
Distribution half-life	1.41 ± 0.5	0.88 ± 0.21	0.91 ± 0.11	0.56 ± 0.07	0.65 ± 0.04
Elimination half-life	13.58 ± 1.31	11.65 ± 0.95	12.29 ± 1.41	9.0 ± 1.81	8.65 ± 0.42
Mean residence time	17.09 ± 1.30	15.57 ± 1.39	16.29 ± 2.04	11.49 ± 2.37	11.48 ± 0.63

From the plasmakinetic study, it was found that both the free as well as the encapsulated indomethacin were cleared from the plasma in a biphasic manner (as shown in figures 5-8). However, at all the time intervals, drug levels were higher with the free drug compared to the encapsulated drug. As we have not estimated the free drug as well as the encapsulated drug in case of liposomal treatment, log plasma concentration Vs time profiles were observed to follow similar trend. However, theoretically it is assumed that the pharmacokinetics of liposomal drug does not resemble with that of the free drug and is directed and dictated by the bilayer composition of the vesicle.

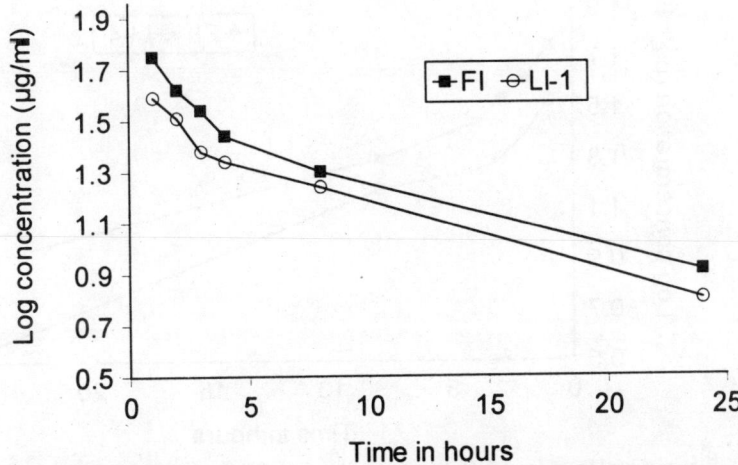

Fig. 5 : Plasma profile of free & lipo- indomethacin following i.v. injection in rats (FI &LI-1)

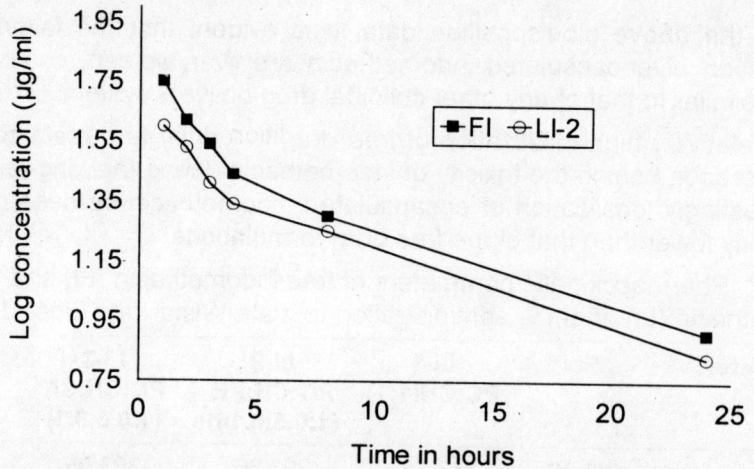

Fig. 6 : Plasma profile of free & lipo- indomethacin following i.v. injection in rats (FI &LI-2)

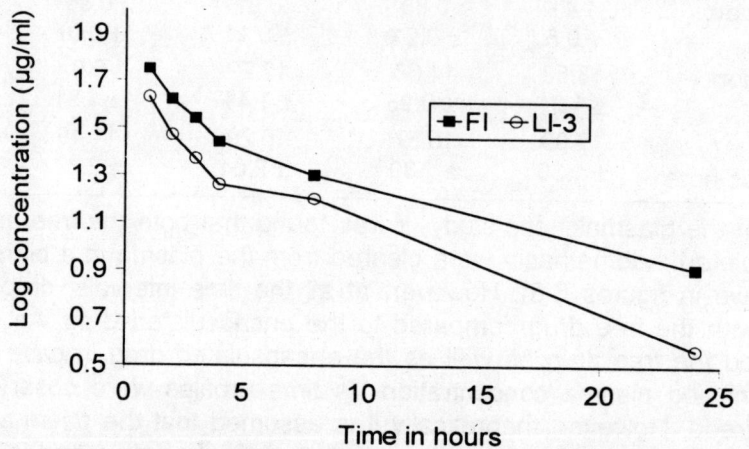

Fig. 7 : Plasma profile of free & lipo- indomethacin following i.v. injection in rats (FI &LI-3)

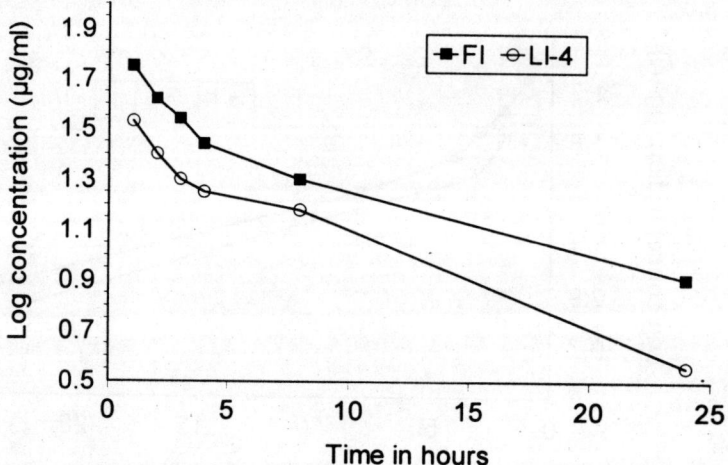

Fig. 8 : Plasma profile of free & lipo- indomethacin following i.v. injection in rats (FI &LI-4)

In table 7, it is shown that distribution half-life of the free drug was higher than all the liposomal formulations studied. This may be because of the rapid clearance of liposomes by RES-rich organs such as liver, spleen and the extravasation at the inflammatory sites. In addition to the preferential localization of the vesicles in some of these organs the slow release of the drug from the localized liposomes could be the reason for the above results. Mean residence time with free drug was slightly higher than the liposomal formulations. Thus, the pharmacokinetics and biodisposition were observed to be changed significantly when encapsulated in liposomes.

CONCLUSION

In conclusion, encapsulation of indomethacin significantly changed the tissue disposition of the injected drug. High accumulation of the drug in inflammatory regions and RES-rich organs such as liver and spleen reflects the targeting potential of liposomes for treating the both rheumatic and non-rheumatic inflammatory conditions. However, unwanted accumulation of the drug in RES-rich organs may lead to saturation of the macrophage system and thus interferes with the immune status of the body. Therefore, attempts have to be made to reduce the RES-uptake of the liposomes.

REFERENCES

1. Srinath, P. and Diwan, P. V. (1994). **Ind. J. Pharmacol.** 26, 179.

2. Love, W.G., Kellaway, I.W. and Williams, B.D. (1993). In :Liposomes in Drug Delivery, Harwood academic publishers, Switzerland, pp. 149.

3. Mizushima, Y. and Igarashi, R. (1992). In : Medicinal Chemistry for the 21st Century, Blacwell Scientific Publishers, London, pp. 381.

4. Shaw, I.H., Knight, C.G., Thomas, P., Phillips, N.C. and Dingle, J. (1979). **Br. J. Exp. Pathol.** 60, 142.

5. Davis, S.C. Howard, R.P. and McHard, M. (1981). **Biochim. Biophys. Acta** 649, 129.

6. Perrett, S., Golding, M. and Williams, P. (1991) **J. Pharm. Pharmacol.** 43, 154.

7. Miquel, P., Monica, L., Montserrat, G., Joan, F., and Joan, E. (1995). **Chem. Pharm. Bull.** 43, 983.

8. Chen, P.S., Joribara, T.Y. and Warner, H. (1956). **Anal. Chem.** 28, 1756.

9. Diwan, P.V., Karwande, I., Margaret, I. and Sattur, P.B. (1989). **Ind. J. Pharmacol.** 21, 1.

10. Graeme, M.L., Fabry, E. and Sigg, E.B. (1996). **J. Pharmacol. Exp. Ther.** 153, (2), 373.

11. Taro, O., Yoshimasa, I., Masahiro, I. and Hidehiko, A. (1989). **J. Pharm. Sci.** 78, 319.

12. Robert, A., Nezamis, J. E., Lancaster, C. and Hanchar, A. (1979). **Gastroenterol.** 77, 433.

16

POLYMERPLIED VESICULAR SYSTEMS FOR CONTROLLED DRUG RELEASE : DEVELOPMENT AND CHARACTERIZATION

N. VENKATESAN, PREETI VENUGOPALAN, PARIJAT KANAUJIA and S.P. VYAS

Department of Pharmaceutical Sciences,
Doctor Harisingh Gour Vishwavidyalaya, Sagar (M.P.) 470 003, INDIA.

- Introduction
- Materials and Methods
- Characterization

- Results and Discussion
- References

INTRODUCTION

Nonionic surfactants of a wide variety of structural types have been found to be useful and cost effective alternatives to phospholipids in formulation of vesicular systems [1]. Nonionic surfactant vesicles (Niosomes), based on alkylglycerol ether surfactants have been studied by Vanlerberghe et al., in 1972 [2]. The potential use of this carrier vesicle has been studied by many for their use in neoplasm, antiinflammatory and antitubercular activity by many researchers [3-8]

Niosomes have been introduced and suggested as a safe vesicular system and advocated to be as an alternative version for liposomes especially for controlled drug delivery purpose. They behave quite similar to liposomes with better stability status. They could prolong the circulation of entrapped drug resulting into an altered distribution and metabolic stability [3,9,10]. However, niosomes are not appreciably stable *in vivo*. Several studies, which have been conducted in, order to improve the stability. The use of polymerizable basic building molecules and their polymerization following vesiculation have been suggested for improvisation of the stability. Polymerizable [11-19] and microencapsulated liposomes [20,21] have also been reported to be stable. Polymerized liposomes have some drawbacks which include co-operative phase transition behaviour, response towards exogenous stimuli [22], disturbances in polymeric chain packing, partial rather than complete polymerization. The limited ability of the highly curved surface of a small unilamellar vesicle to accommodate linear polymers [19] and the intense UV irradiation used to induce polymerization which may extensively degrade the drug [23].

The methods reported earlier discuss the microencapsulation of vesicular dispersion. The reports suggested that these artificial vesicles have close resemblance to biological cells which exhibit permselectivity and other permeation behaviours similar to bio-cells. However, they lack in structural stability for not having any supporting components like cytosterols in bio-animal cells. Any disturbance in the packaging of building block molecules results into destabilisation and as a result reflected a poor trapping efficiency leading to selective opsonization and reticuloendothelial system (RES) mediated clearance *in vivo*.

The reports on studies pertaining to micronecapsulation of liposomes are available. The materials used for microencapsulation were acacia, gelatin and nylon. However, the microcapsules contain vesicular dispersion rather than coating of an individual vesicle. Microencapsulated vesicular dispersion exhibited improved characteristics. Recently, we have reported a method to microencapsulate discrete vesicle [24].

The present study was aimed at polymer coating of niosomes, which could provide distinctive structural integrity and could maintain release profile of drug under osmotic stresses.

MATERIALS AND METHOD

Materials

Span 40, cholesterol (Loba Chemie, India), dicetylphosphate (Sigma, USA), acrylonitrile (Merck, India), diclofenac sodium (Jagsonpal Pharmaceuticals, India). Other materials and reagents were of analytical grade (Qualigens, chemical division of Glaxo (I) Ltd.). The materials were used as received.

Method

Preparation of polymerplied unilamellar vesicles (ULVs)

The niosome forming constituents, i.e. Span 40, cholesterol and dicetylphosphate were taken in different percent mole fractions (see Table 1 and 2) and dissolved in minimum quantity of diethyl ether (5 ml). To this lipid solution, equimolar quantity of polymer coat forming constituent i.e, acrylonitrile, was added. To this solution, 2 ml of phosphate buffer saline (PBS) pH 7.4 was added and the resultant mixture (biphasic) was sonicated at 15,000 Hz frequency (Soniweld, Ultrasonicator) for 3 minutes resulting into an emulsion of high consistency. Finally, the phase inversion was effected by adding 10 ml of PBS pH 7.4 containing drug (5 mg/ml) at 50±2°C. Phase inversion under constant agitation produced unilamellar niosomes of uniform size. On completion of hydration, i.e. after 2 h, the niosomes were harvested using column chromatography (Sephadex G 50 column). The harvested vesicles were redispersed in an aqueous phase of pH 5.8-6.0. Acidification resulted in spontaneous polymerization of acrylonitrile at immediate vesicle/dispersion fluid interface. The polymerization of acrylonitrile completed in 1 h.

Similarly, plain niosomes were prepared as above except for the use of acrylonitrile and pH change.

CHARACTERIZATION

Removal of unentrapped solute/drug

The unentrapped solute was separated from the vesicles by gel chromatography. A 2 ml aliquot of the vesicle suspension was applied to a Sephadex G-50 column and the vesicles were fractionated using PBS pH 7.4 as eluant.

Size and shape

The mean vesicle diameter of the prepared plain and polymer coated vesicles was measured using an optical microscope (Leitz-Biomed, Germany) at 100x magnification with the help of a stage micrometer. The shape of vesicle was also observed using optical microscope. The mean vesicle diameters are reported in table 1 and 2.

Table 1. Percentage Drug Entrapped in Plain Niosomes

Formulation code	Composition - % mole fraction of Span 40:CH:DCP	Mean Vesicle Size (μm)	% Drug Entrapped ± SD
REV-1	95.0:00.0:5	5.92±0.46	58.0±1.8
REV-2	72.5:22.5:5	6.05±0.58	56.5±1.5
REV-3	47.5:47.5:5	6.08±0.32	55.3±1.2
REV-4	22.5:72.5:5	6.13±0.28	53.9±1.0

CH - Cholesterol; DCP - Dicetyl phosphate

Table 2. Percentage Drug Entrapped in Polymerplied Niosomes

Formulation code	Composition -% mole fraction of Span 40:CH:DCP	Mean Vesicle Size (μm)	% Drug Entrapped ± SD
REV-P-1	95.0:00.0:5	6.11±0.39	58.3±1.5
REV-P-2	72.5:22.5:5	6.26±0.27	56.7±1.3
REV-P-3	47.5:47.5:5	6.31±0.50	55.5±1.4
REV-P-4	22.5:72.5:5	6.49±0.32	55.1±1.1

CH - Cholesterol; DCP - Dicetyl phosphate

Encapsulation efficiency

Encapsulation efficiency of plain niosomes was determined by taking 1 ml of the vesicle dispersion to which 1% n-propanol:phosphate saline buffer (pH 7.4) 1:1 mixture was added and allowed to stand for few minutes in order to facilitate disruption of the vesicles. The niosomal suspension was then accurately measured and the volume was diluted appropriately with PBS of pH 7.4 and analysed at 284 nm using a spectrophotometer (Beckman DB-G).

Encapsulation efficiency of polymer coated vesicles was determined by estimating the amount of free drug and deducting it from the total drug added.

Osmotic shock

The effect of osmotic shock on vesicles size and integrity was investigated by monitoring the reduction/expansion in vesicular mean diameter following gradual addition of small volumes (10-100μl) of hypertonic (1M NaI solution), normal saline and hypotonic (0.5% and 0.1% NaCl solution) solution to the vesicular suspension. The results are tabulated in table 3 and 4.

Table 3. Effect of Osmotic Shock on Vesicle Size (plain)

Formulation code	Vesicle size (in µm) after incubation with				
	PBS pH 7.4	1M Nal	0.9% NaCl	0.5% NaCl	0.1% NaCl
REV-1	5.92±0.46	Shrinked	5.90±0.38	7.85±0.52	Ruptured
REV-2	6.05±0.58	Shrinked	6.05±0.29	7.93±0.27	Ruptured
REV-3	6.08±0.32	Shrinked	6.02±0.20	8.04±0.32	Ruptured
REV-4	6.13±0.28	Shrinked	6.20±0.36	8.07±0.40	Ruptured

Table 4. Effect of Osmotic Shock on Vesicle Size (polymerplied)

Formulation code	Vesicle size (in µm) after incubation with				
	PBS pH 7.4	1M Nal	0.9% NaCl	0.5% NaCl	0.1% NaCl
REV-P-1	6.11±0.39	6.00±0.15	6.14±0.16	6.30±0.42	6.34±0.25
REV-P-2	6.26±0.27	6.21±0.38	6.22±0.40	6.34±0.21	6.46±0.18
REV-P-3	6.31±0.50	6.22±0.25	6.25±0.20	6.52±0.32	6.68±0.38
REV-P-4	6.49±0.32	6.40±0.38	6.38±0.26	6.63±0.18	6.75±0.40

In vitro release profile

In vitro release rate was determined using dialysis bag (Sigma, USA). One ml of the dialysed plain/polymerplied vesicle was taken into a dialysis bag with one end tied. After addition, the other end was also tied and placed in a beaker containing 250 ml PBS pH 7.4. The beaker was placed over a magnetic stirrer (York, India) and the contents were stirred at a constant speed at 37±1°C. Aliquots of samples were withdrawn at predetermined time intervals for every 1 h upto 10 h then after 24 h. The drug content in the withdrawn samples was estimated at 276 nm and cumulative percent of drug released was calculated and plotted against time (t) (Fig 1 and 2).

In vivo antiinflammatory studies

Following the in vitro characterisation of various formulations, REV-3 and REV-P-3 were selected for in vivo studies. Antiinflammatory studies were performed using a plethysmometer to measure carageenan induced paw oedema volume following the method of Katare et al. [25]. Twenty four albino rats of either sex (225-250 g) were fasted for 24 h but had free access to water. They were divided into 4 groups of six rats each. First group was used as control. The second group was given plain diclofenac sodium injection. The dose was fixed to be 1 mg/Kg body weight. The niosomal preparation (plain and polymer coated) equivalent to 1 mg/Kg were administered to the selected group of rats through caudal vein. The change in paw volume was measured after 1,2,3,4, 5 upto 24 h (Fig.3).

RESULTS AND DISCUSSION

Size and shape

Microscopic examination of plain and polymer coated niosomes revealed that the vesicles were spherical in shape and the average size of plain vesicles was 6.11µm, while the polymer coated vesicles were measured to be 6.49µ in size. The marginal increase in mean size in the latter case may be attributed to the polymeric coating of the vesicles. The shape of the vesicle however, was found to be spherical with narrow range of distribution. The vesicles were observed microscopically to be unilamellar.

Encapsulation efficiency

Polymercoated vesicles did not show any significant change in encapsulation efficiency as compared to plain vesicles. This clearly reveals that polymerization via pH change after completion of hydration of the vesicle did not affect the encapsulation efficiency. Moreover, the plying of the vesicle could have enhanced the barrier potential of the niosomal membrane thus enhancing the trapping efficiency of the system.

Osmotic shock

Addition of hypertonic salt solution to plain vesicular suspension led to reduction in vesicle diameter this could be attributed to the efflux of the contents in response to the osmotic challenge. While polymer coated vesicles exhibited marginal shrinkage and were noted to recover of shock on readjustment of tonicity. The observations substantiate the structural support of polymeric coat to the vesicles, which could help them out in maintaining the membrane integrity. Similarly, plain vesicles when incubated with hypotonic solution swelled and total rupture was observed. Polymer coated vesicles showed a marginal swelling however, without any disruption of vesicles. The size was restored on readjusting the tonicity.

In vitro release studies

The observations clearly indicate that plain niosomes have faster drug release rate as compared to their polymer coated version. The slower release rate recorded in the case of polymer coated niosomes may probably be related to the additional polymer based diffusion barrier for drug permeation across the membrane (Fig. 1 and 2).

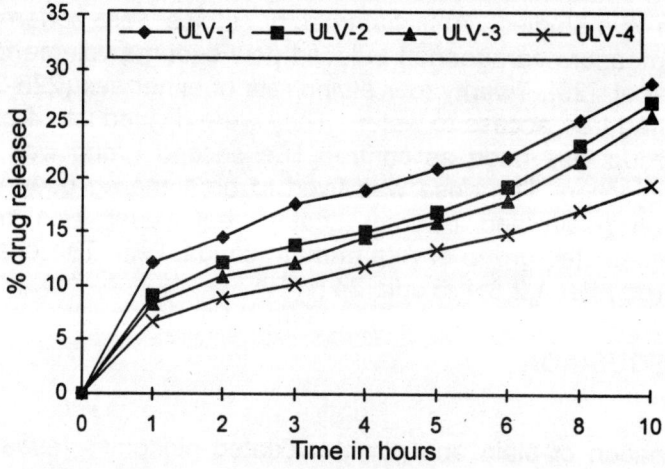

Fig. 1 : *In vitro* release profile of plain vesicles

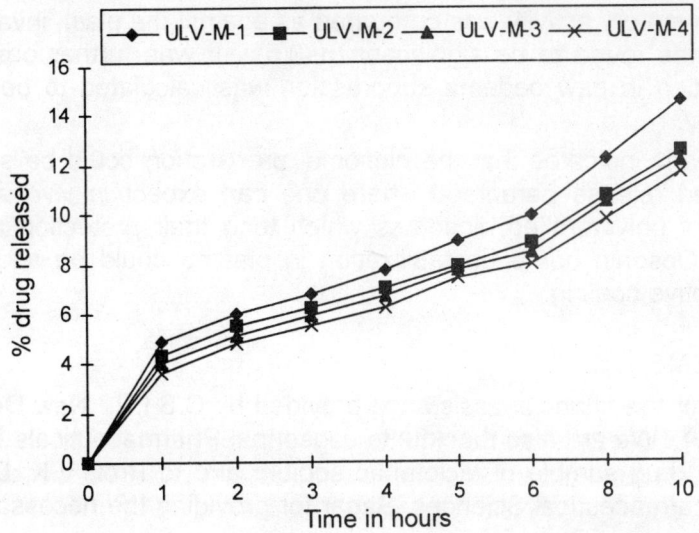

Fig. 2 : *In vitro* release profile of microencapsulated vesicles

In vivo antiinflammatory activity

The percent suppression of paw-oedema volume in first phase of study upto 3 h was recovered and found to be significant in the case of drug administered in the form of aqueous solution (plain) (Fig. 3). This could be related to the drug availability in systemic circulation at sampling time.

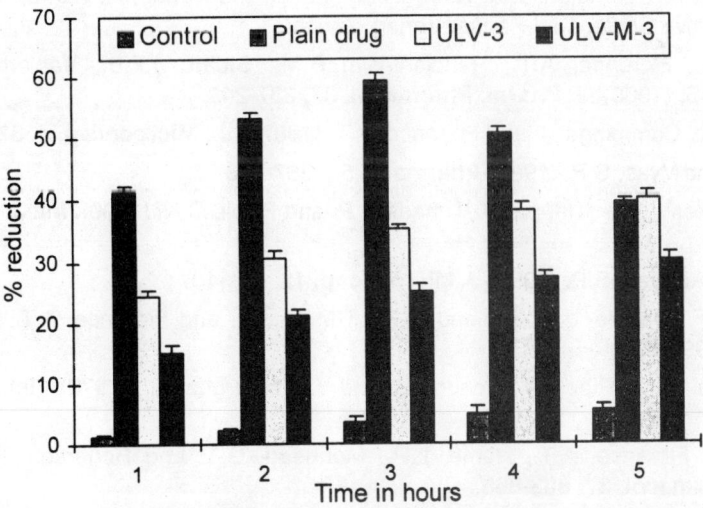

Fig.3 : Percentage reduction in paw volume

In the case of niosomal preparation, the drug could have been available to systemic pool at low concentration level over a prolonged period of time. The drug release rate was retarded and prolonged, accounting for the degree of suppression by the vesicle membrane. Moreover, when observed as time for suppression as therapeutic efficacy, either of the system exhibited better *in vivo* performance. When the drug antiinflammatory activity was compared as against the plain, invariably in all the treatment it was found to be significant ($p < 0.5$). It was further observed that intersubject variation in paw oedema suppression was calculated to be significant ($p < 0.5$) statistically.

The study clearly indicates that the niosomal preparation could be successfully used as controlled release parenteral where one can expect *in yivo* and *in vitro* stability in case of polymerplied niosomes which tend their protection against the osmotic shock. Opsonin borne destabilization in plasma could be addressed via poloxamer adsorptive coating.

ACKNOWLEDGEMENTS

We are thankful for the financial assistance provided by C.S.I.R., New Delhi, to one of the author (N.V). We are also thankful to Jagsonpal Pharmaceuticals Ltd. (India), for providing free drug sample of diclofenac sodium and to Prof. V.K. Dixit, Head, Department of Pharmaceutical Sciences, Sagar for providing the necessary facilities to carry out this work.

REFERENCES

1. Florence, A.T. (1993) Chemistry and Industry 20 Dec.1993, 1000-1004.

2. Vanlerberghe, G., Handjani-Vila, R.M., Berthelot, C. and Sebag, H. (1972). Int. KongreB fur grenzfiachektive Stoffe. Carl Hanser Verlag, Zurich.

3. Azmin, M.N., Florence, A.T., Handjani-vila, R.M., Stuart, J.F.B., Vanlerberghe, G. and Whittaker, J.S. (1985). **J. Pharm. Pharmacol.** 37, 237-242.

4. Rogerson, A., Cummings, J. and Florence, A.T. (1987). **J. Microencap.** 4, 321-328.

5. Jain, C.P. and Vyas, S.P. (1995) **Pharmazie** 50, 367-368.

6. Chandraprakash, K.S., Udupa, N., Umadevi, P. and Pillail, G.K. (1990). **Int. J. Pharm.** 61, R1-R3.

7. Jain, C.P. and Vyas, S.P. (1995) **J. Microencap.** 12, 401-407.

8. Uchegbu, I.F., Double, J.A., Kelland, L.R., Turton, J.A. and Florence, A.T. (1996). **J. Drug Target.** 3, 399-409.

9. Handjani-vila, R.M., Riber, A., Rondot, B. and Vanlerberghe, G., (1979). **Int. J. Cos. Sci. 1,** 303-314.

10. Baillie, A.J., Florence, A.T., Hume, L.R., Murihead, G.T. and Rogerson, R., (1985). **J. Pharm. Pharmacol.** 37, 863-868.

11. Gross, L., Ringsdorf, H. and Schupp, H.(1981). **Angew. Chem, Int. Eng. Ed.** 20, 305-325.

12. Akimoto, A., Dorn, K., Gros, L. and Ringsdorf, H., (1981). **Angew. Chem. Int. Eng. Ed.** 20, 90-91.

13. Johnston, D.S., Sanghera, S., Pons, M. and Chapman, D. (1980). **Biochem. Biophy. Acta** 602, 57-69.

14. Hupfer, B., Ringsdorf, H. and Schupp, H. (1981). **Makromol. Chem.**182, 247-253.

15. Regen, S.L., Czech, B. and Singh, A. (1980). **J. Am. Chem. Soc.** 102, 6638-6640.

16. Takane, M., Shigehara, K. and Tsuchida, E. (1986). **Makromol. Chem.** 187, 853-862.

17. Hasegawa, E., Matsushita, Y., Eshima, K., Ghno, H. and Tsuchida, E. (1986). **Poly. Bull.** 15, 397-403.

18. Hasegawa, E., Matsushita, Y., Eshima, K., Nishide, H. and Tsuchida, E. (1984). **Makromol. Chem. Rapid Comm.** 5, 779-784.

19. Freeman, F.J., Hayward, J.A. and Chapman, D. (1987). **Biochem. Biophy. Acta** 924, 341-351.

20. Yeung, Y.W. and Nixon, J.R. (1988). **J. Microencap.** 5, 331-337.

21. Nixon, J.R. and Yeung, Y.W. (1989). **J. Microencap.** 6, 43-52.

22. Leaver, J., Alonso, A., Durrani, A.A. and Chapman, D. (1983). **Biochem. Biophy. Acta** 732, 210-218.

23. Mehta, R., Hsu, M.J., Juliano, R.L., Krause, M.J. and Regen, S.L. (1986). **J Pharm. Sci.** 75(6), 579-581.

24. Venkatesan, N. and Vyas, S.P. (1998) **Drug Deliv.** 5, 251-255.

25. Katare, O.P., Vyas, S.P. and Dixit, V.K. (1995). **J. Microencap.** 12(5), 487-493.

17

DEVELOPMENT AND CHARACTERIZATION OF POLYSACCHARIDE CAPPED LIPOSOMES FOR ORAL DRUG DELIVERY

V. SIHORKAR and S. P. VYAS
Department of Pharmaceutical Sciences
Dr. H.S. Gour Vishwavidyalaya Sagar, M.P., INDIA

- Introduction
- Materials and methods
- Results and Discussion
- References

INTRODUCTION

Lipid vesicles (liposomes) are self-assemblages of amphiphiles into closed bilayer structures. Hydrated bilayer vesicles however, are not deemed to be thermodynamically stable and are thought to represent a metastable state in that the vesicles possess an excess of energy [1]. Liposomal phospholipids can undergo chemical degradation such as oxidation and hydrolysis. Either as a result of these changes or otherwise, liposomes maintained in aqueous dispersion may aggregate, fuse or leak their contents. Furthermore, method of formulation, nature of amphiphile and encapsulated drug/macromolecules were found to manipulate membrane fluidity/rigidity and permeability characteristics. The leakage of hydrophilic drugs from the aqueous domains of the liposomal bilayers upon storage is an area of considerable interest. The temperature of storage of these dispersions must be strictly controlled. A wide variability in the storage temperature of the system often leads to a change in the fundamental nature of the system [2]. These vesicles are thus predicted to transform into bilayer stacks against the challenges of physicochemical and bio-environment stimuli. To produce a system with an optimal stability requires that these predicted transformations be slowed down to such an extent as to produce a product with a reasonable shelf life. Methods to enhance the stability of liposomes are abounding in the literature [3-6]. The inclusion of a charged molecule in the bilayer shifts the electrophoretic mobility and makes it positive with the inclusion of stearylamine or negative with dicetyl phosphate, thus prevents liposomal fusion/swelling or aggregation [3].

The work described here evaluates the oral delivery potential of polysaccharide appended liposomal system. Polysaccharide has been immobilized on the outer half of the bilayer with the help of hydrophobic anchors adapting palmitoylation and cholesteroyl esterification. Capped liposomes were challenged against harsh environments and physicochemical stimuli to mimic the biological stresses to be encountered in the bio-fluids. The role of partially hydrophobized anchors on the stability and integrity of the coated liposomes has also been discussed.

MATERIALS AND METHODS

Materials

Phosphatidylcholine, cholesterol and dicetyl phosphate was purchased from Lobe Chemi, INDIA. Pullulan from *Aureobasidium pullulans* was obtained from Sigma (St. Louis, MO, USA) and used without further purification. The model drug tetracycline hydrochloride was a gift sample from MAC Laboratories Ltd., Mumbai, INDIA. Other materials and reagents were of analytical grade (Qualigens, Chemical division of Glaxo India Ltd.).

Synthesis of pullulan derivatives

Pullulan was derivatized with O-palmitoyl anchor or cholesterol moiety following the procedure of Hammerling & Westpal [7] and Sato [8] respectively. O-Palmitoyl pullulan (OPPu), in brief, was prepared by reacting pullulan (1.0 g) in dry DMF at 60°C to palmitoyl chloride (0.1 g) in the DMF in the presence of dry pyridine (1.0 ml). The mixture was stirred at 60°C for 6 hours and slowly poured into absolute ethanol (100 ml) under vigorous stirring. The precipitate of OPPu, thus obtained was collected and washed with 50 ml of absolute ethanol and 25 ml of dry diethyl ether, and dried under vacuo at 50±1°C for 1 hour. Cholesterol derivative of pullulan was synthesized as described [8] with appropriate modifications. In brief, carboxymethylated pullulan was obtained by the reaction of pullulan (1.0 g) with sodium monochloroacetate (0.95 g) in 1 M NaOH. Resulting solution was reacted at pH 4.7 with ethylenediamine (1.25 g) in the presence of 1-ethyl-3-(3-dimethylamino) propylcarbodiimide (0.5 g) as a coupling reagent. The aminoethyl carbamylmethyl pullulan, thus obtained was reacted with cholesterol chloroformate (0.5 g) in a water free DMF solution at 60°C for 24 hours and precipitate thus obtained was dried in vacuo at 50°C. The hydrophobized derivatized of pullulan (HP) was subjected to FT-IR and ^{1}H-NMR analysis. The ^{1}H-NMR spectrum was obtained in denaturated DMSO (50 μg/ml) containing tetramethylsilane(TMS) as internal standard operating at a frequency of 425 Mhz (Spectrometer Varion Unity-500). The IR spectrum of OPPu and Pu (1%), incorporated into a KBr disc, was run on a FT-IR single beam spectrometer.

Preparation of liposomes

Phosphatidylcholine, cholesterol and dicetyl phosphate, were taken in different mole fraction ratio (Table 1) and dissolved in minimum quantity of diethyl ether in a rotary flash evaporator. The solvent was evaporated in order to coat the inside surface of the flask of rotary flash evaporator (York, India). After vacuum desiccating the mixture for about an hour, 500 μl of PBS (pH 7.4) containing 10 μg/μl of tetracycline HCl was added at 50°C and dispersion so obtained was allowed for complete hydration at an ambient (30°C) temperature. The prepared vesicles were then dialysed against PBS (pH 7.4) using dialysis tubes (Sigma, USA) for removal of any free drug. The dialysed vesicles were centrifuged at 60,000 g for 60 min. and pellets were resusupendent in PBS (pH 7.4) for polymer capping of the vesicle surface. The liposomal population was harvested and screened for vesicle size and those above 0.88 µm (as retained oversize on ashless hardened Whatman paper, 0.88 µ) were taken for coating and further stability protocols.

Polysaccharide coating of the vesicles

Capping of liposomes with hydrophobized polysaccharide was accomplished by incubation of the vesicle and derivatized pullulan for a period of 6 hours. To the 1000 µl previously prepared vesicular dispersion (total lipid $\cong 3.75 \times 10^{-2}$ µg ml^{-3}) was added hydrophobized pullulan (1:10 volume ratio) dissolved in minimum known volume of mixed phosphate buffers (pH 7.4). This mixture was subsequently kept incubated in a micro-cuvette for an optimized period of 6 hours at ambient temperature followed by at refrigeration temperature for overnight. The surface potential of the vesicles at different time intervals were measured and based upon these observations the incubation time and the amount of protein cloud were optimized. Uncoated liposomes were similarly treated, but without the polymer. The coated liposomes were centrifuged (Beckman L8-55-Ultracentrifuge, 1,50,000g, 15°C, 30 min) to remove unentrapped drug.

Separation of unbound material from the polysaccharide capped vesicles

Isolation of polysaccharide coated liposomes was accomplished by gel chromatographic separation process. Sephadex G-50 column was equilibrated with mixed phosphate buffers and presaturarted with liposomal constituents (Length: 50 cm; diameter: 1.5 cm; flow rate: 150 µl/min.; and fraction volume: 2.0 ml/fraction). Fractions (2.0 ml elute) were collected and aliquots (100 µl) of the fractions were assayed for hydrophobized pullulan (HP) and liposomes (OD at 450 nm) using the established procedures [9,10].

Characterization of the coated liposomes

Vesicular dispersions were appropriately diluted and wet mounted on a haemocytometer and photographed by phase contrast microscope (Leitz, Biomed, Germany). The negatives were projected on a piece of calibrated paper using an enlarger (×1250). Diameter of around 500 vesicles was noted for each system. Predialysed vesicular dispersions were centrifuged at 1,50,000 g for 60 min. as described elsewhere. Pellets thus obtained were resuspended in 0.01 M PBS (pH 7.4) and the process was repeated for 3 times. Vesicles were lysed with 1% n-propanol:PBS (1:1 vol. ratio), centrifuged again and liberated contents were analysed at 274 nm using Shimadzu DB UV/VIS spectrophotometer (Japan). The entrapment efficiency was expressed as the ratio of experimentally measured amount of the drug in the dispersion and the added amount of the drug intended for encapsulation (Table 1).

In vitro release profile in simulated fluids having different pH and compositions

The medium for the released study was designed to simulate gastrointestinal fluids. Because the gastric fluid has a pH around 1.2-2, one set of release media contained 0.01 N hydrochloric acid and was adjusted to be isotonic using sodium chloride (model gastric medium). However the composition of the simulated gastric fluid has been selected to accommodate the aggressive species of the intestinal tract specially bile salts and phospholipases. Consequently a second set of release media simulating intestinal fluid (model intestinal medium) was chosen: 10mmol/litre of sodium taurocholate, 5 U/ml of phospholipases A2, and 3 mM calcium chloride in pH 6.8 phosphate buffered isotonic saline. Pellets from uncoated and OPPu and CHPu coated liposomes (500 µl) were suspended in 2.5 ml of simulated gastric (SGF) and simulated intestinal fluids (SIF), and placed in a Sigma dialysis bag at 37±1°C. The bags were incubated at 37±2°C in a metabolic shaker (York, India). Samples of 25µl were removed at various time intervals up to 24 hours, centrifuged (10,000 rpm, 25°C, 10 min.) and the supernatants were analysed at 274 nm for the released drug.

In a parallel experiment the stability of vesicle encapsulated tetracycline and of vesicles against simulated bile salt solution was appraised by measuring the amount of intact (unchanged) drug associated with vesicles at the end of six-h incubation. The experiment was conducted with sodium taurocholate dissolved in phosphate buffered saline to concentrations below, at and above critical micelle concentrations and monitored for the percent initial content at 37°C. At an incubation time of 2 h aliquots of vesicular dispersion were removed, centrifuged as earlier and supernatnat analysed for the drug content and from the data so obtained, the percent of initial content was calculated.

Osmotic stress studies

Effect of osmotic challenge on vesicle size and structural integrity was investigated by monitoring the variations in vesicle size, i.e., reduction or expansion of vesicular mean diameter (Phase contrast microscope, Leitz, Biomed, Germany) following the incubation of small volumes (100-500µl) of different tonicity (molar solutions of NaCl to the vesicular dispersion, 1.0 ml, in glass ampoules flushed with nitrogen). Aliquots of samples withdrawn over a period of 24 hours, were diluted appropriately and estimated for mean vesicle size.

Long term stability studies

Vesicular dispersions were kept in an amber colored bottle tightly capped in a nitrogen atmosphere, and samples were withdrawn at different time intervals to check the visual appearance as vesicle shape, size, integrity and % drug leaching. The remaining drug per unit of surfactant per unit time was estimated at different time intervals (Drug latency).

Vesicular dispersions of various compositions (2.0 ml) were stored in glass ampoules, flushed with nitrogen, and stored for a period of six months at an ambient temperature. Stability of the liposomes were checked (during storage) by their visual appearance with respect to aggregation and mean vesicle size, vesicles remaining per cu mm, and by measuring the released drug as a function of time at an ambient temperature. At different incubation times, aliquots of liposomal dispersions were removed, centrifuged at 60,000g for 60 min., and supernatant was analysed for released drug at 274 nm. The maximum level of drug leaching was measured after the addition of 0.1%w/v Triton X-100.

RESULTS AND DISCUSSIONS

Sunamoto and co-workers [11,12] succeeded in assembling an artificial cell wall on outermost surface of liposomes by using hydrophobized polysaccharides and reported an effective trapping of water soluble fluorescent marker probe, against the bio-environmental challenges of plasma, serum and elevated temperatures. In addition, the enzymatic lysis by phospholipase D, was arrested and addressed as ascertained by the fluorescence quenching based experiments. These results encouraged us to employ polysaccharide net over liposomal membrane to make an improved and stable (as compared against liposomes they are more chemically and mechanically stable and osmotically active) vehicle, especially for oral delivery of drugs/macromolecules.

Characterization of hydrophobized polysaccharides (HP)

Pullulan is a linear α-glucan, produced by the yeast like fungus *Pullunaria pullulans*, in which about 480 maltotriose units are linked by $\alpha(1{\rightarrow}6)$ glycosidic bonds. Like other naturally occuring polysaccharides, pullulan is known to protect plasma membranes against physico-chemical stimuli, such as osmotic pressure and ionic strength. However, when adsorbed on to the vesicular surface, it is easily desorbed on dilution or mechanical agitation [13]. However, chemically modified pullulans (hydrophobized pullulans) were found to strongly interact with the vesicles [14]. In this study, pullulan was chemically modified with O-palmitoyl anchor or cholesteroyl anchor using the procedures of Hammerling and Westpal and Sato [7,8] respectively with minor modifications. Pullulan was appanded on the preformed vesicles (OPPu) or otherwise as a chol-pullulan derivative (CHPu) gets inserted/interdigitalized in to the bilayer as a part of it. The derivatization products were subjected to characterization using IR and ^{1}H-NMR. The derivatization procedures employed to prepare OPPu and CHPu has a degree of substitution of 1.57 palmitoyl chains and 0.71 cholesterol molecules per hundred saccharide units of pullulan as estimated by ^{1}H-NMR.analysis. Hydrophobized pullulans were also characterized by IR spectroscopy to identify carbonyl groups, and thus, to ascertain that pullulan is covalently bound to palmitoyl or cholesteroyl anchors. A frequency shift of most characteristics C=O stretching vibration (original band at 1735 cm^{-1}) was found, which could be ascribed to a consequence of intramolecular hydrogen bonds between carbonyl and hydroxyl groups, which lower the stretching force vibration of the C=O band (1645 cm^{-1} for OPPu and 1690 cm^{-1} for CHPu). These observations are suggestive of an ester bond between pullulan and hydrophobic moieties indicating that they are not just physically admixed.

Characterization of polysaccharide coated liposomes

An artificial cell wall consisted of hydrophobic palmitoyl and cholesteroyl anchors was assembled on the outer surface of liposomes. When added to liposomes the hydrophobic anchors interact with the outer half of the bilayer orienting and projecting hydrophilic portion towards the aqueous bulk. In this way a two dimensional network of polymers is framed around the liposomal membranes. The conductivity of the vesicles measured till stabilized to ensure the completion of the coating. Simultaneously conductometric measurements were used to optimize the hydrophobized polysaccharide to surfactant ratio. The results suggest that the conductance of the vesicles stabilized at lower ratio of CHPu to surfactant (0.01:1) than of OPPu to surfactant (0.1:1) when measured the current with an applied voltage of 10 mV to the dispersion. This could be due to the fact that CHPu could have filled the locus of defects by becoming a part of the liposomal membrane, thus establishing equilibrium at lower concentration of coat material. Optimized time for the coating of the liposomal bilayer was found to be 6 hours, as no change was recorded in the conductance of coated systems at an applied voltage of 10 mV, beyond this time period (data not shown).

Liposomes derivatized with hydrophobized pullulans were subjected to vesicle type, shape and size analysis with the help of phase contrast and electron microscopic techniques (table 1). Vesicles were found to be spherical and multilamellar with a mean vesicle diameter of 2.5-3.0 μ. Opacity of the system revealed that coated vesicles were relatively larger in mean size, as compared to plain liposomes (uncoated). This may be accounted to the polymeric capping, a dual barrier on the liposomal surface. Encapsulation efficiency of drug in CHPu and OPPU compositions were 27.5±0.75 and 30.1±0.7 respectively, revealing that CHPu and OPPu coatings didn't affect significantly the initial levels of encapsulation (35.5±0.1 recorded for plain vesicles) (Table 1). Further, the decrease in encapsulation efficiency was statistically insignificant when compared with other (P>0.05) in a rank sum test manner.

Table 1. Various formulations with their characterization parameters

Composition (molar ratio)	Shape (phase contrast microscope)	Average vesicle size	Encapsulation efficiency
PC:CH (7:3)	Multilamellar, bifringes visible	2.5±0.57	32.7±1.2
PC:CH:DCP (7:3:0.5)	Multilamellar, bifringes visible	2.7±0.9	35.5±0.8
(PC:CH:DCP):OPPu (7:3:0.5):0.1	Lamellarity indistinguishable; opaque appearance	3.1±1.4	27.8±0.6
(PC:CH:DCP):CHPu (7:3:0.5):0.1	Lamellarity indistinguishable; opaque appearance	3.1±2.1	30.4±0.6

Influence of hydrophobized pullulan anchors for membrane stabilization

In vitro stability studies revealed that by coating of the outermost surface of liposomes with a naturally occurring polysaccharide bearing hydrophobic substituents (capable anchoring into the bilayer membrane) imparts stability to the liposomes. The first apparent effect of webbing hydrophobized pullulan on to the liposomal membrane, was the protection against simulated gastric and intestinal fluids with compositions mimicking pH, bile salts and lipases present in the bio-environment after oral delivery. The liposomal coating with hydrophobized polysaccharides (HPs) retarded the leakage of entrapped drug in simulated gastric (SG) and simulated intestinal (SI) fluids. Moreover, the release profile remained the same as in either case it followed bi-phasic release kinetics. Fig. 1 presents % drug released as a function of time recorded over various time intervals (1, 6, and 12 hrs.). The efficacy of the system has been assessed in terms of % drug latency (drug remaining associated with the vesicles). It could be seen that in the model intestinal medium (SIF, pH 6.8) CHPu coated liposomes were able to retain 90.5±0.7 percent of the drug, whilst OPPu coated liposomes showed 82.9±0.1 drug latency at the end of the experiment.

As the incubation periods increase the drug release also increase in the case of plain liposomes. For the coated systems, however, a biphasic release profile was observed. After the initial release, a sustained and slower second phase was observed. However, the rate and extent of drug release was comparatively higher from the OPPu coated liposomes than in CHPu coated liposomes. The results recorded in terms of drug release are significantly better than plain liposomal system which could retain 22.5±0.5% of the drug under the same experimental conditions. The drug release profiles followed more or less the same trend in the SG fluids (Fig. 1A vs. 1B) where the % latency for the plain liposomes was found to be 17.5±1.7%. However the relative drug release was slightly higher (as compared to SIF) in the case of from polymer coated vesicles (17.6±0.12 and 25±0.1 respectively from OPPu and CHPu coated liposomes). Comparatively faster and higher release in the case of CHPu coated liposomes (reverse to the SG fluid) could be ascribed to the leaching of the intervening cholesterol anchor (Fig. 1B). To gain more information about the interaction of the delivery systems in the harsh environments of biofluids, polysaccharide coated liposomes were subjected to various stability studies.

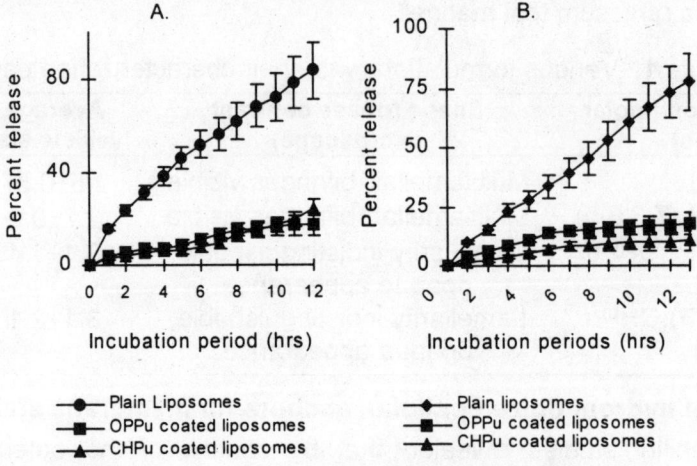

Fig. 1: *In vitro* release recorded with polysaccharide coated and plain liposomes in simulated gasric fluid (A) and simulated intestinal fluid (1B)

In order to explore the role of different molar concentrations of bile salts on the integrity of the bilayered membrane, % of initial content was recorded for plain and coated system after challenging with sodium taurocholate. Stability of liposomal formulations were tested by incubating with different mM concentration of taurocholate (below, above and in the vicinity of CMC) at 37°C for a period of 2 hours. No significant changes in the vesicle size, integrity and drug content were observed for coated liposomes as compared against plain versions over 2-hr incubation period at low concentrations. It could be seen from fig. 3 that at salt concentrations below and at CMC the drug content was not affected much in the case of coated liposomes, but at higher concentrations of bile salts (above CMC) a reduction in the % of initial content was recorded. This reduction however was significantly lower than that observed for plain liposomes.

The solubilization of bilayer via the build up of CMC of taurocholate molecules within the liposomal membrane, followed by micellization could be proposed as the possible mechanism for residual drug content at higher bile salt concentrations. Dual diffusion barrier of coated liposomes was instrumental in its exceptional stability against the bile salt.

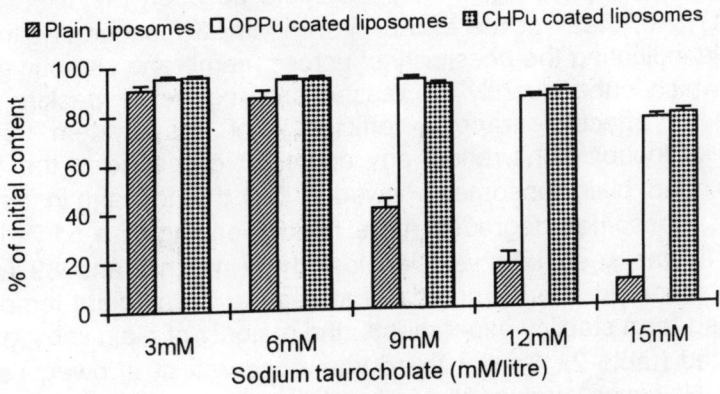

Fig. 2 : Interaction of different coated and plain liposomal formulations with sodium deoxycholate

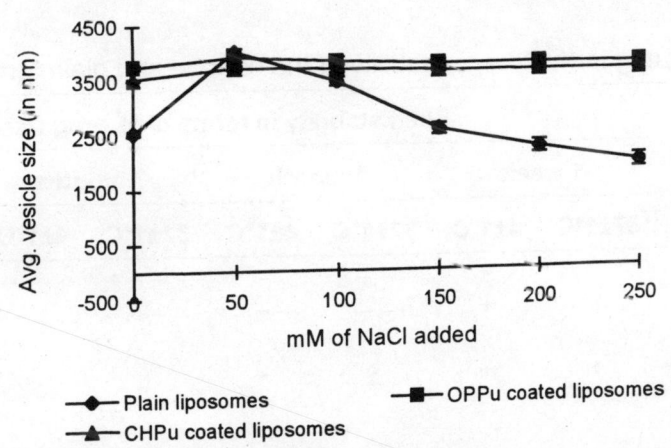

Fig. 3 : Assessment of osmotic challenge against coated and plain liposomal formulations

The vesicle integrity of hydrophobized polysaccharide coated liposomes was further assessed following osmotic stress under increasing concentrations of different molar solutions of sodium chloride. Pullulan capped vesicles were found to resist the tonicity gradiance. As evident from figure 3, the average vesicle size was found to increased in hypotonic environment, whilst under hypertonic conditions a marginal shrinkage and resultant decrease in the average size was observed. At hypotonic environments (50 mM and 100 mM) the plain vesicles show an increase in the vesicle size, whereas at hypertonic environments (200 mM and 250 mM) the vesicles shrink due to the osmotic variation in the surrounding fluids. It is evident that except of a marginal increase in response to the hypertonic media, no appreciable change has occurred in the case of polymer capped systems. Insignificant change in the vesicles size in the pullulan coated liposomes, reflected the better vesicle integrity offered by the polysaccharide cap against the osmotic challenges.

Long term stability of liposomes was examined by measuring the % drug remaining associated with the liposomal dispersions as a function of time at an ambient temperature (% drug latency). It could be seen that HP coated vesicles recorded a 17.5±0.1 leak at the end of first month. Subsequently, the loss of drug was negligible indicating the possibility of across membrane osmotic gradiance to be operational which subsequently decreases allowing better packing of membrane resulting in to effective trapping efficiency of the system. The nature of hydrophobized anchor didn't reflect any appreciable change in the stability profile. On the other hand, plain liposomes showed 18.3±1.5 % leakage in first 7 days, but in next 21 days, liposomes degraded more rapidly leading to a 51.7±1.5% leak after first month. It was seen that vesicles lost their integrity and 89.1±4.1% of drug leakage was recorded after 3 months of storage at an ambient temperature. At the end of the long-term stability experiments, the majority of plain liposomes were found to be disrupted (table 2). Similar trend was observed at a lower, i.e., 4°C storage experiments. However, an over all comparatively slow leaching profile was recorded, as appreciated due to higher stability of the vesicular membranes at a lower temperatures.

Table 2. Long term storage stability of the capped and plain formulations

Liposomal composition	Shelf stability in terms of % drug latency							
	1 week		1 month		3 months		7 months	
	37±1°C	4±1°C	37±1°C	4±1°C	37±1°C	4±1°C	37±1°C	4±1°C
PC:CH (7:3)	−	±	− −	−	− − − −	− − −	− − − −	− − − −
PC:CH:DCP (7:3:0.5)	±	+	− −	±	− − − −	− −	− − − −	− − −
(PC:CH:DCP): CHPu (7:3:0.5):0.1	+	+	±	+	±	+	±	+
(PC:CH:DCP): OPPu (7:3:0.5):0.1	+	+	±	+	±	+	±	+

All results are recorded in terms of % drug leaching values. * Leakage criteria are related to the amount of liposome bound metronidazole at day zero or at the start of the incubation, (+) leakage within accepted limits, 0-10%; (±) 10-25%; (-) 25-50%; (- -) 50-75%; (- - -) above 75% (- - - -) vesicles disrupted and released their contents.

The hydrophobized pullulan coated liposomes exhibited exceptional stability profile against the challenge of pH, ionic strength, osmotic pressure, simulated enzymatic solutions and long term stability, it could be inferred that palmitoyl or cholesteroyl moieties act as hydrophobic anchor groups for the lipids of the liposomal bilayer. The system can be exploited for the delivery of drugs to either gastric or intestinal tract or otherwise for oral delivery of peptides or proteins. The system could also be equally useful in targeting the loaded antimicrobial agents to the bacterial bio-film upon oral administration.

ACKNOWLEDGEMENTS

The authors are thankful to CSIR, New Delhi, India for providing financial assistance to one of the author (VS). The facilities provided by the Head, Department of Pharmaceutical Sciences is also duly acknowledged.

REFERENCES

1. Lasic, D. D. (1990). **J. Colloid Interface Sci.** 140, 302.

2. Chiang, C. M. and Weiner, N. (1987). **Int. J. Pharm.** 37, 75.

3. Larrabee, A.L. (1979). **Biochemistry** 18, 3321.

4. Leaver, J., Alonso, A., Aziz, A.D. and Chapman, D. (1983). **Biochim. Biophys. Acta** 732, 210.

5. Weinstein, J.N., Klausher, R.D., Innerarity, T., Ralston, E. and Blumenthal, R. (1981). **Biochim. Biophys. Acta** 647, 270.

6. Crowe, L.M., Womersley, C., Crowe, J.H., Reid, D., Appel, L.and Rudolph, A. (1986). **Biochim. Biophys. Acta** 861, 131.

7. Hammerling, U. and Westpal, O. (1967). **Eur. J. Biochem.** 1, 46.

8. Sato, T. and Sunamoto, J. (1992). **Prog. Lipid Res.** 31, 345.

9. Katare, O.P., Vyas, S.P. and Dixit, V.K. (1991). **J. Microencap.** 8, 1.

10. Venkatesan, N. and Vyas, S.P. (1998). **Drug Deliv.** 5, 1.

11. Sunamoto, J., Goto, M., Iida, T., Hara, K., Saito, A. and Tomonaga, A. (1984). in: Receptor mediated targeting of drugs (Gregoridis, G., Ed.) NATO ASI Ser., Plenum Press, London, Vol. 82, pp. 359.

12. Sunamoto. J. and Iwamoto, K. (1986). **CRC Crit. Rev. Ther. Drug Carrier Syst.** 2, 117.

13. Sunamoto, J. and Sato, T. (1989). **J. Chem. Soc. Jpn.** 161, 34.

14. Mollerfield, J., Prass, W., Rignsdorf, H., Hamazaki, H. and Sunamoto, J. (1986). **Biochim. Biophys. Acta** 857, 265.

18

INSULIN DELIVERY THROUGH THE OCULAR ROUTE

R. SRINIVASAN and S.K. JAIN
Department of Pharmaceutical Sciences,
Dr. Harisingh Gour Vishwavidyalaya, Sagar (M.P.) 470 003

- Introduction
- Materials and Methods
- Preparation of Liposomes

- Characterization
- Results and Discussion
- References

INTRODUCTION

Many problems remain associated with insulin therapy due to its rapid enzymatic degradation on oral administration. This leads to short biological half-life and ineffectiveness of the drug. Moreover, the membrane permeability is often low due to lack of lipophilicity and high molecular weight [1]. Hence, there is the need to develop a system that could effectively deliver the drug in a controlled manner for prolonged periods of time. An assortment of delivery systems has been developed for prolonged and efficacious delivery of insulin [2-4]. However, none of these alternatives have yet been adopted for the treatment of diabetes.

The eye has potential as an excellent route for peptide administration, including insulin [5,6]. Blood glucose levels of test animals can successfully be lowered on instillation of insulin in the eye [7-9].

When the peptide is instilled into the precorneal area of the eye, it can have four possible fates [10-12]. It can:-

1. exist in precorneal area as overflow associated with high level of tearing.
2. absorb through the cornea into the intraocular chamber
3. enter the systemic circulation on absorption from the conjunctiva
4. exit the precorneal area through the nasal lachrymal drainage system and enter the systemic circulation on absorption from the nasopharyngeal mucosa

The overflow of the drug through the tear may be reduced by use of liposomal systems. Liposomes enhance the intracorneal and transcorneal penetration of water as well as lipid-soluble drugs and offer advantages over most ophthalmic preparations because of their complete biodegradation and nontoxicity [13,14]. Positively charged liposomes with known charge affinity may be adsorbed at the corneal surface and transfer the drug directly to the corneal epithelial cell membrane and blood circulation, thus facilitating drug transport across the cornea. The drug may reach the systemic circulation via nasolacrimal route as some of the liposomes drain through punctae into the nasolacrimal duct.

In recent years, the most preferred route of insulin administration has been subcutneous. The major drawback of insulin therapy is that it cannot be given orally because of its enzymatic degradation [15] and its inability to cross the intestinal mucosa [16]. Although the subcutaneous route of administration is effective in controlling blood glucose level and diabetic complications such as retinopathy in IDDM patients, it is not convenient for patients who require daily pricking with insulin needle. Therefore, it would be more convenient if the insulin could be administered by other non-invasive routes. Various routes have been studied for this purpose including duodenal [17], rectal [18], nasal [17,19,20], vaginal [21], pulmonary [22-24] transdermal [25,26], and buccal [27]. These routes exhibited low bioavailability of the insulin as compared to subcutaneous administration. It is suggested that ocular route can successfully be used for systemic administration of insulin and for controlling the blood glucose level with the help of adjuvants [28,29]. Liposomes enhance the systemic bioavailability of drug administered through the ocular route because of the bioadhesive nature of liposomes. Positive-charged liposomes were preferred as they show charge affinity with ocular tissue or corneal membrane and therefore change their residence time [30].

In this study, the effectiveness of a liposomal system bearing insulin was studied on ocular administration and compared to other formulations administered via various routes. The effect of charged lipids and penetration enhancers on ocular penetration of insulin was also studied.

MATERIALS AND METHODS

Egg phosphatidylcholine, cholesterol, stearylamine, sodium deoxycholate, sodium taurocholate, sodium glycocholate, and polyoxyethylene-9-lauryl ether (POE) were purchased from Sigma (St. Louis, MO, USA), Pork insulin (25 U/mg) was received as gift from M.J. Pharmaceuticals (Baroda, India). Other chemicals and reagents were of analytical grade.

PREPARATION OF LIPOSOMES

Multilamellar liposomes were prepared using the cast film method reported by Bangham, et al. [31]. The phospholipids (egg PC/DPPC:CH:SA/DCP) in different weight ratios (Table 1) were dissolved in a 5 ml chloroform:methanol mixture (2:1) in a 250 ml round bottom flask. A thin film of lipid was casted on the inner wall of the flask by constantly rotating the flask under vacuum under an inert atmosphere of nitrogen using rotary flask evaporator. The film was hydrated with 5 ml phosphate buffer saline (PBS), pH 7.4, containing insulin (20 mg/ml). After hydration, the contents of the flask were centrifuged at 60,000 rpm to remove the free drug. The sediment was lyophilized and stored under nitrogen atmosphere in amber-coloured vials.

CHARACTERIZATION

Size, Shape and Charge

The shape and size of the liposomes were determined using a phase-contrast microscope (Wild-Leitz, Germany) and ocular micrometer at x1000 magnification. The charge of the vesicles was determined by observing the movement of vesicles in the electrical field of zeta meter (Appelex 35, France).

Table 1a. Composition and characterization of various liposomal products

Product code	Composition					Charge
	EggPC	DPPC	CH	SA	DCP	
In-L-1	70	-	30	-	-	N
In-L-2	60	-	30	-	10	-ve
In-L-3	60	-	30	10	0	+ve
In-L-4	-	70	30	-	-	N
In-L-5	-	60	30	-	10	-ve
In-L-6	-	60	30	10	-	+ve

Table 1b. Characterization of various liposomal products

Product code	Av. Size (µm)	%drug entrapment	Captured Vol. (mL/g) of lipid	% drug leakage (10h)
In-L-1	3.8	24 ± 1.0	3.0	8.5 ± 0.4
In-L-2	5.7	38 ± 1.5	4.7	15.6 ± 0.6
In-L-3	8.8	42 ± 1.3	5.3	11.8 ± 0.5
In-L-4	3.6	28 ± 1.8	3.5	14.2 ± 0.7
In-L-5	4.9	34 ± 2.0	4.3	17.4 ± 1.0
In-L-6	7.5	46 ± 1.7	5.2	16.4 ± 0.8

Encapsulation efficiency and captured volume

The percent entrapment efficiency and capture volume (V_{cap}) was calculated (Table 1) using the following equations [32].

% entrapment efficiency = [TAE/TAA] x 100 ; Where,
TAA = total amount of insulin used (by weight)
TEA = total amount of insulin entrapped in liposomes (by weight) and

Captured volume (V_{cap}) = % entrapment efficiency x [TVA/TAP] x 100; Where,
TVA = total volume of insulin solution applied
TAP = total amount of phospholipid in final preparation determined using the method reported by Stewart [33].

The drug-loaded liposomal pellets were resuspended in simulated lachrymal fluid (pH 7.4). The final insulin concentration in the preparation was determined using the following equation:

Drug concentration in liposomes = V_{cap} x LC x DC; Where,
V_{cap} = captured volume (5 ml/mg)
LC = Lipid concentration in the preparation (100 mg/ml)
DC = concentration of drug used for the hydration of lipid film 1000 U/mL

Drug leakage

Liposomal formulations were centrifuged at 60,000 rpm for 30 min. at 0°C. The pellet formed was resuspended in 10 ml of PBS (pH 7.4), filtered and analyzed spectrophotometrically at 276 nm [31] (Table 1b).

In vitro drug release

The drug-release study was performed using a Franz diffusion cell (Crown Glass, NJ, USA). The treated cellophane membrane was clamped between donor and receptor compartments of the cell to support the liposomal formulation. The receptor compartment contained artificial tear solution (ATS) of pH 7.4 as diffusion medium, and the temperature was maintained at $37\pm1°C$ with the help of a circulating water bath. Samples were withdrawn periodically and assayed for drug content (Fig. 1).

In vivo performance : Effect of charged lipid

In vivo studies were performed by monitoring the blood glucose levels in rabbits. Twelve rabbits (male 2-2.5 Kg) were divided into three groups of four animals in each. The first group received plain insulin solution (300 U/ml; PI), the second group received liposome-bearing insulin (IN-L-3), and third group was given temperature-sensitive liposome-bearing insulin (In-L-6). All the preparation contained the same amount of insulin and were instilled in the eye with the help of a calibrated eye dropper. The blood samples were collected from the ear marginal vein at scheduled time intervals for 48 h and analyzed for blood glucose content using an Ames glucometer and dextrostrix. The blood glucose level of each animal was also monitored before instillation of the formulation in the eye that served as control. The effect of temperature was observed by increasing the eye temperature using warm water bags placed on eyelids every 4 h (Fig. 2).

In vivo performance: Effect of penetration enhancer and route of administration

Albino rabbits weighing 2.5-3.0 Kg were fasted overnight before the experiments. The experiments were performed to study the effect of the route of administration of insulin solution on its bioavailability and the effect of permeation enhancers and liposomal systems on the penetration of insulin through corneal membrane following ocular instillation of insulin preparation.

The rabbits were separated into four groups, each having 6 rabbits. The insulin solution was administered via intravenous (i.v.) (0.5 U/Kg), subcutaneous (s.c.) (0.8 U/Kg) and through ocular (10 U/Kg) routes to the first, second and third group of animals, respectively [34]. The animals of the fourth group were kept as control. Blood samples were collected at pre scheduled time intervals and analyzed for blood glucose concentration.

In the next study, the effect of permeation enhancers was observed by first testing their ocular compatibility. One eye of each healthy rabbit was treated with penetration enhancers separately by instillation of two drops of various concentration (0.2-1.0% w/w) of penetration enhancers, while another eye was kept as a control (two drops of simulated lachrymal fluid, pH 7.4 was instilled). Then, the eyes were tested for the degree of blinking, tear flow, and redness. On the basis of this eye compatibility study, 0.8% w/w penetration-enhancer concentration was selected to study its effect on insulin penetration through corneal membrane on ocular instillation. The solution of different penetration enhancers (0.8% w/w), i.e., sodium glycocholate, sodium deoxycholate, sodium taurocholate and polyoxyethylene-9-lauryl ether (POE), was first instilled separately into the eye of the animals of the first, second, third, and fourth groups, respectively. Then, 5 minutes later, the insulin solution (10 U/Kg) was instilled into an eye of each animal and the resulting fall in blood glucose level was measured.

Finally, the effect of liposomal system bearing insulin was studied for insulin penetration through the corneal membrane. The drug-loaded liposomal system was instilled into one eye of each animal of the first group; the second group of animals received ocularly the drug-loaded liposomal system along with penetration enhancer (POE, 0.8% w/w). The fall in blood glucose level was recorded periodically.

Blood samples were withdrawn periodically from the canula (Intracath No. 26) inserted into the marginal ear vein of the rabbits and analyzed for glucose concentration using an autoanalyser (Miles, India) and Dextrostrix. Data were recorded ± SEM. The sensitivity of glucose assay was 0.5 mg/ml. The inter- and intra run variations in the glucose assay were estimated to be 4 and 8% respectively.

RESULTS AND DISCUSSION

Normal and temperature-sensitive liposomes were prepared using the cast film method reported by Bangham et al. [31]. They were characterized by various attributes, viz., type of vesicles, size, charge, entrapment efficiency, captured volume and drug leakage (Table 1a and 1b). The liposomal formulation (In-L-1) composed of egg phosphotidylcholine:cholesterol (70:30) exhibited aggregation, while liposomes containing charged components showed no aggregation. A higher drug-entrapment efficiency (42±1.5 and 46±2.0%) was observed with positively charged liposome formulations (In-L-3 and In-L-6, respectively). This could be accounted for the large aqueous space between bilayers of MLVs due to repulsion of similar charges. Drug-leakage profiles revealed maximum leakage with the product In-L-5 (DPPC:CH:DCP; 60:30:10) and minimum with product In-L-1 (eggPC:CH: 70:30). This could be ascribed to the loosening of bilayers due to the repulsion of negatively charged bilayers.

The liposomes composed of dipalmitoylphosphatidylcholine (DPPC) exhibited sensitivity to temperature as these liposomes changed from an ordered gel to a more disordered fluid (crystalline liquid) with varying temperature from 30 to 55°C. The release of insulin was observed due to change in the fluidity of liposomes (Table 2). The ruptured bilayers of liposomes were observed under the microscope at higher temperature that enhanced the drug release. Therefore, a pulsatile delivery of the drug may be achieved according to need by providing a temperature stimulus.

The *in vitro* drug-release data exhibited a linear relationship between the log of drug release versus the log of time, with the slope of 0.96 that is very near to one. This is an indication of near zero-order release kinetics. Further, it was confirmed by plotting a graph between cumulative drug released versus time. A straight line showed that the drug release from the liposomal products follow near zero-order kinetics (Fig.1). The release of drug was found to be higher for products In-L-3 and In-L-6, which could be due to the high degree of repulsion between bilayers and loosening of the bilayers configuration.

Table 2. Effect of temperature on liposomes

| Product | Temperature effect after 30 min | | | | | |
| | 30°C | | 40°C | | 55°C | |
	% drug released	Shape	% drug released	Shape	% drug released	Shape
In-L-1	0.4	+	2.6	±	6.1	±
In-L-2	0.7	+	4.8	+	10.5	-
In-L-3	0.9	+	3.7	+	8.6	-
In-L-4	0.5	+	20.0	-	36.2	-
In-L-5	1.0	+	32.0	-	52.4	-
In-L-6	0.8	+	26.0	-	48.3	-

Note : Drug content at time zero was taken as 100%, ± Aggregated: + unchanged, - irregular or ruptured

Products In-L-3 and In-L-6 were selected for *in vivo* performance studies because they showed comparatively high *in vitro* drug release and positive charge affinity for corneal membrane [32,35]. The blood glucose level was monitored periodically after the instillation of the product into the animal's eye. The blood glucose level was presented as a percentage of time zero where each animal served as its own control.

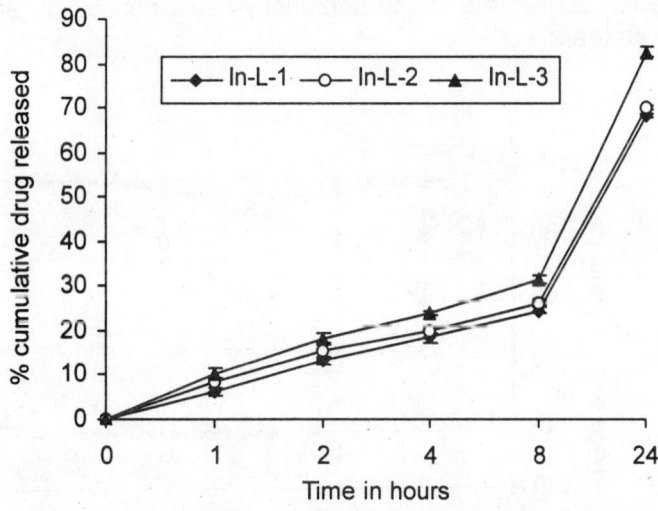

Fig. 1 : *In vitro* release profile of various liposomal formulations

The *in vivo* performance revealed that no significant effect in reduction in blood glucose level was observed when the buffered insulin was instilled into the eye (Fig. 2). The plain liposome bearing insulin decreased the blood glucose level to a minimum of 29±2% in 4 h and showed prolonged effect due to slow drug release.

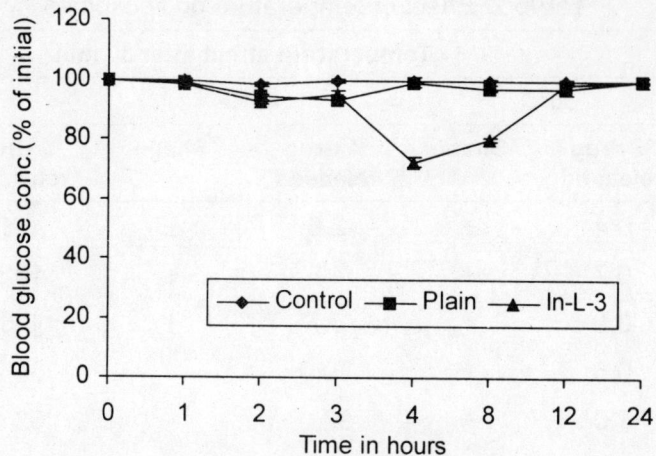

Fig. 2 : Blood glucose concentration versus time plot following ocular administration of insulin formulations

The effect of the route of administration of insulin solution (0.8 U/Kg body weight) on the systemic bioavailability of insulin was studied by periodically measuring the fall in blood glucose level. The i.v. route showed faster fall in blood glucose level (58±7% in 15 min.) than the s.c. route (59±6% in 45 min.), which could be due to direct delivery of insulin to the blood stream (Fig. 3). The insulin administered through the ocular route did not show a significant effect at 10U/Kg concentration because of the limited volume of the conjunctiva sac, i.e., 50 µL and draining of the drug solution with tears.

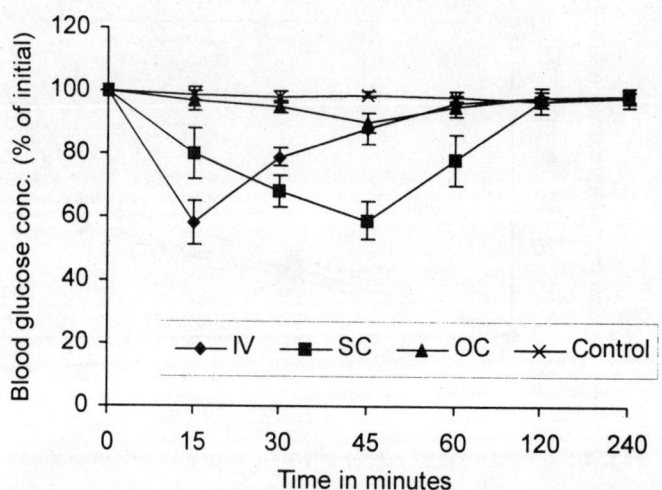

Fig. 3 : Blood glucose concentration time profiles following insulin solution administration by various routes

Because of poor permeability of insulin through the corneal membrane from its solution, the various penetration enhancers were used to enhance insulin permeability through the ocular route. Among various concentrations of penetration enhancers, the 0.8% w/w concentration was found to be most suitable, since it did not affect the degree of eyelid blinking, tear flow and eye redness; above 0.8% w/w penetration enhancers, the degree of eye lid blinking and tear flow increases. Therefore, an 0.8% w/w concentration of penetration enhancer was used to enhance insulin penetration through the corneal membrane. Among the various penetration enhancers, the maximum increment in insulin penetration was observed with POE as it reduces the blood glucose level to 65±5.3% of base line in 15 min. on ocular instillation of insulin solution (Fig. 4).

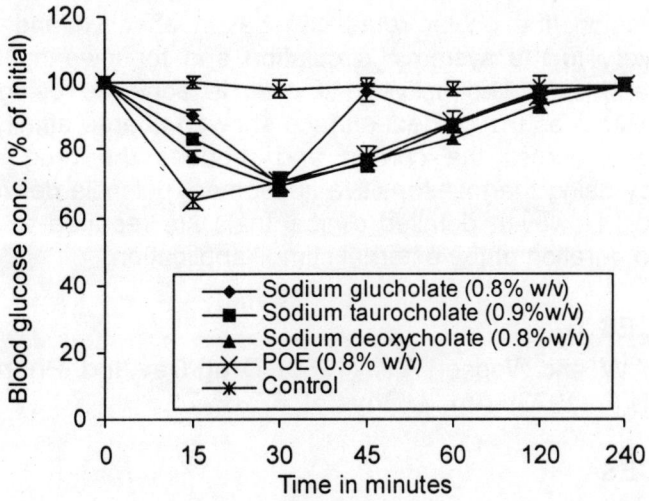

Fig. 4 : Blood glucose concentration time profiles after ocular administration of insulin solution in the presence of penetration enhancer

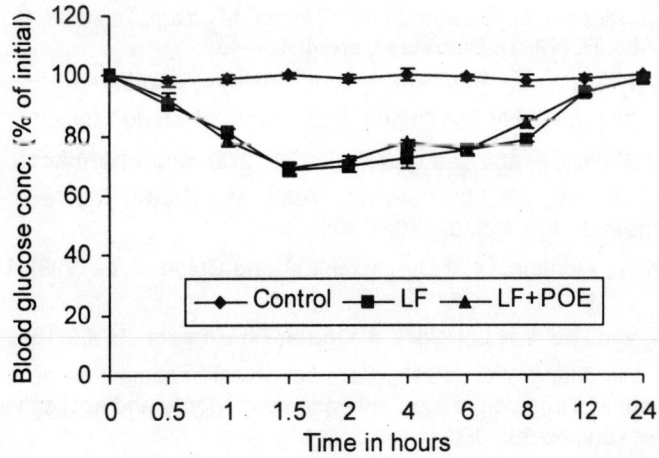

Fig. 5 : Blood glucose time profiles after ocular administration of liposomal formation bearing insulin

Further, the blood glucose level decreases to 65-70% from the base line in 90 min. on instillation of the insulin-loaded liposomal system (Fig. 5), which is similar to s.c. administration of plain insulin solution (Fig. 3) or instilling drug solution with penetration enhancer (Fig. 4). But the liposomal system exhibited this reduction up to 5 h from the onset of action. This could be due to positive charge affinity of the corneal membrane, which reduced drainage of liposomal product with tear flow and facilitated drug transport through the corneal membrane and the nasolachrymal passage.

It could be concluded that positively charged liposomes bearing insulin could be utilized effectively for ocular administration of insulin and management of blood glucose level.

In conclusion, the ocular route can be an effective and convenient route for insulin delivery to the systemic circulation and for lowering blood glucose. The prolonged and controlled delivery of drug is achieved using a positive charged liposomal system as the corneal surface showed charge affinity, and thus facilitates drug transport across the cornea and reduces the drug drainage with tears. Moreover, by using thermal-sensitive liposomes, pulsatile delivery of the drug could be achieved. However, detailed clinical trials are required to establish the dosage regimen and duration of the external stimuli application.

REFERENCES

1. Chien, Y.W. and Wagner, A.K. (1989). **Drug Dev. Ind. Pharm.** 15, 1601-1634.
2. Fisher, N.F. (1923). **Am. J. Physiol.** 67, 65-71.

REFERENCES

1. Chien, Y.W. and Wagner, A.K. (1989). **Drug Dev. Ind. Pharm.** 15, 1601-1634.

2. Fisher, N.F. (1923). **Am. J. Physiol.** 67, 65-71.

3. Wisley, F.M., Londono, J.A., Wood, S.H., Shipp, J.C. and Waldmoan, R.H. (1971). **Diabetes** 20, 552-556.

4. Yamaski, Y., Shirehiri, M., Kawamori, R., Kikuchi, M., Yagi, T., Aarai, S., Tohdo, R., Nakui, N., Oji, N. and Abe, H. (1981). **Diabetes Care** 4, 454-458.

5. Chiou, C.Y. (1991). **Annu. Rev. Pharmacol. Toxicol.**, 31, 457-467.

6. Chiou, C.Y., Chauang, C.Y.and Chang, M.S. (1988). **Diabetes Care** 11, 750-751.

7. Chiou, C.Y., Shen, Z.F. and Zheng, Y.Q. (1990). **J. Ocular Pharmacol.**, 6, 233-241.

8. Pillion, D.J., Bartlett, J.D., Meezan, E., Yang, M., Crown, R.J. and Grizzle, N.E. (1991). **Invest. Opthalmol. Vis. Sci.** 32, 3021-3027.

9. Segwade, N.D., Albritton, IV, F.D., Liu, S.X.L. and Chiou, C.Y.(1993). **Drug Delivery** 1, 139-142.

10. Chang, S.C. and Lee, V.H.L. (1987). **J. Ocular Pharmacol.** 3, 159-169.

11. Chiou, C.Y. and Zheng, Y.Q. (1993). Permeation enhancement for ocular route of polypeptide administration, In: Drug permeation enhancement:Theory and applications (Hsiegh, D.S. Ed.), Dekker, New York, pp 385-395.

12. Robinson, J.R. (1980). Opthalmic Drug delivery System, American Phamaceutical association, Washington DC, 57.

13. Ahmed, I. and Patton, T.F. (1985). **Invest. Ophthalmol. Vis. Sci.** 26, 584-587.

14. Schaeffer, H.E. and Krohn, D.L. (1982). **Invest. Opthalmol. Vis. Sci.** 21, 220-227.

15. Tobey, N., Heizer, W., Yeh, R., Huang, T.L. and Hoffner, C. (1985). **Gastroenterology** 88, 913.

16. Ziv, E., Lior, O. and Kidlron, M. (1987). **Biochem. Pharmacol.** 36, 1035.

17. Moses, A.C.and Flier, J.S. (1987). Unconventional routes of insulin administration, In: The Diabetes Annual (Alberti, K.G.M.M. and Krall, L.P. Eds) Elsevier, New York, 107-120.

18. Kawamori, R. and Shichiri, M. (1982). **Diabetes** 315-322.

19. Frauman, A.G., Cooper, M.E., Partsons, B.J. Jerums, G. and Louis, W.J. (1987). **Diabetes Care** 10, 573-578.

20. Nagai, T., Nishimoto, Y., Nambu, N., Suzuki, Y. and Sekine, K. (1984). **J. Control. Rel.** 1, 15-28.

21. Okada, H., Yamazaki, I., Yashiki, T. and Mima, H. (1983). **J. Pharm. Sci.** 72, 75.

22. Yoshida, H., Okumura, H., Hori, R. Anmo, I. and Yamaguchi, H. (1979). **J. Pharm. Sci.** 68, 670.

23. Kohlert, D., Enzmann, F. and Kerp, L. (1984). **Diabetes** 33(Suppl) 75A.

24. Salzman, R., Manson, J.E. and Griffing, G.T. (1985). **New Eng. J. Med.** 312, 1078.

25. Kari, B. (1986). **Diabetes** 35, 217.

26. Siddiqui, O., Sun, Y., Liu, J.C. and Chien, Y.W. (1987). **J. Pharm. Sci.** 76, 341.

27. Nagai, T. (1985). **J. Control. Rel.** 2, 121.

28. Nomura, M., Kubota, M.A., Kawamori, Y., Yamasaki, T. and Kamada, H. (1994). **J. Pharm. Pharmacol.** 46, 768.

29. Yamamoto, Y., Luo, A.M. and Lee, V.H.L. (1989). **J. Pharmacol. Exp. Ther.** 249, 249.

30. Klyce, S.D. (1972). **J. Physiol.** 226, 407.

31. Bangham, A.D., Standish, M.M. and Watkins, J.C. (1965). **J. Mol. Biol.**, 13, 138.

32. Guo, L.S.S., Radhakrishnan, R. and Redmann, C.T. (1989). **J. Liposome Res.** 3, 319-333.

33. Stewart, J.C.M. (1959). **Anal. Biochem.** 104, 10.

34. Jizomoto, H. and Hirano, K. (1989). **Chem. Pharm. Bull.** 37, 3066.

35. Jeong, S.Y., Kim, S.W., Eenink, M.J.D. and Feijen, J. (1984). **J. Contr. Rel.** 1, 57-66.

19

GENERAL APPROACHES FOR ENHANCEMENT OF DRUG ENTRAPMENT IN LIPOSOMES

MONICA GULATI[1] and SARANJIT SINGH*

National Institute of Pharmaceutical Education and Research (NIPER),
Sector 67, S.A.S. Nagar 160 062.
[1]University Institute of Pharmaceutical Sciences,
Panjab University, Chandigarh 160 014.

Tel. +91 172 673848; Fax +91 172 677185; e.mail niper@chd.nic.in

- Introduction
- Approaches for enhancement of drug entrapment in liposomes

- Conclusion
- References

INTRODUCTION

Liposomes are delivery systems with good potential. They are one of the most researched means of drug delivery. The efforts made over the last three decades have resulted in their coming out of stage of obscurity and a few of the liposomal formulations have already reached the market place. The marketed liposomal preparations, AmBisome™ (amphotericin B), DaunoXome™ (daunorubicin citrate), and Doxil™ (doxorubicin), have proved to be superior in comparison to their conventionally delivered presentations. Currently, liposomal delivery systems of several drugs, toxins, enzymes, protein/peptides and even the genetic material are in an advanced stage of development. The day is not very far when these tiny vesicles will take a prominent place in delivering the modern drugs.

The reason why it has taken so long for these delivery systems to come to the market place has been the problem of stability of the liposomal vesicle as such. The stability problem of lipids and that of the vesicle has been resolved to an extent, due to which these systems have become marketable. However, a hitch remains with respect to their high cost which, apart from technology development costs, is primarily due to costly phospholipids which form their backbone. Hence for making these systems economical, it is imperative that the drug:phospholipid ratio in a liposomal formulation is kept maximum in the favour of the former.

There is another aspect that is important with respect to incorporation of drugs in liposomes. Drugs that are incompletely entrapped are associated with added complications, as the drugs remain in the continuous aqueous phase of liposomes in their free form. The presence of free drug defeats the entire purpose of liposomal delivery, resulting in exposure of the non-target sites to the drug and hence the therapeutic disadvantage. The procedures employed for the removal of the unentrapped drug, such as dialysis and passage through exclusion columns are often time-consuming, tedious and expensive.

Thus, to get a maximum economic as well as therapeutic advantage from the liposomal formulations, it is necessary that the drug incorporation in liposomes is optimised. The factors effecting microencapsulation of drugs in liposomes, in general, were reviewed by Kulkarni et al. [1]. This chapter specifically discusses the various approaches to enhance incorporation of drugs in liposomes.

APPROACHES FOR ENHANCEMENT OF DRUG ENTRAPMENT IN LIPOSOMES

If one looks at a liposomal vesicle from the angle of incorporation of a drug, one can identify three elements that can be considered important. The first is the liposome itself, that is primarily composed of lipid bilayers and the aqueous milieu, the second is the drug that is sought to be incorporated and the third is the method of preparation of drug loaded liposomes. So when the goal is to formulate liposomes having maximum entrapment of the drug, one has to consider optimising the type of liposomes, liposomal lipid and aqueous phase characteristics, drug properties, and the technique of preparation of liposomes.

Choice of type of liposomes

Liposomes are formed in different types (Table1). Among these, the most common type, MLVs, have largest lipid load and maximum number of bilayers. Their aqueous volume, however, is very low. Hence owing to these characteristics, they can understandably incorporate hydrophobic drugs better than the hydrophilic drugs. However, for hydrophobic drugs the type and size of liposomes is not a critical issue as these remain entrapped in lipid bilayers. In contrast, however, for hydrophilic drugs unilamellar liposomes can be considered more suitable because the ratio of aqueous phase/lipid phase is in favor of the former. Therefore, in general, it is better to incorporate hydrophobic drugs in MLVs & water-soluble hydrophilic drugs in unilamellar type of liposomes.

Table 1. Various types of liposomes

	Type	Size
MLV	MulitiLamellar Vesicles	>500 nm
OLV	OligoLamellar Vesicles	100-1000 nm
UV	Unilamellar Vesicles	All sizes
SUV	Small Unilamellar Vesicles	20-<100 nm
MUV	Medium-sized Unilamellar Vesicles	50-250 nm
LUV	Large Unilamellar Vesicles	60->1000 nm
GUV	Giant Unilamellar Vesicles	>1000 nm
MVV	MultiVesicular Vesicles	>1000 nm

Optimization of the liposomal lipid and aqueous phases

The drug entrapment can be influenced by properties of both the lipid and aqueous phases of liposomes. Hence, phospholipid bilayer composition as well as the aqueous phase needs to be optimised in favor of maximum possible entrapment.

Phospholipid bilayer composition

The phospholipids forming the bilayer of liposomes are amphipathic molecules, containing a phosphatidyl group and a hydrophilic polar head (Fig.1). These are available in a large number of types, containing different head groups and different hydrophobic chain lengths (Table 2).

Table 2. Naturally occurring phospholipids and their subtypes with varying chain lengths

Phospholipid with different head groups	Subtypes with varying chain length
Phosphatidyl Choline (PC)	Dilaureoyl Phosphatidyl Choline (DLPC), Dimyristoyl Phosphatidyl Choline (DMPC), Dipalmitoyl Phosphatidyl Choline (DPPC), Disteroyl Phosphatidyl Choline (DSPC), Dioleoyl Phosphatidyl Choline (DOPC), etc.
Phosphatidyl Glycerol (PG)	DLPG, DMPG, DPPG, DSPG, DOPG, etc.
Phosphatidic Acid (PA)	DLPA, DMPA, DPPA, DSPA, DOPA, etc.
Phosphatidyl Inositol (PI)	DLPI, DMPI, DPPI, DSPI, DOPI, etc.
Phosphatidyl Serine (PS)	DLPS, DMPS, DPPS, DSPS, DOPS, etc.
Phosphatidyl Ethanolamine (PE)	DLPE, DMPE, DPPE, DSPE, DOPE, etc.

The entrapment of drugs, accordingly, depends upon the type of phospholipid and other factors, including the charge on the phospholipid, the use of combination of phospholipids and the presence of sterols and other additives. These are discussed below.

The type of phospholipid

Under this heading the important factors are variation in chain length (R in Fig. 1), nature of the head group (X in Fig. 1), etc

Chain length: The effect of chain length of the phospholipid on entrapment of drugs in liposomes varies with the nature of the drug being entrapped. For hydrophobic and biphasic soluble drugs, the entrapment generally increases with the increase in chain length but with water soluble drugs, no such fixed behavior has been observed.

Ma et al. [2] found that increase in chain length of the phospholipids increased the partitioning of the lipophilic esters of p-amino benzoic acid into the bilayers. Similarly, the entrapment efficiency of colchicine, which is highly soluble in both aqueous as well as organic solvents, is reported to increase with an increase in the chain length of the phospholipids [3]. The effect of chain length on the entrapment efficiency of the hydrophilic drugs is reported to differ from one drug to another. For example, an increased entrapment of propanolol was observed with an increase in chain length. Similarly, the entrapment of glutathione was found to increase in the order of DSPC>DPPC>DMPC [4]. However, the entrapment of suramin increased in the reverse order of DLPC>DMPC>DPPC>DSPC [5]. This specific behavior is explained on the basis of a decrease in net Van der Waals interaction and increase in bilayer intermolecular spacing with decrease in the length of the acyl chain. There also exist examples of water-soluble drugs where no significant influence of chain length of the phospholipid has been observed. Carboxyfluorescein did not show any significant change when soya PC was replaced by DPPC and DSPC [6]. Similar behavior is reported for insulin [7].

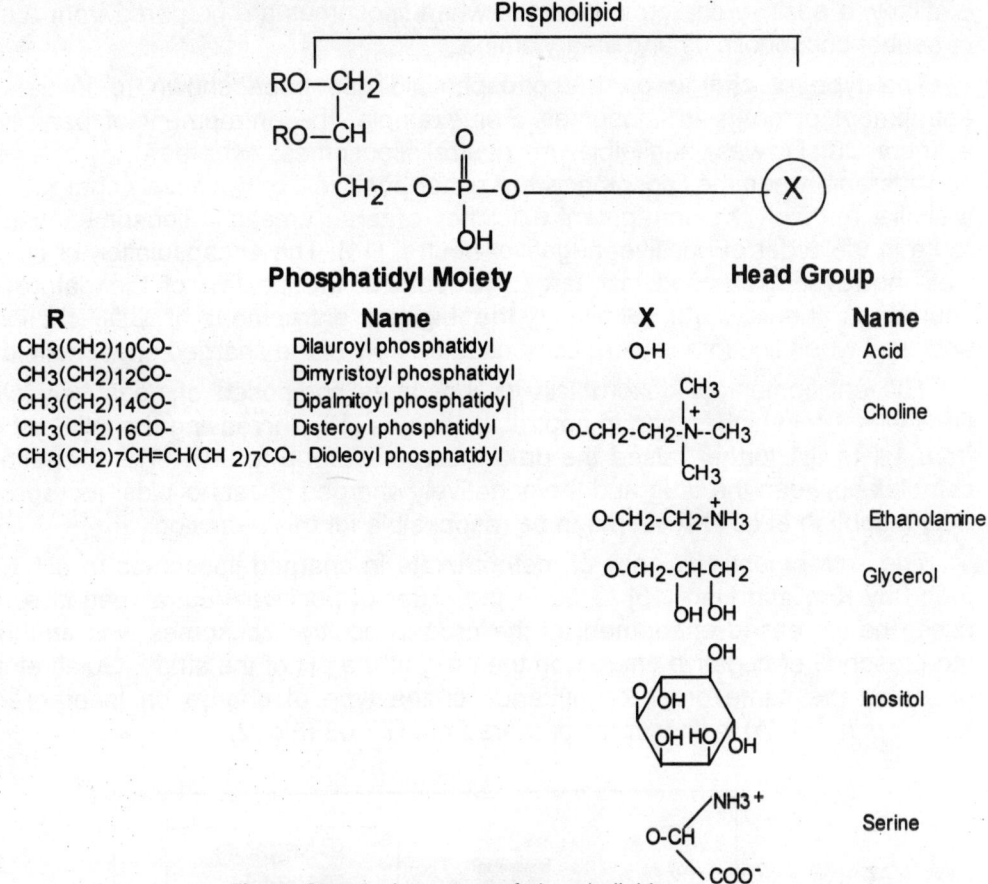

Fig. 1: Chemical structure of phospholipids

Nature of head groups: Among the naturally occurring phospholipids (Table 2), the most widely used are those which contain two types of head groups, choline and glycerol. The problems with other types are the high cost, non-availability in pure form and toxicological considerations.

A different degree of drug encapsulation may result when a phospholipid with one type of head group is changed with another. For example, the entrapment of citicoline has been reported to be three times higher in liposomes prepared with DMPA in comparison to those prepared with DPPC [8]. In a similar manner, use of PG has been found to result in higher entrapment of erythromycin A and azithromycin, as compared to liposomes prepared with PC or PE [9].

Charge: With the exception of phosphatidylcholine and phosphatidyl ethanolamine that are neutral, all other phospholipids are negatively charged as the charge on the phosphate group is not neutralized by the head group. Therefore, negatively charged liposomes are obtained when anionic phospholipids, e.g., cardiolipin, phosphatidic acid, phosphatidyl glycerol, phosphatidyl ethanolamine, phosphatidyl serine, etc., are employed for formation of bilayers. Negative charge in liposomes is also induced when dicetyl phosphate is added in conjunction with the neutral phospholipid. Similarly, a positive charge is inducted when liposomes are prepared from a mixture of neutral phospholipids and stearylamine.

The type of charge on the phospholipid has been shown to influence the entrapment of drugs in liposomes. For example, the entrapment of penicillin and actinomycin D was negligible in neutral liposomes, whereas the same was considerable when the liposomes were either positively or negatively charged [10]. In a similar manner, the entrapment efficiency of tartar emetic in liposomes was found to be in the order of positive>negative>neutral [11]. The encapsulation of colchicine was, however, increased in charged liposomes, irrespective of the nature of the charge on the lipid [3]. Similarly, the highest entrapment of CDP-choline was achieved when liposomes were composed entirely of the charged phospholipids [12].

The entrapment of doxorubicin in liposomes composed of negatively charged DPG was 4-fold higher than in neutral liposomes [13]. Increasing the DPG:drug ratio from 1:1 to 5:1 further raised the drug incorporation up to 90%. The formation of a complex between the drug and the negatively charged phospholipids, as reported by Goormaghtigh et al. [14] seems to be responsible for this behavior.

The entrapment efficiency of methotrexate in charged liposomes at pH 7.4 was found by Kim and Han [15] to be in the order of positive>neutral>negative. In this case, the increased entrapment of the drug in positive liposomes was attributed to the presence of negative charge on the drug at the pH of the study. Gulati et al. [16] observed the same order of influence of the type of charge on incorporation of azathioprine (AZA) in liposomes prepared at pH 7.03 (Fig. 2).

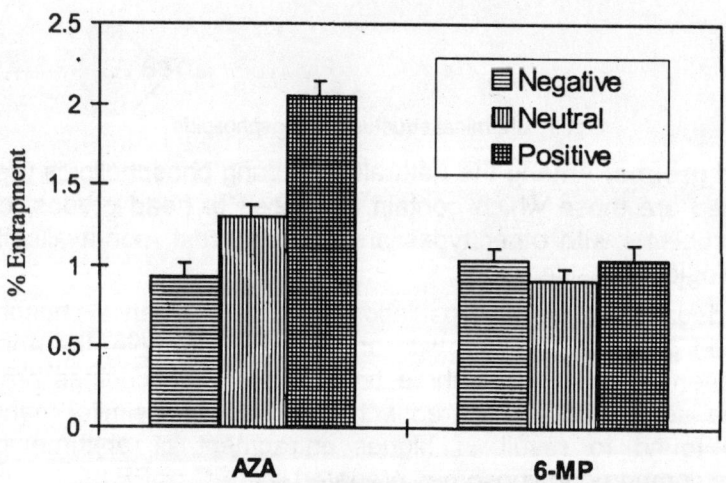

Fig. 2 : Effect of charge on per cent entrapment of AZA and 6-MP in MLVs at pH 7.03; n=3, except neutral liposomes where n=4; drug strength= 4×10^{-5} M.

The drug exists partially in an anionic form at pH 7 (pKa = 8.15) and the charge effect was, accordingly, ascribed to the ionic interaction between the anionic drug and positively charged stearylamine. Another example is that of sodium cromoglycate, where also the entrapment of negatively charged drug was higher in the positively charged liposomes [17]. Examples of an opposite effect involving negatively charged liposomes and positively charged drugs also exist in literature. Positively charged hydroxocobalamin hydrochloride [18] and polymyxin B sulphate [19] have been shown to give maximal entrapment in negatively charged liposomes. For charged drugs, therefore, apparently the 'rule' is that entrapment efficiency is increased by the presence of oppositely charged lipids in the bilayer. However, in rare situation, one may not observe enhanced entrapment even when charged drug is incorporated in liposomes prepared with oppositely charged lipid. Gulati et al. [16] interestingly observed no influence of charge on encapsulation of 6-mercaptopurine (6-MP), when the study was done at pH 7.03, similar to AZA. The comparison of profiles is shown in Fig. 2. This was the case despite the fact that 6-MP is slightly more acidic (pKa = 7.77) than AZA, and was expected to give higher entrapment in positively charged liposomes. The difference is explained based on the intramolecular H-bonding (Scheme 1) between the 6-S group and the N-7 proton of 6-MP that renders the anionic 6-S group unavailable for interaction with the positively charged stearylamine. In AZA, the 6-S group is blocked by the imidazole moiety and hence no intramolecular H-bonding is possible. Therefore, when no charge effect is seen despite the drug and lipid being oppositely charged in the pH conditions of the study, it is desirable that one should look more deeply into the state of charge on the drug molecule.

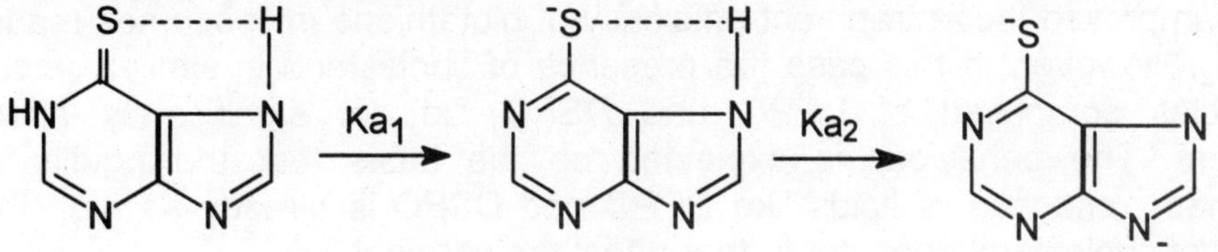

Scheme 1

In general, the viable mechanism by which neutral drugs are better entrapped in charged lipids is the increase in the interlamellar space created by electrostatic repulsion of charged phospholipids within the bilayers. The enhancement of entrapment of charged drugs in oppositely charged liposomes occurs due to stronger and closer packing, owing to electrostatic attraction between opposite charged drug species and the substrate.

Use of combination of phosopholipids

The use of a mixture of phospholipids for the preparation of liposomes has also been found to help in optimization of the properties of liposomes, including drug entrapment. A two to three times better entrapment of citicoline was observed by Puglisi et al. [8] in liposomes formed from the use of DMPC in conjunction with either DPPA or DPPS. Perez-Soler and Khokher [20] observed an increase in encapsulation of liposomal neodecanoato-trans-R,R-1,2-diaminocyclohexane-platinum II (L-NDDP) on incorporation of DMPG along with DMPC. The increase in incorporation was directly proportional to the amount of DMPG in the bilayer and was attributed to the formation of an active complex between DMPG and NDDP. Amselem et al. [21], similarly, observed a higher entrapment of doxorubicin in liposomes composed of a bilayer containing lecithin and phosphatidyl glycerol, than when the bilayer was formed from the two alone.

Presence of steroids and other additives

Steroids. incorporation of steroids like cholesterol and α-tocopherol into the liposome bilayers can bring about major changes in their properties. These additives impart rigidity to the membrane, making it less permeable to the solutes. To cite an example, Mayhew et al. [22] observed a marked reduction in leakage of ARA-C on addition of cholesterol to a phospholipid combination of PC and PG. The profile is shown in Fig. 3. The authors postulated that the presence of cholesterol decreased the permeability of the liposomes, increasing their physical stability, resulting eventually in better retention of the drug within the vesicle.

This mechanism of increase in entrapment efficiency applies particularly to water-soluble drugs which otherwise are rapidly leaked out of liposomes. A few of the examples of hydrophilic drugs, where addition of cholesterol has helped in increasing entrapment, include sodium ioxitalamate [23], methotrexate [15] and sodium cromoglycate [17]. Among other examples, a maximum entrapment of CDP-choline was achieved when equimolar concentrations of cholesterol and DPPC were present in the membrane [8]. Similarly, incorporation of equimolar cholesterol increased the encapsulation of dideoxyinosine triphosphate in liposomes prepared using DMPC [24]. In the same manner, incorporation of 30 mol % cholesterol markedly improved the entrapment efficiency of glutathione in liposomes made from DMPC [4]. However, in this case the presence of cholesterol in similar amounts in the vesicles composed of DPPC and DSPC did not significantly affect the entrapment. The behaviour is explained on the basis that the rigidity of the membranes composed of lipids like DPPC and DSPC is already so high that the presence of cholesterol does not further affect the permeability.

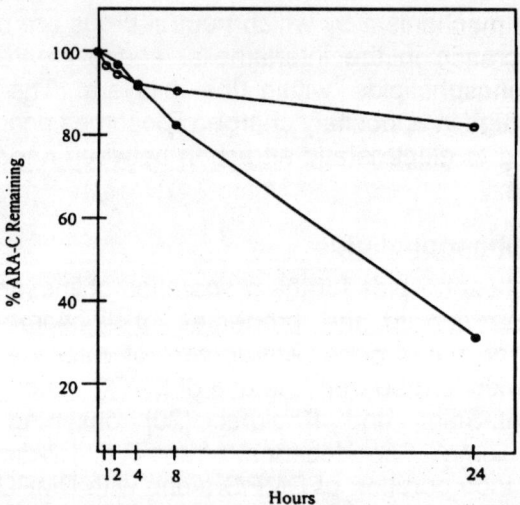

Fig.3 : Profile showing the effect of presence of cholesterol on per cent retention of Ara-C. Key:
PG:PC; 1:4 (•) and PG:PC:Chol; 1:4:5(o) . Adapted from [22].

Interestingly, the increase in entrapment of drugs in liposomes on addition of steroids is not restricted to water-soluble drugs alone. The same has even been reported for hydrophobic drugs. The mechanism here, of course, is different. Hydrophobic drugs are targeted to the vesicle bilayer and as cholesterol increases the lipohilicity of the bilayer, an increased quantity of the lipophilic drug is taken up. This has been the observation for hydrophobic alkyl p-amino benzoates [2] and also hydrophobic steroids [25].

In some cases, presence of cholesterol in the membrane has been shown to rather decrease the drug entrapment. This type of behaviour has been observed in those drugs where entrapment is a result of interaction with the head groups of the phospholipids. For example, doxorubicin interacts with negatively charged phospholipids and a decrease in entrapment was found on addition of increasing amounts of cholesterol in negative liposomes [26]. Through a similar mechanism, addition of 50 mol % of cholesterol caused a significant reduction in entrapment of suramin [5].

Reports also exist in literature showing no effect of the presence of cholesterol on drug entrapment. Examples include salbutamol [27] and amphotericin B [28].

The effect of presence of cholesterol on the entrapment efficiency of some of the drugs is summarised in Table 3.

Table 3. Effect of the presence of cholesterol on the entrapment efficiency of various drugs

Drug	Effect on entrapment efficiency	Mechanism	Reference
CDP choline	Increase	Decrease in permeability of the bilayer	12
Dideoxyinosine triphosphate	Increase	Decrease in permeability of the bilayer	34
Sodium ioxitalamate	Increase	Decrease in permeability of the bilayer	23
Methotrexate	Increase	Decrease in permeability of the bilayer	15
Sodium cromoglycate	Increase	Decrease in permeability of the bilayer	17
Alkyl -p-amino benzoates	Increase	Increase in hydrophobicity of the bilayer	2
Steroids	Increase	Increase in hydrophobicity of the bilayer	25
Doxorubicin	Decrease	Decrease in drug-phospholipid interaction	26
Suramin	Decrease	Decrease in drug-phospholipid interaction	5

Glycolipids: Glycolipids is another class of additives which when incorporated into the bilayer at the time of formation of liposomes may help to increase encapsulation of the drugs. For example, galactocerebroside has been shown to increase the entrapment of mitoxantrone in proportion to the concentration of glycolipid added [29]. The reported mechanism is that the hydrophilic head groups of glycolipids orientate towards the aqueous phase and in this process the hydroxyl groups are exposed outside and the drugs may bind to these groups by hydrogen bonding.

Optimisation of the aqueous phase

An increased entrapment of drugs in liposomes can be achieved by optimising the aqueous phase with respect to pH, ionic strength, etc.

pH

The ionizable drugs exist in different forms at different pH values. The pH at which the ionization state of the drug is most favourable for its entrapment gives the best results. Liposomal entrapment of thioguanine was studied as a function of pH and maximum entrapment was observed at pH 4.7. At this pH, the drug exists as a neutral species and shows highest apparent partition coefficient [30]. Similarly, for clofibric acid and chlorphentermine, the highest liposomal binding was obtained under the conditions where drugs existed in their uncharged forms [31]. Another example is that of tin-mesomorphin which was entrapped to an extent of 90% at pH 5 and to a mere 10% at pH 7.0 [32]. In an opposite effect, mitoxantrone, which is an amphipathic drug, showed an increase in the entrapment efficiency with increase in pH. The order of entrapment was found to be pH 5.7 > 5.1 > 4.5. Similarly, 6-MP and AZA, the two biphasic insoluble drugs, were found by Gulati et al. [16] to be entrapped increasingly with an increase in pH. The pH-entrapment profiles for these two drugs are shown in Fig. 4.

These examples illustrate that for ionizable drugs, one shall study the pH-entrapment profile and select the optimum pH for drug entrapment.

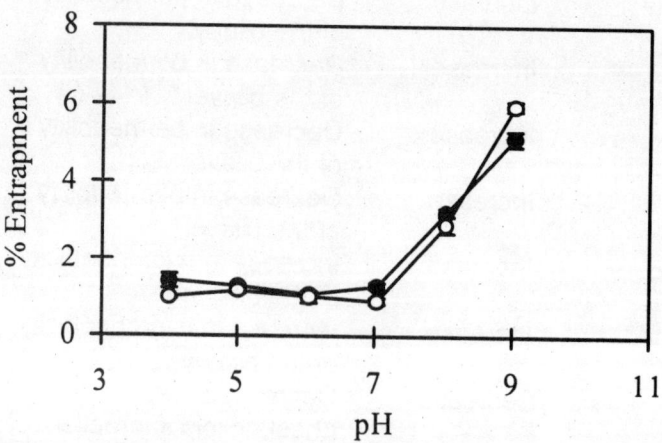

Fig. 4 : Profile showing the effect of pH on per cent entrapment of AZA (●) and 6-MP (o)in MLVs

Ionic strength

The entrapment efficiency of a liposomal preparation may depend on ionic strength of the aqueous phase. For example, a clear-cut effect of ionic strength was observed on entrapment of mitoxantrone [29]. The entrapment was found to increase with an increase in ionic strength from 0.067 to 0.154. A report also exists, where an ionic substance, tetra ethyl ammonium perchlorate (TEAP), helped to achieve high solute entrapment in liposomes prepared by the freeze-thaw method [33]. Because of the permanent and ionic nature of tetraethyl ammonium cation and perchlorate ion, TEAP acts as an osmotic balancer and allows higher gradients of solutes to be maintained.

Alteration in drug properties

The physicochemical properties of the drug itself, especially solubility and partition coefficient, are important determinants of the extent of its incorporation in liposomes. Dependent upon whether the drug is hydrophobic, hydrophilic, amphiphilic or biphasic insoluble, the encapsulation efficiency may vary from 0-100%. The behaviour of liposomal entrapment of various categories of drugs is expressed in fig. 5.

The water-soluble drugs (log P<-0.3) are entrapped in the liposomal aqueous compartment to a theoretical maximum entrapment efficiency of 70%. The remaining 30% counts towards the unencapsulated volume left in the void space due to the curvature of the liposomes [34]. These drugs, apart from limited entrapment, have other associated problems when incorporated into the aqueous milieu of liposomes. They show bilayer dependent leakage and hydrolytic instability.

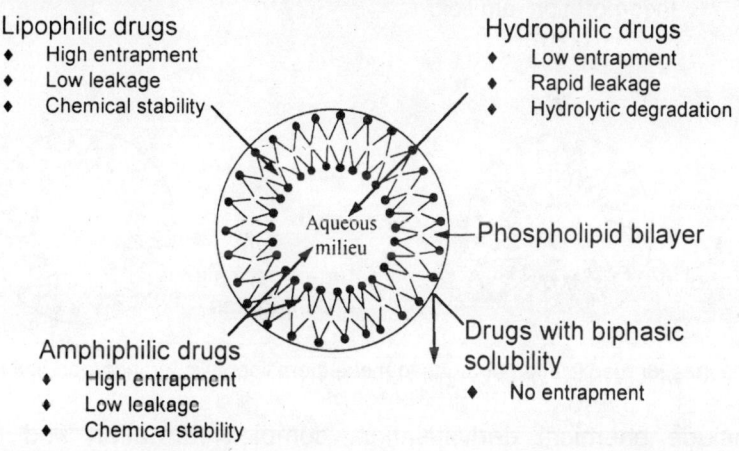

Fig. 5 : Types of drugs and their behaviour of incorporation in liposomes.

Amphiphilic drugs enter both aqueous and lipid phases and due to their biphasic solubility they are rather well entrapped in liposomes. However, the problem with these drugs is that the liposomal membrane constitutes no barrier for their passage from inside to outside. Such drugs leach out very fast and are entrapped in the liposomes only if they form complexes with the membrane lipids, e.g., actinomycin D [35]. The another category of drugs, those with poor biphasic solubility, e.g., 6-mercaptopurine, azathioprine, azaguanine, 5-fluorouracil, etc., are the poorest candidates for liposomal entrapment. All these drugs show only meagre uptake by liposomes [36]. The fourth category of drugs, i.e., lipophilic drugs with log P>5, are incorporated in the phospholipid bilayer of liposomes and it is only with these drugs that entrapment efficiencies as high as 100% are achieved. For example, cyclosporin shows almost complete entrapment [37]. These drugs neither face leakage nor chemical stability problems.

Therefore, one good way of increasing entrapment of drugs and for solving other drug related problems of liposomal incorporation is to change the hydrophilic, amphiphilic and biphasically insoluble drugs into their lipophilic forms and target them into lipophilic bilayers of liposomes. In the last three decades, three approaches have emerged for doing this (Fig. 6).

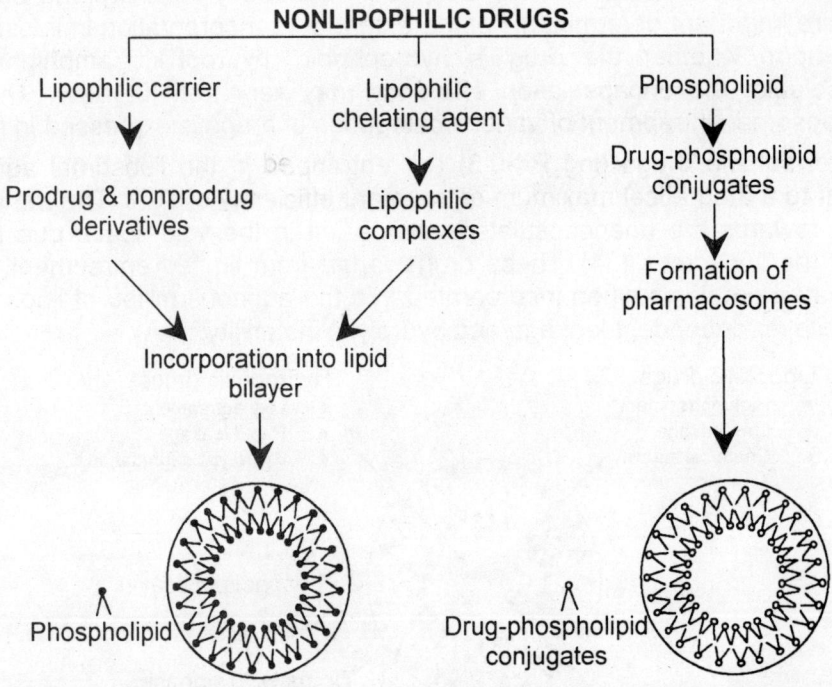

Fig. 6 : Approaches for modification of drugs to make them lipophilic for incorporation into bilayer of liposomes

These include chemical derivatisation, complex formation and formation of pharmacosomes, that are colloidal dispersion of drugs linked covalently to lipids. A good number of anticancer, antiviral, steroids and diagnostic aids with incorporation problems have been altered and their incorporation into lipid bilayers of liposomes has been studied. At least three lipophilic drug derivatives are currently in the stage of clinical trials. These include MTP-PE [38], NDDP [39], and annamycin [40]. The structures of these drugs are given in Fig. 7. Liposomal formulations of several other drugs are in development stages.

The details of these are not discussed here, as a full chapter in this book is separately devoted to this topic. The subject has also been recently reviewed [41].

Method of preparation

During the preparation of liposomes, a number of variables are involved, a change in any of which can bring about a marked change in the drug encapsulation. These variables depend upon on the technique of preparation, and need to be optimised for obtaining maximum entrapment.

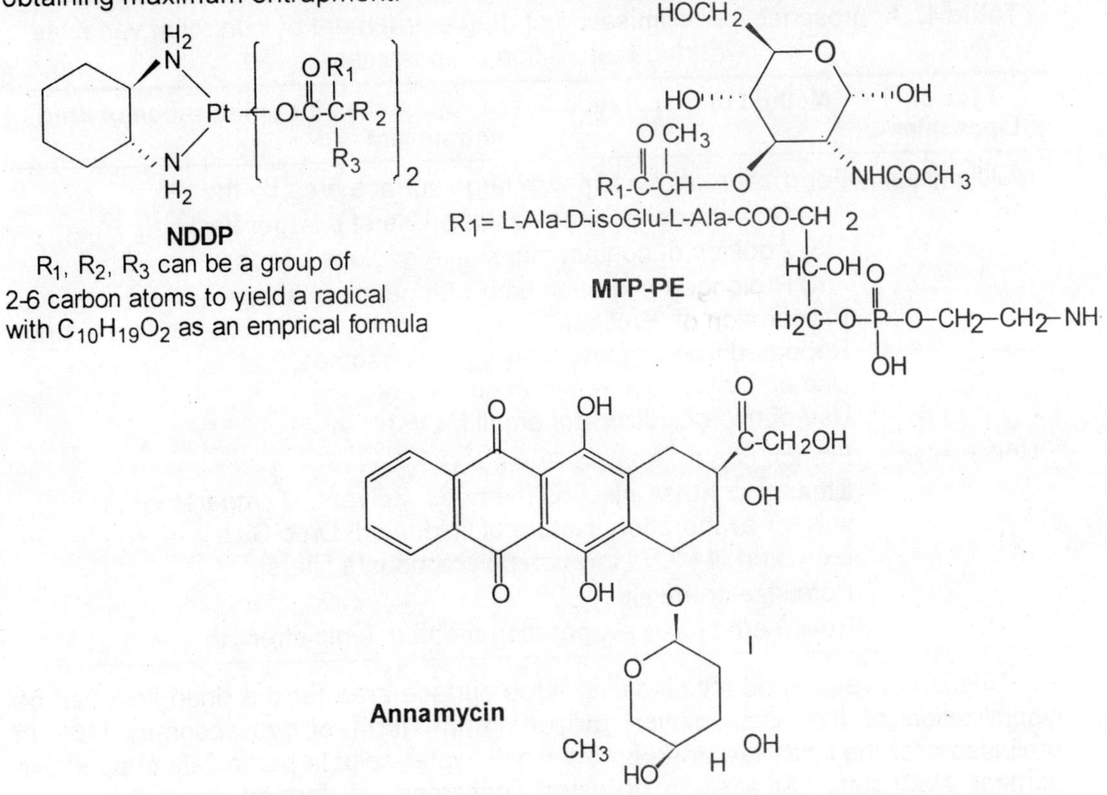

NDDP

R_1, R_2, R_3 can be a group of 2-6 carbon atoms to yield a radical with $C_{10}H_{19}O_2$ as an emprical formula

R_1= L-Ala-D-isoGlu-L-Ala-COO-CH$_2$

MTP-PE

Annamycin

Fig. 7 : Structures of lipophilic drug derivatives whose liposomal preparations are presently in clinical trials.

Influence of the technique

A number of techniques of generating liposomes are documented in literature [42]. Different methods of preparation yield different types of liposomes that exhibit a large variation in entrapment efficiency. In case of each method, it is possible to get higher entrapment by standardisation of the variables. Table 4 gives the summary of approaches in this respect.

The MLVs prepared by the dispersion method of Bangham et al [43] contain only a small proportion of the aqueous volume. This method, therefore, is wasteful for water-soluble compounds [44] but gives good entrapment with lipophilic substances [45]. Even the MLVs prepared by the shake-flask method vary markedly in their entrapment efficiency. One of the major factors affecting the drug entrapment is the lipid hydration, which in turn is mainly dependent upon the surface area available for the lipid/water contact. One common means of increasing the lipid surface area is the addition of inert beads at the time of formation of the lipid film. The advantage of this approach is exemplified by the study done by Amselem et al. [21] on doxorubicin. The level of free drug in the final preparation was reduced from 40% to

16% when the liposomes were prepared using glass beads. Similarly, the use of beads during film formation was found to give better incorporation of colchicine [3].

Table 4. Approaches for optimisation of drug entrapment by control of variables during preparation of liposomes

Type of Liposomes	Method of preparation based approaches for optimisation of drug entrapment
Multilamellar	Forrmation of thin film with large surface area by the : (1) Use of pear shaped flask (2) Use of a larger flask (3) Addition of contact masses (e.g. glass beads) (4) Prolonged hydration time with gentle shaking Preparation of Proliposomes using finely divided particulate support Repeated freezing and thawing of liposomes, Use of dehydration/rehydration method Use of microfluidizer (for small MLVs)
Unilamellar	French press: Applied Pressure, Ethanol or Ether injection methods: Solvent, Temperature of solvent evaporation, Nature of lipid used, Drop Size Extrusion of MLVs through polycarbonate filters: Pore size of the filter, Reversed–phase evaporation method: Ionic strength

An alternative method for obtaining large surface area for the dried lipid can be lyophilization of the lipid solution utilized in the form of proliposomes [46]. In proliposomes, the lipids are dried onto a highly water-soluble particulate support like sorbitol, NaCl, etc. On addition of water, liposomes are formed when hydrophilic support gets dissolved. However, the method is applicable mostly to hydrophobic drugs [46].

MLVs with high trapping efficiencies can also be obtained by the use of reverse phase evaporation (REV) procedure [17,47]. The dehydration-rehydration vesicles (DRVs) prepared by Kirby and Gregoriadis [6] and Deamer and Barchfeild [48] have been reported to give liposomes capable of enclosing a wide variety of materials with entrapment values up to 80%. A comparison between these methods for the preparation of liposomes of amikacin and teicoplanin showed a higher encapsulation in DRVs as compared to the REVs for both the drugs [49].

As regards the time for hydration, which is another critical factor, slow hydration has been shown beneficial, as it enables longer contact between the phospholipid bilayers of the liposomes and the drug. A study on the dependence of encapsulation on the time of hydration was made by Olson et al. [50]. The entrapment efficiency was reported to increase in the order of 20h > 2 h >30 min.

In comparison to MLVs, LUVs contain considerable internal aqueous volume and, therefore, are more suitable for higher entrapment of hydrophilic drugs [51]. LUVs are either prepared by the ether injection method or through extrusion of MLVs through filter membranes. LUVs with as large as 60% trapping efficiencies were produced when MLVs were extruded five to ten times through membranes of pore size 0.1μm or less [52].

In situ active drug trapping procedures

Certain active trapping procedures have been employed for incorporation of solutes to achieve >90% entrapment efficiency in liposomes. Table 5 lists the approaches, and the variable factors that influence the extent of loading.

Table 5. Active loading techniques for getting liposomes with high entrapment of solutes

Procedure	Variable factors	Solutes incorporated	Ref.
Transmembrane pH-gradient method for charged, amphipathic drugs	Lipid composition, lipid quality, medium composition, temperature, pH of incubation mixture, and pKa and hydrophobicity of the solute	Doxorubicin, Vincristine, Ciprofloxacin	54, 65-68
Ionic gradient	Lipid composition, lipid quality, medium composition, temperature, and pKa and hydrophobicity of the solute	Acridine Orange, Doxorubicin, Safranine, Dibucaine, Dopamine, Serotonin, Epinephrine etc.	57-60, 69, 70
Remote loading	Concentration of the chelating agent, pH of incubation mixture, and concentration and type of transporter	^{111}In, ^{67}Ga	61, 62, 71
In situ complexation	Concentration of the chelating agent and concentration and type of transporter	Gd-DTPA complex	72

The first type is loading of drugs through generation of trans-membrane pH gradients. This subsequently leads to accumulation of the drug inside the liposomes. Liposomes are prepared in low pH buffer and the transmembrane gradient is established by setting the exterior pH to 7 or higher. The drug is taken up on simple addition after a short incubation at elevated temperature with intermittent stirring. For a pH gradient of three units, a 1000-folds higher interior concentration than the exterior can be achieved by this method [53]. An example is that of doxorubicin, where an entrapment efficiency of 98% was achieved. Similarly, ciprofloxacin was entrapped with 90% efficiency compare to only 9% with the conventional methods [54]. However, on storage of liposomes prepared by this method, rapid efflux of the loaded drug was observed for some of the drugs, e.g., metaproterenol sulphate [55], verapamil and prochlorperazine [56]. A survey of the drugs loaded by the pH gradient method indicates that many compounds, including vincristine, vinblastine, quinidine, diphenhydramine, quinine and chloroquine, leak from liposomes during extended periods [56]. This is attributed to the collapse of the gradient resulting in the efflux of drug from the interior of the liposomes.

Just like pH gradient, ion gradient has also been exploited for the active liposomal entrapment for a large number of drugs. Ammonium sulphate gradient was utilized by Haran et al. [57] to achieve high loading of doxorubicin. The method has been successfully employed to increase the entrapment of other drug molecules like safranine [58], dibucaine [59], dopamine, serotonin, epinephrine [60], etc.

Novel *in situ* approaches have been employed to load high amounts of paramagnetic ions in liposomes. The ions are used as agents for magnetic resonance imaging. The problem with these cations is that they are rapidly leached out of the vesicles. One of the approaches to keep them retained is to use a carrier moiety. Acetylacetone, a lipophilic chelate, was used to entrap high levels of Indium(III) (>90%) into liposomes [61,62]. In this case, a remote *in situ* technique was employed that involved three stages,

i)   preparation of liposomes,

ii) encapsulation of water soluble chelating agent (nitriltriacetate) and,

iii) incubation with acetylacetone-indium complex, just prior to administration.

Hwang et al. [62] used 8-hydroxyquinolone instead of acetylacetone to incorporate ^{111}In and also ^{67}Ga in liposomes. In a related technique, Tilcock et al. [63] entrapped gadolinium using an ionophore A23187 that was employed to help transport the ions into aqueous mileu of SUVs. Once inside, the ions were chelated by passively entrapped diethylenetriaminepenta-acetic acid (DTPA). The *in-situ* formed lipophilic chelate was resistant to leaching and helped retain the cations for several days at room temperature.

The general design considerations for the vesicle associated MR contrast agents based on paramagnetic chelates, either entrapped within the vesicle interior or attached to the membrane surface, have been discussed by Tilcock et al. [63].

Dependence on initial solute concentration

The drug loading in liposomes has been shown to be dependent upon the concentration of drug used at the time of preparation of liposomes. In general, the entrapment efficiency increases with increase in the drug concentration. Beyond a certain concentration, a plateau is reached due to the saturable nature of the process. For example, in the case of mitoxantrone, increase in the solute concentration was found to result in an increase in the entrapment efficiency upto a specific concentration, after which the solute concentration had no effect on the loading capacity [29]. Similar behavior was also observed with a number of other solutes like KCl and NaCl [6], cytosine arabinoside and doxorubicin [21]. Sometimes even a small fall in the entrapment has been observed after the plateau [16]

However, the effect of solute concentration on the entrapment efficiency is also dependent on the method employed for the preparation of liposomes. When the effect of the concentration of sucrose on its entrapment efficiency was studied in the liposomes prepared by the freeze-thaw extrusion process, the entrapment was found to first increase with increase in the concentration and then a decline was observed [33]. However, in case of liposomes prepared by dehydration-rehydration technique, the percentage entrapment was found to decrease with increase in the solute concentration [6]. In case of suramin, the absolute values of entrapment decreased with increase in solute concentration throughout the concentration range tested, but the specific entrapment (mol of suramin/mol of phospholipid) showed a corresponding increase [5].

CONCLUSION

Liposomes are capable of incorporating a wide spectrum of materials ranging from highly lipophilic molecules like tacrolimus [64] to highly hydrophilic compounds like sucrose [33]. The tiny vesicles have even been used for entrapment of ionic compounds, like paramagnetic ions. As discussed above, a variety of approaches have been employed to get maximum entrapment of different types of solutes with diverse structures. These approaches can be exploited for optimising the liposomal entrapment of the compounds of interest.

REFERENCES

1. Kulkarni, S.B., Betageri, G.V. and Singh, M. (1995). **J. Microencapsul.** 12, 229-246.

2. Ma, L., Ramachandran, C. and Weiner, N.D. (1991). **Int. J. Pharm.** 70, 127-140.

3. Kulkarni, S.B., Singh, M. and Betageri, G.V. (1997). **J. Pharm. Pharmacol.** 49, 491-495.

4. Jurima-romet, M. and Shek, P.N. (1991). **J. Pharm. Pharmacol.** 43, 6-10.

5. Chang, H.C. and Flanagan, D.R. (1995). **J. Pharm. Sci.** 84, 1078-1082.

6. Kirby, C. and Gregoriadis, G. (1984). **Biotech.** 2, 979-984.

7. Weingarten, C., Moufti, A., Delattre, J., Puisieux, F. and Couvreur, P. (1985). **Int. J. Pharm.** 26, 251-257.

8. Puglisi, G., Fresta, M., La Rosa, C., Ventura, C.A., Panico, A.M. and Mazzone, G. (1992). **Pharmazie** 47, 211-215.

9. Stuhne-Sekalec, L., Stanasev, N.Z. and Djokic, S. (1991). **J. Microencapsul.** 8, 171-183.

10. Gregoriadis, G. (1973). **FEBS Lett.** 36, 292-296.

11. El-Ridy, M., Akbarieh, M., Kassem, M., Sharkawi, M. and Tawashi, R. (1989). **Int. J. Pharm.** 56, 23-27.

12. Fresta, M., Puglisi, G., Panico, A.M., DiMarco, S. and Mazzone, G. (1993). **Drug Dev. Ind. Pharm.** 19, 558-585.

13. Gabizon, A., Dagan, A., Goren, D., Barenholz, Y. and Fuks, Z. (1982). **Cancer Res.** 42, 4734-4739.

14. Goormaghtigh, E., Chatelain, P., Caspers, J. and Ruysschaert, J.M. (1980). **Biochim. Biophys. Acta** 597, 1-14.

15. Kim, C.K. and Han, J.H. (1995). **J. Microencapsul.** 12, 437-446.

16. Gulati, M., Grover, M., Singh, M. and Singh, S. (1998). **J. Microencap.** 15, 485-494.

17. Taylor, K.M., Taylor, G., Kellaway, I.W. and Stevens, J. (1990). **Int. J. Pharm.** 58, 49-55.

18. Alpar, O.H., Bamford, J.B. and Walters, V. (1981). **Int. J. Pharm.** 7, 349-351.

19. Lawrence, S.M., Alpar, O.H., McAllister, S.M. and Brown, M.R. (1993). **J. Drug Target.** 1, 303-310.

20. Perez-Soler, R. and Khokhar, A.R. (1992). **Cancer Res.** 52, 6341-6347.

21. Amselem, S., Gabizon, A. and Barenholz, Y. (1990). **J. Pharm. Sci.** 79, 1045-1052.

22. Mayhew, E., Rustum, Y.M., Szoka, F. and Papahadjopoulos, D. (1979). **Cancer Treat. Rep.** 63, 1923-1928.

23. Benita, S., Poly, P.A., Puisieux, F. and Delattre, J. (1984). **J. Pharm. Sci.** 73, 1751-1755.

24. Betageri, G.V. (1993). **Drug Dev. Ind. Pharm.** 19, 531-539.

25. Kulkarni, S.B. and Vargha-Butler, E.I. (1996). **Int. J. Pharm. Adv.** 1, 408-413.

26. Ganapathi, R. and Krishan, A. (1984). **Biochem. Pharmacol.** 33, 698-700.

27. Farr, S.J., Kellaway, I.W. and Carman Meakin, B. (1989). **Int. J. Pharm.** 51, 39-46.

28. Lopez-Berestein, G., Mehta, R., Hopfer, R., Mehta, K., Mersh, E.M. and Juliano, R. (1983). **Cancer Drug Del.** 1, 37-42.

29. Law, S.L., Chang, P. and Lin, C.H. (1991). **Int. J. Pharm.** 70, 1-7.

30. Foradada, M. and Estelrich, J. (1995). **Int. J. Pharm.** 124, 261-269.

31. Mohr, K. and Struve, M. (1991). **Biochem. Pharmacol.** 41, 961-965.

32. Cannon, J.B., Martin, C., Drummond, G.S. and Kappas, A. (1993). **Pharm. Res.** 10, 715-721.

33. Chapman, C.J., Erdahl, W.E., Taylor, R.W. and Pfeiffer, D.R. (1991). **Chem. Physics Lipids** 60, 201-208.

34. Betageri, G.V., Jenkins, S.A. and Parsons, D.L. (1993). Industrial applications of liposomes. In : Liposome Drug Delivery Systems, Technomic Publishing Co., Pennsylvania, pp. 109-125.

35. Defrise-Quertain, F., Chatelain, P., Delmelle, M. and Ruysschaert, J. (1984). Model studies for drug entrapment and liposome stability. In : Liposome Technology : Incorporation of drugs, proteins and genetic material (Gregoriadis, G. Ed.), CRC Press, Boca Raton, pp. 183-204.

36. Tsujii, K., Sunamoto, J. and Fendler, J.H. (1976). **Life Sci.** 19, 1743-1750.

37. Vadiei, K., Lopez-Berestein, G., Perez-Soler, R. and Luke, D.R. (1989). **Int. J. Pharm.** 57, 133-138.

38. Gano, J.B. and Kleinerman, E.S. (1995). **Oncol. Nurs. Forum** 22, 809-816.

39. Chase, J., Wood, J., Pazdur, R., Khokhar, A.R., Perez-Soler, R., Siddik, Z.H. and Roh, M. (1991). **Proc. AACR** pp. 420.

40. Wasan, K.M., Ng, S. and Cassidy, S.M. (1997). **J. Pharm. Sci.** 86, 872-875.

41. Gulati, M., Grover, M., Singh, S. and Singh, M. (1998). **Int. J. Pharm.** 165, 129-168.

42. Cullis, P.R., Mayer, L.D., Bally, M.B., Madden, T.D. and Hope, M.J. (1989). **Adv. Drug. Del. Rev.** 3, 267-282.

43. Bangham, A.D., Standish, M.M. and Watkins, J.C. (1965). **J. Mol. Biol.** 13, 238-252.

44. Gruner, S.M., Lenk, R.P., Janoff, A.S. and Ostro, M.J. (1985). **Biochemistry** 24, 2833-2844.

45. Habib, M.J. and Rogers, J.A. (1987). **Drug Dev. Ind. Pharm.** 13, 1947-1971.

46. Payne, N.I., Timmins, P., Ambrose, C.V., Ward, M. and Ridgeway, F. (1986). **J. Pharm. Sci.** 75, 325-329.

47. Szoka, F. and Papahadjopoulos, D. (1978). **Proc. Nat. Acad. Sci.** 75, 4194-4198.

48. Deamer, D.W. and Barchfield, G.L. (1982). **J. Mol. Evol.** 18, 203-206.

49. Ravaoarinoro, M., Toma, E., Agbaba, O. and Morisset, R. (1993). **J. Drug Target.** 1, 191-195.

50. Olson, F., Hunt, C.A., Szoka, F., Vial, W.J. and Papahadjopoulos, D. (1979). **Biochim. Biophys. Acta** 557, 9-23.

51. Deamer, D.W. and Bangham, A.D. (1976). **Biochim. Biophys. Acta** 443, 629-634.

52. Mayer, L.D., Hope, M.J. and Cullis, P.R. (1985). **Biochim. Biophys. Acta** 858, 161-168.

53. Mayer, L.D., Bally, M.B. and Cullis, P.R. (1986). **Biochim. Biophys. Acta** 857, 123-126.

54. Oh, Y.K., Nix, D.E. and Straubinger, R.M. (1995). **Antimicrob. Agents Chemother.** 39, 2104-2111.

55. Vemuri, S. and Rhodes, C.T. (1994). **J. Pharm. Pharmacol.** 46, 778-783.

56. Murray, S.W., Wheeler, J.J., Bally, M.B. and Mayer, L.D. (1995). **Biochim. Biophys. Acta** 1238, 147-155.

57. Haran, G., Cohen, R., Bar, L.K. and Barenholz, Y. (1993). **Biochim. Biophys. Acta** 1151, 201-215.

58. Bally, M.B., Hope, M.J., van Echteld, C.J.A. and Cullis, P.R. (1985). **Biochim. Biophys. Acta** 812, 66-76.

59. Mayer, L.D., Wong, K.F., Menon, K., Chong, C., Harrigan, P.R. and Cullis, P.R. (1988). **Biochemistry** 27, 2053-2060.

60. Bally, M.B., Mayer, L.D., Loughrey, H., Redelmeier, T., Madden, T.D., Wong, K.F., Hope, M.J. and Cullis, P.R. (1988). **Chem. Physics Lipids** 47, 97-107.

61. Beaumier, P.L. and Hwang, K.J. (1982). **J. Nucl. Med.** 23, 810-815.

62. Hwang, C.J., Merriam, J.E., Beaumier, P.L. and Luk, K.F.S. (1982). **Biochim. Biophys. Acta** 716, 101-109.

63. Tilcock, C.P.S, Ahkong, Q.F., Koenig, S.H., Brown, R.D., Davis, M. and Kabalka, G. (1992). **Magn. Reson. Med.** 27, 44-51.

64. Lee, M.J., Straubinger, R.M. and Jusko, W.J. (1995). **Pharm. Res.** 13, 1055-1059.

65. Mayer, L.D., Bally, M.B. and Cullis, P.R. (1990). **Biochim. Biophys. Acta** 1025, 143-151.

66. Nichols, J.W. and Deamer, D.W. (1990). **Biochim. Biophys. Acta** 455, 269-271.

67. Harrigan, P.R., Wong, K.F., Redelmeier, T.E., Wheller, J.J. and Cullis, P.R. (1993). **Biochim. Biophys. Acta** 1149, 237-244.

68. Boman, N.L., Mayer, L.D. and Cullis, P.R. (1993). **Biochim. Biophys. Acta** 1152, 253-258.

69. Gabizon, A., Shiota, R. and Papahdjopoulos, D. (1989). **J. Natl. Canc. Inst.** 81, 1484-1488.

70. Gabizon, A., Barenholz, Y. and Bialer, M. (1993). **Pharm. Res.** 10, 703-708.

71. Arien, A., Goigoux, C., Baquey, C. and Dupuy, B. (1993). **Life Sci.** 53, 1279-1290.

72. Tilcock, C.P.S., Ahkong, Q.F. and Parr, M. (1991). **Invest. Radiol.** 26, 242-247.

20

PRODRUG MESOPHASES BASED LYMPHOTROPHS OF PROPRANOLOL HCl FOR IMPROVED ORAL ABSORPTION

PARIJAT KANAUJIA, VIKAS JAITELY, R. SRINIVASAN and S. P. VYAS

Department of Pharmaceutical Sciences
Dr. Harisingh Gour Vishwavidyalaya
Sagar (MP) 470 003

- Introduction
- Materials
- Synthesis and characterization of prodrug
- Preparation of formulations of prodrug
- Characterization and evaluation of formulations
- Results and discussion
- Conclusion
- References

INTRODUCTION

Propranolol HCl is one of the most commonly used β-blocker available in the market. When it is orally administered, it gets metabolised and partially inactivated due to extensive hepatic first pass metabolism [1]. According to the reports in literature some of the serious drawbacks of drugs could be effectively circumvented by covalent linkage of the drug to fatty acids [2]. The resulting lipidised prodrug could be used for its effective lymphatic transportation for systemic delivery after oral administration. These lipidic prodrugs if provided with some surface-active properties tend to form supramolecular assemblages (liquid crystalline to micellar) in the aqueous media. Supramolecules are defined as the self-assemblages, whose functions and properties are determined by the molecular orientation of the assembling units [3]. Vizoglu and Speiser, [4] have previously reported Pindolol glycerolmonostearate and buperinol hydrochloride glycerol dipalmitate esters with self-dispersion properties.

Various vesicular systems including liposomes [5] and niosomes [6] have demonstrated their potential for their applicability in effective drug delivery. Pharmacosomes have been introduced as relatively recent version of novel drug delivery systems with well identified advantages. Drug covalently bound to lipid may exist as a colloidal dispersion or ultrafine-vesicular micellar or hexagonal aggregates, which are referred to as pharmacosomes or prodrug mesophases. Thus the pharmacosomes combine the properties of the active drug principle (pharmacon) and the carrier (soma). Contrary to various classical vesicular drug delivery systems, problems of drug incorporation and leakage from the carrier are effectively alleviated in the case of pharmacosomes [7, 8].

Any drug possessing a free carboxyl group can be esterified with the hydroxyl group of a lipid molecules (glyceride, phosphatide etc.); similarly, the drugs that with active hydrogen atom i.e., -OH or -NH etc. can be esterified. Synthesis of such compounds results into strongly amphiphilic molecules that facilitate trans-membranes transfer. These amphipathic prodrug mesogens may serve as building blocks by participating in supramolecular assemblages thus acquire a colloidal state. The later may possibly offer a modified newer *in-vivo* fate to the derivatised drug(s).

The present work was undertaken with an intention to enhance the oral absorption of poropranolol HCl as it is extensively metabolised during the first pass hepatic metabolism nearly 50-60% of administered dose suffers first hepatic elimination [1] therefore a major portion of drug remains pharmacodynamically unavailable. Propranolol HCl has been derivatised so as to obtain an ampiphathic prodrug with a long hydrophobic chain, and hydrophilic head group. The prodrug could orient to form supramolecular nanoconstructs. The later may be expected to absorb well via lymphatics transportation or at-least display some modified absorption and distribution characteristics.

MATERIALS

Propranolol HCl was obtained as gift sample from Cipla India Ltd. Phosphatidyl choline and olive oil was obtained from Sigma USA, Dimethyl aminopyridine fromMerck, India and palmitoyl chloride from Fluka, Switzerland. All other chemicals and solvents were obtained from BDH, a division of E. Merck India Ltd. (Mumbai).

SYNTHESIS AND CHARACTEIZATION OF PRODRUG

Palmitoyl propranolol hydrochloride (PPH) was synthesised by the esterification of propranolol hydrochloride with palmitoyl chloride employing the procedure specified by Pech et al., [9] replacing timolol maleate with propranolol HCl in same schicometric ratios. The obtained compound was purified using column chromatography (Keislgur, Mobile phase of diethyl ether:acetic acid (95:5)) and characterised using NMR and IR spectroscopy.

Identification of the prodrug

IR and NMR spectroscopic analysis were conducted to confirm the synthesis of the prodrug using a Shimadzu (Japan) IR and Perkin Elmer NMR (360 MHz) systems.
IR- 2910 (C-H stretching vibration CH_3), 2830 (C-H stretching vibration CH_2), 1730 (C=O stretching vibration), 1612 (NH bending vibration CH_3), 1575 (band due to phenyl ring), 1385 (C-H bending vibration CH_3), 1225 (C-O-C stretching vibration), 1155 (C-O stretching vibration), 924 (C-H out of playing vibration in aromatic region)
NMR- ($CDCl_3$) δ in ppm values 0.82 (3H, H_3-16), 0.9 (7 H, s, $CH(CH_3)_2$), 1.2 (24 H, s H_2-15), 1.57 (m, H_2-3), 2.33 (m, H_2-2), 3.12 (1H, m, H'-γ), 3.48 (1H,d, H''-γ) 4.2 (2H, m $OCOCH_2$), 5.9 (1H, w, H-α), 6.8-7.8 (5 medium peaks due to aromatic ring)

Physicochemical characterisation of the prodrug

The physicochemical parameter viz., melting point, partition coefficient and solubility of the prodrug were determined and the data were compared with propranolol.

Propranolol content

Accurately weighed prodrug was hydrolysed using 0.1N HCl by heating at 90^0C for 2 hrs. The solution was filtered and following appropriate dilution with phosphate saline, estimated spectrophotometrically (λmax. 290 nm) using Systronics 119 UV/VIS spectrophotometer for propranolol content [10].

Hydrolysis profile

The hydrolysis profile of the prodrug was followed in simulated gastric fluid (SGF) and simulated intestinal fluid (SIF). The standard dialysis method was applied using Sigma dialysis tubes. The samples were withdrawn periodically and analysed for propranolol content spectrophotometrically as described earlier (Systronics 119 UV/VIS spectrophotometer at λmax. 290 nm)(Fig. 1).

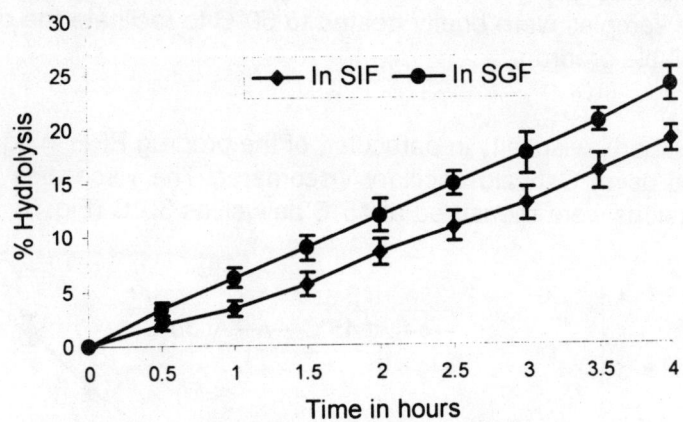

Fig. 1 : *In vitro* hydrolysis of palmitoyl propranolol hydrochloride

Tensiometric studies

The samples of different concentrations of PPH were prepared in a concentration range of 0.1, to 0.001 w/w in phosphate saline buffer (pH 7.4). The surface tension was recorded at ambient temperature over different time intervals up to 30 minutes [11]. Different concentrations of palmitoyl propranolol hydrochloride (PPH) were prepared (0.5, 0.1, 0.05, 0.01, 0.005, 0.001, 0.0005 % w/w) for the determination of critical aggregation concentration and the measurements were recorded until equilibrium was attained. The results are presented in figure 2 (a) & (b).

Microscopic examination

The liquid crystalline phases were observed under polarized microscope. The textures and morphology of liquid crystals was identified as described by Rosevear [12]. Dispersion of prodrug in water was studied between 90° and 0.05% w/w at

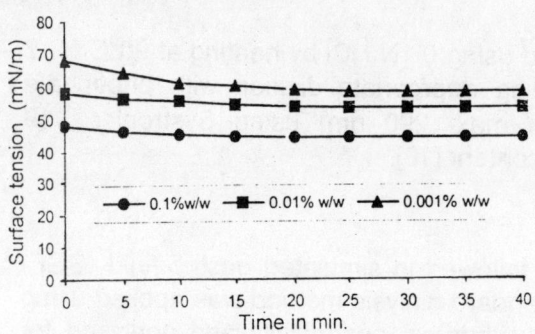

Fig. 2a : Change in surface tension with time for different concentration of PPH

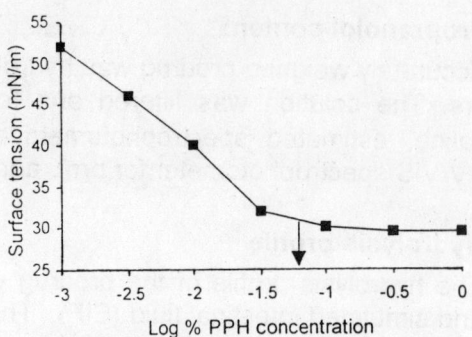

Fig. 2b : Plot used for determination of critical micellar concentration of PPH

ambient temperatures using a Nikkon (Japan) microscope equipped with crossed polarisers. The samples were briefly heated to 50°C to facilitate the dispersability of poorly water soluble prodrug.

Viscosity

A rheological property, viscosity in particular, of the prodrug PPH in aqueous medium was determined using Ostwald capillary viscometer. The viscosities of the prodrug aqueous dispersions were measured at 45°C as well as 30°C (Fig. 3).

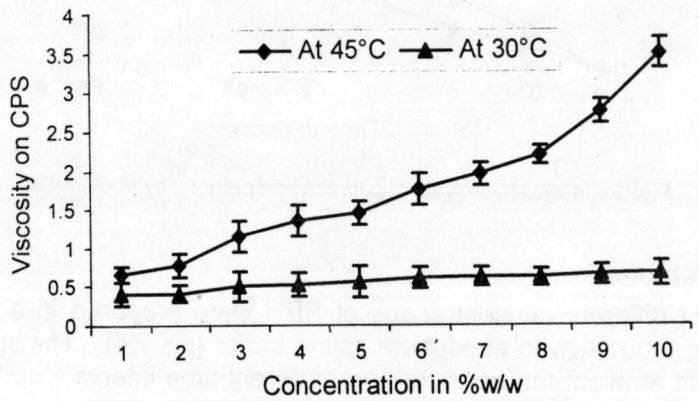

Fig. 3 : Change in viscosity with concentration at different temperatures

PREPARATION OF PRODRUG FORMULATIONS

Liquid crystalline dispersion

A 10% w/v liquid crystalline dispersion of PPH [PLCD] was prepared using the method described by Jaitely and Vyas, [13]. The dispersion was heated to 60°C so as to achieve the isotropic phase and slowly cooled to ambient temperature under continual stirring in order to achieve its anisotropic phase. The self assembled liquid crystalline phase of PPH was surface stabilized by incubating it at 40°C with phosphatidyl choline (PC) (10% w/w with respect to the weight of PPH). The preparation was used as such its without any further processing.

Lipid solution

A lipid solution of PPH [PLS] was prepared in olive oil. PPH equivalent to 2mg of propranolol content in 1ml of oil was introduced into olive oil and sonicated briefly to obtain a clear solution.

CHARACTERIZATION AND EVALUATION OF FORMULATIONS

In-vitro release profile

The *in-vitro* release profiles of the PLCD and PLS was determined using dialysis method. The accurately weighed dispersions (PLCD or PLS) were placed in the dialysis tubes (Sigma USA) and the tubes were placed in the dialysing medium (SGF pH 1.2 or SIF pH 7.5) under constant stirring maintained at 37±2°C. The samples were withdrawn periodically and were estimated spectrophotometrically for drug content (Systronics 119 UV/VIS spectrophotometer at λmax. 290 nm). Each time the withdrawn sample was replaced with an equal volume of respective dialysing medium (Fig 4).

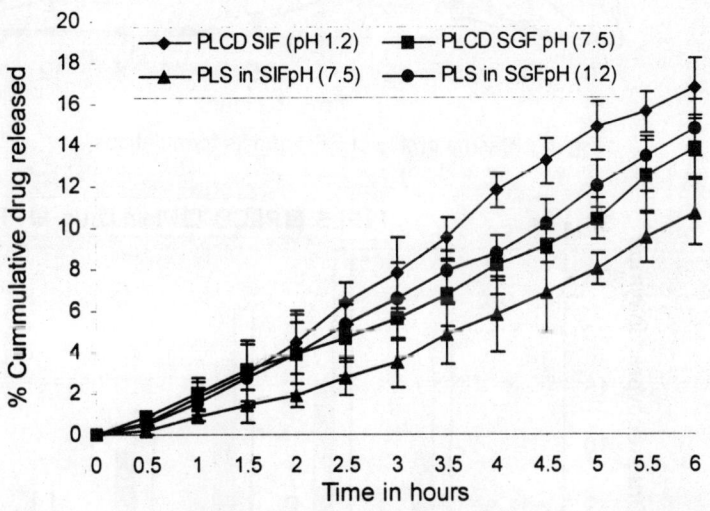

Fig. 4 : *In vitro* release rate profile

In vivo performance evaluation

The albino rats of either sex were weighed (250-300gms) and divided into five groups of six animals each. All the animals were kept for overnight fasting but given free access to water. All the animals of group 1 were given an oral dose of PLCD; group 2 was given orally the dose of lipid dispersion; animals of group 3 were given orally aqueous dispersion of prodrug (PPH) and group 4 were given aqueous solution of propranolol HCl, in equivalent doses, whereas the 5th group served as control (doses for all the formulations were calculated to be equivalent for propranolol).

All the animals were anesthesized by urethane injection (1.2 g/Kg body weight). The animals were dissected and thoracic duct was cannulated as described by Warshaw A. L. [14]. Simultaneously, jugular vein was also cannulated. All the animals were kept in supine position and infused with normal saline solution at the rate of 4 ml/hr/kg. Lymph and blood samples were collected periodically and analysed for the propranolol content using the fluorometic method for determination of propranolol as reported by Trivedi B.M. et.al. [15] (Fig 5 & 6).

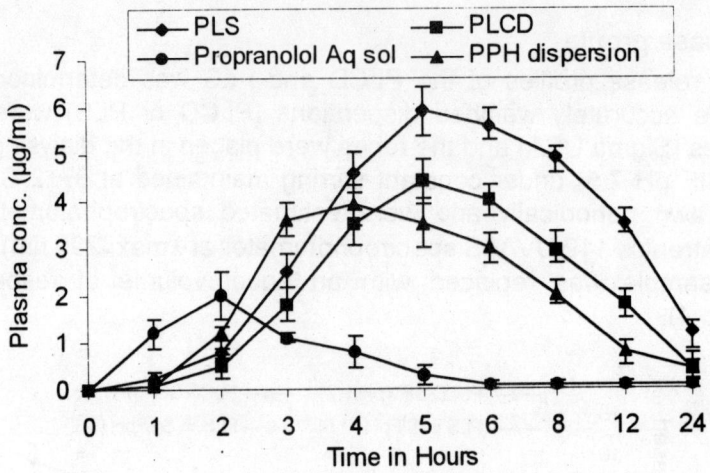

Fig. 5 : Plasma profile of PPH and its formulations

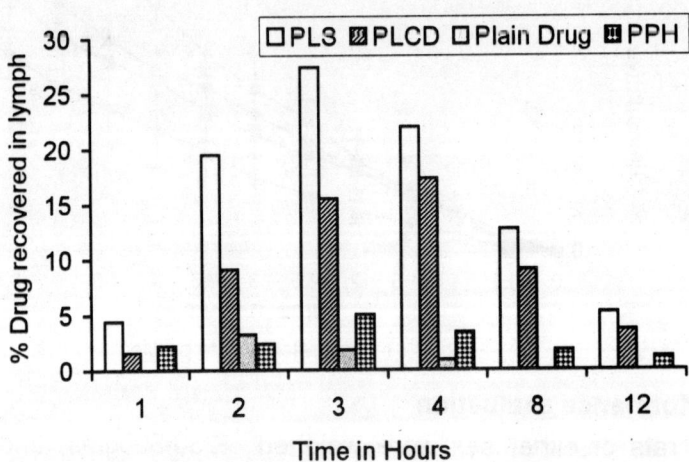

Fig. 6 : *In vivo* lymphatic uptake of various formulations

RESULTS AND DISCUSSION

Supramolecular assemblages are described as ordered orientation that molecules adopt to attain a thermodynamically stable state [16]. The formation of assemblages is attributed to the architectural behaviour of the molecules ascribed to the intrinsic properties of the molecule in a particular solvent; like amphiphilic compounds (e.g. sodium lauryl sulphate, cetyl triammonium bromide) have been known to form ordered assemblages. The formation of these ordered assemblages for drug molecules leads to the modifications in the pharmacokinetic and pharmacodynamic behaviours of drug molecules in biological milieu. The assembleges offer protection against bioenvironmental challenges through supramolecular orientation [17].

Propranolol HCl is a water-soluble β-blocker, which on oral administration metabolised extensively during first hepatic pass as well as partially inactivated during intestinal absorption in gastrointestinal tract [1]. Nearly 75% of the administered dose is inactivated (metabolised) by liver during first hepatic passage. Leading to a low bioavailability of propranolol on oral administration. The present work was undertaken with an intention to increase the overall oral bioavailability of Propranolol HCl utilising intestinal lymphatics transportation.

The prodrug of propranolol HCl was prepared by esterification at the secondary alcoholic group with palmitoyl chloride by the method described by Pech et. al. [9]. The product obtained was purified using column chromatography.

The isolated prodrug was studied for its chemical structure with the help of IR and NMR spectroscopy. The IR spectra for the synthesised prodrug O-palmitoyl propranolol hydrochloride (PPH) when compared against that of propranolol HCl, clearly revealed a peak for OH bending vibration at 1400 cm^{-1} and a prominent peak at 1100 cm^{-1} for alcoholic C-O stretching vibration disappeared. In addition, an additional peak at 1740 cm^{-1} appeared. The later peak corresponds to C=O vibration of the ester group formed depicting the esterification of propranolol HCl with palmitoyl chloride. The presence of ester linkage was further confirmed by NMR spectroscopy (peaks previously indicated). The probable structure that explains for newer peaks is given following structure.

Structure of palmitoyl propranolol HCl

The synthesised prodrug (PPH) was studied for its physicochemical parameters. The melting point of the prodrug was found to be 49±0.5°C. The amphiphilic nature of the prodrug was realised by the solubility determination. It was found that PPH was differentially soluble in polar as well as in non-polar solvents however, it demonstrated higher solubility in the organic solvents. The partition coefficient in octanol/water system was 1.857 ± 0.045 indicating an amphiphilic nature of PPH however; the hydrolysis of PPH was affected in SGF and SIF. Figure 1 clearly suggests that the propranolol ester was quite stable at acidic as well as at basic environments. The hydrolysis, at the gastric pH was found to be relatively faster as compared to the rate of hydrolysis at intestinal pH. At the intestinal pH, the formation of N-palmitoyl propranolol as derivatised base could be one mechanism, of degradation, which avoids ester hydrolysis.

The self-assembling nature of PPH was established with the help of tensiometric studies. The amphiphilicity of PPH can be appreciated by measuring the surface tension of dispersion against time by drop volume method using stalagmometer [18] as illustrated in figure 2 (a) & (b) at pH 6.5. It was found that the surface tension decreased with increasing concentration of PPH (equilibrium surface tension of 0.1%, 0.01% and 0.001% w/w solution were 44mN/m, 53mN/m and 58 mN/m). The concentration also significantly affected the kinetic profile, for lower concentrations the initial surface tension values decreased slowly till equilibrium surface tensions were attained [Fig. 2 (a)].

The aggregation concentration was determined from a plot prepared between surface tension and concentration (log scale) [Fig. 2 (b)]. It was found that after an initial linear decrease, the surface tension was almost constant. The point of variation was denoted as critical aggregation concentration, which was found to be 0.06% w/w (corresponding log value -1.22). The observation further substantiates the amphiphatic nature of the PPH. This could be attributed to the presence of a hydrophobic palmitoyl chain and an intrinsic hydrophilic group of propranolol (quaternary ammonium salt). The amphiphilicity and the presence of a long hydrophobic chain of the prodrug may be attributed to the assemblage of PPH molecules with a particular orientation leading to the formation of a composite aggregated system.

The anhydrous state of the prodrug (PPH) at room temperature exhibited an amorphous form with typical birefringent microcrystals scattered in all directions appearing spherulitic in shape with irregular maltase crosses. In the temperature range of 45-55°C complete isotropic melting was observed. However, the liquid crystalline phase reappeared on cooling with a typical radiant pattern. On reheating, melting occurred regularly at 48°C. The crystalline phase of PPH existed below 35±1°C. Above 50±2°C the isotropic melting of PPH was observed.

Smectic type liquid crystalline phases, which are referred to as 'lamellar phase', were observed in the preparation. These 'lamellar phases' were identified by the presence of myelinic systems with characteristic labyrith like patterns. These myelin systems are clearly visualized that resemble closely to that of phospholipids. The cylindrical structures of myelinic systems showed various alterations and narrowings are also seen. These shapes are the result of subsequent deformations in the myelinic structures and lamellar textures.

At 30°C and above up to 35°C the PPH dispersion was observed microscopically to be heterogeneous distinctively marked by the existence of solid crystals and liquid crystalline phase, whereas below 30°C mainly solid crystals rich phase was seen. Similarly, in the microscopic observation made at 45°C and above, an explicit phase transition from solid crystalline state to an absolutely liquid crystalline phase was recorded. Simultaneously, the viscoelastic studies were conducted at 30°C and 45°C. The prepared system displayed typical temperature dependent viscoelastic behaviour as suggested by Kirwet, et al. [19]. The viscosity enhanced at a lower temperature i.e. 30°C presumably due to the presence of solid crystalline phase. It was observed to be independent of concentration of PPH. At higher temperature i.e. 45°C the system however demonstrated a linear increase in viscosity with the increasing concentration of PPH. The intrinsic viscosity measurement was found to be $[\eta]=2.5\phi$, corresponding to spherical to cylindrical assemblages [19]. Moreover, the conversion of isotropic phase to the anisotropic phases with a concomitant change in temperature from 45°C and above witnessed by varying viscoelastic behaviour. It further suggests for formation of lamellar liquid crystalline phases of PPH as it was also optically observed under the stated temperature conditions with the help of polarised microscope. The presence of liquid crystals supports the viscoelastic behaviour and findings are in accordance with those suggested by Chang and Bodmier, [20] for monoglycerides.

The overall oral bioavailability of the prodrug (PPH) was determined following its oral administration in various formulations i.e., in assembled (dispersion) as well as solution forms. The PPH was found to convert to its anisotropic forms due to specific amphiphilic properties and microscopic phase behaviour under varying temperature conditions. The PPH was restricted to its liquid crystalline aggregated supra-molecular phase using phophatidylcholine as the surface stabiliser as well as to protect it from G.I. environmental challenges as suggested by Satpardar et al. [21] for the preparation of nanocrystals [PLCD]. The lipid solution of PPH was prepared in olive oil in order to study the effect of lipid vehicle and lipophilicity of drug on its lymphatic transportation.

The *in vitro* release profile obtained (Fig. 4) in SGF and SIF indicates that all the formulations of PPH are fairly stable throughout the gastric environment. 13.8±0.25% of the free drug released in the SGF in 6hrs whereas 16.83±0.354% of the drug was estimated in SIF in the case of PLCD. However, only 10.2±0.25% and 12.83±0.54% of drug was released in SGF and SIF respectively in the case of PLS. It indicates the high shielding effect offered by the molecular geometry of aggregated system as well as surfacial phospholipid layer highlighting the suitability of their use as carrier for intestinal delivery of drugs.

The *in vivo* performance evaluation of the prodrug solution and in form of its supramolecular aggregates or dispersion was conducted on albino rats. The rats were given an initial oral dose of soybean oil in order to swell its lymphatic duct to make it accessible for cannulation. A double cannulated anaesthetised rat model was used to investigate the potential lymphatic transportation of PPH in its supramolecular assemblages. Periodically collected plasma and lymph were estimated for propranolol content. Figure 6 shows the plasma profile. The data obtained were subjected to appropriate statistical treatment. The bioavailability of propranolol following various treatments was determined by computing area under the curve of drug plasma profile. The area under the curve (AUC) was determined employing trapezoidal rule. A significantly higher bioavailability of propranolol HCl following the administration of PPH was recorded as compared against drug plasma profile and AUC recorded after to plain drug administration, a significant statistical difference was recorded ($p < 0.05$) (Table I). Similarly the bioavailability estimated for PLCD was much higher than the others, whereas it was maximum amongst the various treatments in the case of PLS. The AUC recorded were 292.83 ± 0.25 µg/ml/hr and 326.34 ± 0.78 µg/ml/hr (n=6) for PLCD and PLS respectively which were significantly higher (p < 0.05) than AUC's recorded for plain and prodrug treatments. Thus on the basis of multiple statistical competitive evaluation the preparation based on prodrug of propranolol in the form of self aggregated supramolecular forms demonstrated the best results by producing significantly higher propranolol blood plasma levels and overall AUC reflecting better bioavailability too.

Table I. Comparative bioavailability of various formulations

S. No.	Formulation	Area under the curve (AUC)
1.	Propranolol HCl aqueous solution	218.46 ± 1.09 µg/ml/hr
2.	Palmitoyl Propranolol HCl dispersion in water	276.77 ± 1.24 µg/ml/hr
3.	Liquid crystalline dispersion [PLCD]	292.83 ± 0.25 µg/ml/hr
4.	Lipid solution of PPH [PLS]	326.34 ± 0.78 µg/ml/hr

In the case of supramolecular PLCD as well as PLS an initial lag phase was observed. This is suggestive of the mechanism, which are operative in uptake and trafficking of the drug to systemic circulation via lymphatics as well as by normal systemic absorption. The lymph was simultaneously collected and periodic lymphatic drug concentration profile was generated figure 8 to support the absorption mechanism.

The lymphatic drug concentration profile indicates that lymphatic uptake and trafficking of the PPH are apparently responsible for increased oral bioavailability. The effects, one contributed by the lipophilicity and other by supramolecular assemblage of PPH are seemingly responsible for an increased lymphatic uptake which would have been further enhanced by presence of lipidic vehicle. The increased bioavailability in case of oral administration of PPH contained in lipid vehicle could be attributed to the effect of vehicle, which reportedly enhances the enterocyte production, and in turn chylomicron expression. The latter is well-documented process of lipid uptake [22]. Obviously, the lipid vehicle digestion may at large be attributed to better uptake of PPH, which is more lipophilic as compared to its drug molecule. The relatively better systemic absorption via lymph in case of supramolecular assemblages of PPH tensiogen may be accounted for its chylomicron mimicking architecture, surface stabilised with phospholipid is critical in negotiating its lymphatic transportation. However, a well-designed study protocol should be followed in order to establish the exact mechanism that operates for better availability.

The intestinal lymphatics are characterised by a centrally located vessel; a lacteals within the intestinal villi which join a plexus of lymphatic capillaries in the mucosa and sub mucosa and drain via the mesenteric lymph vessels into the cisterna chyli. The lymph from cisterna chyli is drained by the thoracic lymph duct, which empties directly into the general circulation at the junction of left internal jugular and left subclavian veins, thus avoiding hepatic first pass metabolism [23]. Therefore, lymphatic transportation could be at large ascribed to the higher bioavailability of PPH after oral administration. The avoidance of hepatic first pass extraction is seemingly a pivotal factor that could be accounted for improved bioavailability.

CONCLUSION

It could be concluded from the study that the palmitoyl prodrug of propranolol having an amphiphilic nature is tensiogeneic mesogens that assemble to form supramolecules convertible to its liquid crystalline states. The nanoconstructs restricted to this particular orientation by surface stabilisation are susceptible to lymphatic uptake and transportation to systemic pool and bypass liver, which as a result enhances the availability. Furthermore, the major constraint related to propranolol ester i.e. aminolysis could be effectively arrested when a supramolecular assemblages are utilised. Hence the supramolecular aggregates could serve as effective lymphotrophs exploitable for effective drug delivery for better bioavailability of the drugs which undergo extensive first hepatic pass metabolism.

ACKNOWLEDGEMENTS

We are thankful to CSIR, New Delhi for financial assistance to two authors (VJ & PK) as well as to Cipla laboratories, Mumbai for kindly providing the gift sample of propranolol HCl to carry out the study.

REFERENCES

1. Dvornik, D., Kraml, M., Duvue, J., Coelho, J., Novello, L. A., Arnold, J. D. and Mullane, J. F. (1983) **Curr. Therap. Res.** 39, 595-605.

2. Mantellp, S., Speiser, P. and Hauser, H. (1985) **Chem. Phys. Lipids** 37, 329-43.

3. Wolf, K.L. and Wolf, R. (1948) **Angewandte Chemie** 61, 191.

4. Vizoglu, O. and Speiser, P. (1992) **Eur. J. Pharm. Biopharm.** 38, 1-6.

5. Gregoriadis, G. and Florence, A. T. (1993) **Drugs** 45, 15-28

6. Baillie, A. J., Florence, A. T., Hume, L., Muirhead, G. T. and Rogerson, A. (1985) **J. Pharm. Pharmcol.** 37, 863-868.

7. Viazoglu, O. and Speiser, P. (1986) **Acta Pharm. Suec.** 23, 163-172.

8. Goymann, C. M. and Hamann, H. J. (1991) **Eur. J. Pharm. Biopharm.** 37, 113-117.

9. Pech, B., Duval, O., Richomme, P. and Benoit, J. P. (1996) **Int. J. Pharm.** 128, 179-188.

10. Clark, E. G. C. (1969) Isolation and Identification of drugs, Pharmaceutical Press London, Vol I, 521.

11. Pech, B., Proust, J. E., Bouloguand, Y. and Benoit, J. P. (1997) **Pharm. Res.** 14(1), 37-41.

12. Rosevear, F. B. (1954) **J. Am. Oil Chem. Soc.** 31, 628-639.

13. Jaitely, V. and Vyas S. P. (1999) **J. Drug Targeting** 6(5), 315-322.

14. Warshaw, A.Z. (1972) **Gut** 13, 66.

15. Trivedi, B. M., Gohel, M. and Chawa, H. (1986) **Ind. J. Pharm. Sci.** 48, 142-143.

16. Vyas, S. P., Jaitely, V. and Kanaujia, P. (1997) **Die Pharmazie** 52(4), 259-267.

17. Kataoka, K., Kwon, G. S., Yokoyama, M., Okano, T. and Sakuri, Y. (1993) **J. Control. Rel**. 24, 119-132.

18. Davis, J. T. and Ridear, E. K. (1963). Surface Chemistry: The Physics of Surface, Academic Press, New York.

19. Kirwet, K. and Muller-Goymann, C. C. (1993) **Eur. J. Pharm. Biopharm.** 39, 234-238.

20. Chang, C. M. and Bodmier, R. (1997) **J. Pharm. Sci.** 86, 747-752.

21. Satpadar, P., Bruno, J., Liversidge G., Meriske-Liversidge, E., Shaw, J., Mattes, K., Cobett, T., Polin, L., Jhones, J. and Rake, J. (1993) **Gorden Conference on Chemotherapy of Experimental and Clinical Cancer**, Oct 3-8, 1993, Isee, Germany.

22. Palin, K. J. and Wilson, C. G. (1984) **J. Pharm. Pharmacol.** 36, 641.

23. Granger, D. N., Korthius, R. J., Kvietys, P. R. and Tso, P. (1988) **Am. J. Physiol.** 255, G690.

21

LECTINIZED LIPOSOMES: A NOVEL APPROACH FOR INTRAPERIODONTAL POCKET DRUG DELIVERY

P.K. DUBEY, V. SIHORKAR, V. MISHRA, Y.K. KATARE and S.P. VYAS
Department of Pharmaceutical Sciences
Dr. Harisingh Gour Vishwavidyalaya, Sagar 470 003

INTRODUCTION

The existence of membrane lectins as carbohydrate specific receptors on the bio-membranes, which recognize carbohydrate epitopes also, present on membrane glyco-sphingolipids and glycoproteins, suggests a clear role in cellular adhesion and recognition process. The lectin-carbohydrate interaction constitutes the basis of carbohydrate mediated cellular interactions. One of the most relevant techniques is to conjugate a lectin to the liposomal surface and to engineer up a proteoliposome. Lectin appended liposomes interact selectively with the sugars expressed on bacterial cell surface as glyco-conjugates. The specificity and affinity of lectins to bind to a particular cell type (s) has led to their appreciation as site directing modules for targeted delivery of anti-microbial agent via glycocalyx mediation.

Bacteria develop in the periodontal pocket as a plaque (bio-film) behave rather differently in their pharmacological and metabolical manifestations, thus making their eradication difficult [1]. In the present study lectin (Con-A) was immobilized on liposomal surface adapting a novel procedure. The system was checked for the affinity and specificity of the ligand after immobilization on liposomal surface using competing studies. Developed system was finally evaluated for its targeting potential *in vitro* against cultured *Streptococcus mutans*.

MATERIALS AND METHODS

Materials

Egg phosphatidylcholine (EPC) and distearoyl phosphatidylcholine (DSPC) were purchased from Sigma (St. Louis, MO, USA) and used as supplied. Cholesterol (Chol), dicetyl phosphate (DCP), stearoylamine (SA) and bovine submaxillary mucin (BSM) were from Fluca chemicals, Switz. Concanavalin A (Con-A) from *Concanavalis easoniformis* was from sigma. All other chemicals used were of analytical grade, unless otherwise mentioned and were obtained from Qualigens (Glaxo India Ltd.). *Streptococcus mutans* bacteria (NCTC 7447) were obtained from Institute of Microbial

Technology (IMT, Chandigarh, India) as bacterial strips. The metronidazole MIC was determined by the dilution susceptibility test as described by Banker and co-workers [2]. Metronidazole MIC_{50} for *Streptococcus mutans* was recorded to be $\approx 18\,\mu g/ml$ as estimated with triplicates of representative experiments. The metronidazole dose is 50% of the MIC of free drug in plain and coated preparations as well as in plain drug.

Preparation of concanavalin-A coated vesicles

Plain (protein free) liposomes were prepared by first removing the solvent using a rotary flash evaporator from a 250 µ mole mixture of EPC and/or DSPC, Chol and charge imparting constitutive lipids to form a thin film on the inner wall of round bottom flask. The casted film was hydrated using mixed phosphate buffer of different pH values and the contents of the flask (vesicular dispersion) vortexed for about an hour to get the lipids off from the wall of the flask of flash evaporator into the dispersion. The drug metronidazole was dissolved in the aqueous phase (phosphate buffer) and incorporated at concentration level that corresponds to 1:5 weight ratio of total lipid. These vesicles were centrifuged thrice (1,00,000g) for 60 min to remove any unentrapped metronidazole. The liposomal population were harvested and screened for vesicle sizes and those above 1 µm (as retained oversized on Acrodiscs, Gelman, 1.2 µm) were taken for coating and subsequent stability protocols. Coating of liposomes with lectin (Con-A) was accomplished by charge induced interaction of the protein over the oppositely charged lipid bilayer. The zwitterionic behavior of concanavalin A was exploited. Lectin acquires different charge status above and below and in the vicinity of its isoelectric point [3]. To the whole vesicular dispersion so obtained (total lipid $\cong 5.1 \times 10^{-3}\,\mu g\,ml^{-3}$) 100 µg of Con-A dissolved in minimum volume (just sufficient to dissolve) of mixed phosphate buffers of varied pH was added. The pH of the dispersion was adjusted to pH 7.4 in the case of stearoylamine based formulations and to pH 6.0 in the case of dicetyl phosphate based formulations using mixed phosphate buffers. The dispersions so obtained were kept incubated for an optimized period of 6 hours. Measuring the resultant surface potential of the vesicles at different intervals, the incubation time and protein concentrations were optimized. Charge induced anchoring of Con-A on to the liposomal surface was measured by recording the change in turbidity using a nephelometer (York, India).

In vitro characterization

Vesicle characterization for size and shape was performed using transmission electron microscopy (TEM). Phosphotungstic acid (1%) was used as a negative stain (JEM 1200, EX 11, JEOL, JAPAN). Carbon coated samples were treated with albumin to render the surface hydrophilic, placed over a copper grid and subjected to TEM analysis. Vesicle size distribution was also assessed using a phase contrast microscope (Leitz, Biomed, Germany). The surface charge of the vesicles was calculated using zeta potential measurements. Liposomes with an average diameter of 3.1±0.9µ was calculated using Smoluchowski's equation from their mobility in PBS (pH 7.4, 0.001 M) using a zeta-potentiometer [4]. The probe reflected 25-40 mV of potential on either side of the grid depending upon the formulations. The % entrapment was determined and expressed as the percentage of added drug incorporated in the vesicles. The yield was referred to as the ratio of experimentally measured amount of the drug in the dispersion and the theoretical amount used. Predialysed vesicular dispersions were centrifuged at 1,00,000 g for 60 minutes. Pellets thus obtained were resuspended in 0.01M PBS (pH 7.4) and the process repeated for 3 times. Vesicles were lysed by adding 1.0 ml of 0.1% v/v triton X-100, centrifuged and the liberated contents were analyzed for metronidazole on a silica gel 60 F HPLC column at a detection wavelength of 254 nm [5]. Liposomes were assessed in terms of total lipid phosphorus. The concentration of phospholipids was determined by measuring inorganic phosphate after acid hydrolysis at 180 °C in 70 % $HClO_4$ [6,7]. Percent entrapment was expressed as % entrapment/mg of lipid.

In vitro ligand activity studies

The developed system was evaluated for carbohydrate specificity and *in-vitro* ligand activity. The affinity towards exogenously provided bovine submaxillary gland mucin (BSM) was used as a measure of activity [8]. BSM is a glycoprotein containing saccharides as oligosaccharide chains consisted of six different sugars namely, N-acetylglucosamine (168.0 µg/mg BSM); N-acetylgalactosamine (69.2 µg/mg BSM); galactose (15.2 µg/mg BSM); mannose (2.07 µg/mg BSM); fucose (9.53 µg/mg BSM) and sialic acid (16.9 µg/mg BSM). Different mM of Ca^{++} was added to the reaction mixture to activate binding specificity of immobilized lectin with carbohydrates [9]. The *in vitro* biological activity of the lectinized system was determined by mixing 1.0 ml of BSM solution in phosphate buffer (0.5 mg/ml) with the same volume of dispersion of the lectinized liposomes in phosphate buffer (50 µg of liposome surface bound lectin per ml). After incubation for 60 min., the samples were centrifuged for 30 minute at 1,00,000 g, aliquots of supernatant were taken, and analysed for Con-A using Wang and Smith modified Lowry assay, 1975 [10]. Assessing the difference between the total (reference system) and the residual BSM in the clear supernatant, the amount of interacted BSM was calculated. The reference system consisted of the same amount of BSM as in the sample (250 µg/ml in saline buffer), centrifuged as described earlier.

For specificity studies, α-methyl mannoside (50 mM) was added to the BSM bulk solutions in saline buffer and the interaction studies with the lectinized liposomes were conducted following the same protocol as used to characterize the plain (non ligand) system.

In vitro targeting elucidation

In order to assess the targetability of the developed system to the bacterial film(s) (of periodontal pocket) bacterial cell-liposome interaction was studied *in-vitro* taking axenically grown broth culture of *Streptococcus mutans* species as model bacterial cell lines. % Bacterial growth inhibition (%GI) was studied.

Percent growth inhibition study

Streptococcus mutans bacterial strips were used to inoculate agar plates prepared from Brain heart infusion, BHI (3.7g) in double distilled water (100 ml) to which was added bacteriological agar (1.5 g). The plates were inoculated by streaking and the inverted streaked plates were incubated at 37°C for 18 hours. The resulting colonies were used to inoculate aliquots (10 ml) of nutrient broth prepared by mixing BHI (3.7g) and yeast extract powder (0.39g) in double distilled water (100 ml). These were incubated in coated bottles at 37°C for 18 hours after which the bacterial suspensions were centrifuged (200 rpm, 15 min.), the supernatant was discarded and the separated pellets were re-suspended in sterile PBS. The centrifugation and re-dispersion were repeated three times and the bacterial cell concentration appropriately adjusted by dilution with phosphate buffer for measuring the absorbance at 550 nm.

To study the effect of metronidazole bearing lectinized liposomes on *Streptococcus mutans*, 4.5 ml of broth (BHI) was inoculated with 2.5×10^8 colony forming units (CFU) of the organism, obtained from an early stationary phase of a broth culture at 37°C as discussed earlier. Different systems (plain and protein coated) were added to the tubes to a final volume of 5.0 ml per sterile tube, and the tubes were incubated under constant agitation at $37 \pm 1°C$; bacterial growth was monitored spectrophotometrically at 550 nm against blank (uninoculated broth) at different time intervals. Every experiment was conducted in triplicate maintaining aseptic conditions. The effect of different formulations on bacterial growth was investigated. The formulations include free metronidazole, control liposomes with buffer, plain liposomes and protein coated liposomes. Control tubes contained metronidazole free plain (Control 1) and lectinized (Control 2) liposomal system filled with buffer and incubated with bacteria to check any antimicrobial activity of the constitutive lipids or immobilized lectin. The drug alone in a final concentration that corresponds to 50% of MIC was added in the sterile tubes. Similarly in another set of experiment an equivalent amount of drug (MIC_{50}) was added from the metronidazole bearing liposomal system. After incubation of bacteria-vesicle mixture for the stated period of time, the growth inhibition was measured periodically for different formulations. The growth was recorded by measuring optical density (550 nm) of the dispersion mix using Shimadzu 1601A UV/VIS DB spectrophotometer [11].

Statistical analysis

The anti-microbial activity of liposome encapsulated metronidazole against S. sanguis in fluid phase was compared with that of plain drug and controls (placebo formulations) using a rank sum test. The significance was evaluated at 5% probability level (P<0.05 denoting significance).

RESULTS AND DISCUSSION

The binding specificity of lectins for sugars [12] make them an interesting alternative for targeting liposomes to the glycocalyx of the membrane surface and other bio-surfaces [13]. Lectins have been used as mediators in the targeting of liposomes to erythrocytes by either physically coating the liposome or by physically coating the erythrocytes with lectin [14].

Assemblage of Con-A on the surface of liposomes lend the vesicles mechanically stable and offer them stability against external stimuli vis ≠ vis suppressed leakage of water soluble drugs. Plain liposomal dispersion was surface appended with Con-A using charge induced interaction manipulating with ionic behavior of the lectin.

Liposomes (stearoylamine based) were coated with Con-A at the physiological pH (7.4) and were used in the further experiments. Dicetyl phosphates based liposomes also showed significant coating with Con-A at pH 6.0, but were not used in further studies as Con-A is reported to exhibit maximal polysaccharide specificity at pH 6.5 to 8.0 [3]. However, it clearly signifies that a charge-induced interaction could work for the coating of Con-A using its zwitterionic characteristics. Unconjugated Con-A was separated from the lectinized liposomes using three cycles of centrifugation (1,00,000g) of 30 min each, after which a plateau of Con-A concentration (estimated using Wang and Smith modified assay) was recorded. Subsequent cycles did not result in any increase in the unconjugated Con-A concentration, signifying not only the separation of the unconjugated Con-A, but also its resistivity towards delodging under mechanical agitation.

Protein-coated liposomes were characterized for vesicle size, shape, surfacial charge, vesicle size distribution and % entrapment. Plain liposomes were found to be multilamellar and spherical in shape with vesicles ranging from 1.5μm to 6.5 having a mean vesicular diameter of 2.5-3.0±0.5 μm. No significant change was observed in mean vesicle size of the coated vesicles as compared against plain liposomes (average vesicle size 2.9±0.9 μm). However, the lectinized vesicles appear opaque and this may be accounted to protein coating, which resulted into a dual diffusion barrier on the liposomal surface. % Entrapment was recorded to be marginally decreased in the coated vesicles from an average of 27.5±2.5% to 22.5±1.5%. The decrease could be attributed to the residual drug leakage from the vesicles during the incubation time lag employed for anchoring of lectin to the outer half of the liposomal bilayers. Lectinized liposomes with their *in vitro* characterization parameters are presented in Table 1. Surface charge of the vesicles prior to and after the coating of the vesicle suggests for charge-induced coating and quenching. A zeta potential of 5±2°C mV recorded even after coating of Con-A could be attributed to the residual charge contributed by the dispersion.

Table 1. *In vitro* characterization of various coated and plain liposomal formulations

Composition	Molar ratio	Average size[1]	Entrapment[2] (%)	Surfacial charge[3]
PC:Chol:SA	(7:2:1)	2.9±1.2	27.1±0.8	+++
PC:DSPC:Chol:SA	(5:2:2:1)	2.7±1.4	28.8±0.3	+++
(PC:Chol:SA):Con-A	(7:2:1):0.01	2.9±0.9	22.4±0.6	++
(PC:Chol:SA):Con-A	(7:2:1):0.1	3.1±0.9	22.4±0.6	+
(PC:DSPC:Chol:SA):Con-A	(5:2:2:1):0.01	2.9±1.1	22.8±0.8	++
(PC:DSPC:Chol:SA):Con-A	(5:2:2:1):0.1	3.2±0.1	22.8±0.8	+

1. Average vesicle size of previously screened and oversized (1.2μm) population was obtained using phase contrast microscope, coupled with calibrated eye-piece.
2. %Entrapment was analyzed using classical dialysis format.
3. Characterization of the protein modified system as compared to the plain system. * Zeta potentiometer readings have been graded as (+) 0-5 mV; (++) 6-25 mV; and (+++) above 25 mV

Analogous to previous study, which describes that chemical modification of Con-A does not lead to any significant changes in lectin affinity towards saccharide [15], no change in the ligand affinity of Con-A (immobilized on liposomal bilayer) was detected in our study. This was estimated with α-methyl mannoside, taking it as a competing sugar in the solution of bovine submaxillary mucin. Further, ligand activity was also found to be unaffected as deduced from bovine submaxillary binding assay. The ligand related activity was evaluated and established by bovine-maxillary-gland mucin interaction with lectinized liposomes (Fig. 1). The addition of mM Ca^{++} to the reaction mixture is a prerequisite for the Concanavalin A-sugar recognition and is already established [16]. Ca^{++} activates metalloprotein lectins in carbohydrate binding assay. Experiments were carried out in the absence (for the study of *in vitro* activity) or in the presence of the specific sugar α-methyl mannoside for Con-A (for the study of *in vitro* specificity). In the absence of α-methyl mannoside, lectinized system showed more than two folds interaction with BSM as compared against the interaction with unmodified or plain liposomes (used as control).

Percent BSM interaction recorded by plain liposomes could be ascribed to non-specific adsorption of protein (BSM) over the vesicle surface. With no significant changes in the levels of BSM binding were recorded after the addition of α-methyl mannoside, it clearly signifies the nature of the non-specific adsorption. These results clearly indicate that surface appended lectin remained functionally active even after its coupling to lipid vesicles.

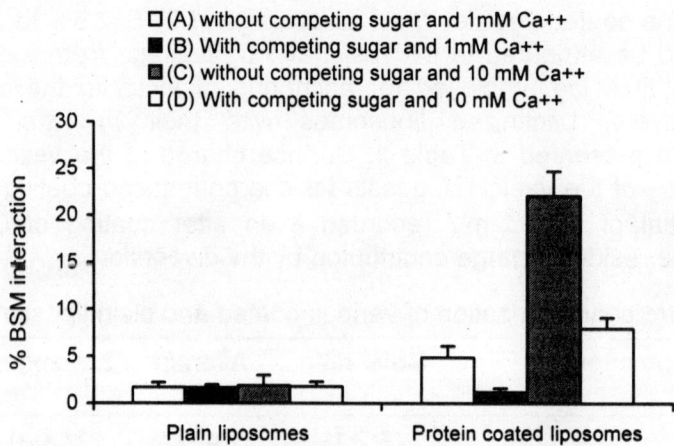

□ (A) without competing sugar and 1mM Ca++
■ (B) With competing sugar and 1mM Ca++
▨ (C) without competing sugar and 10 mM Ca++
□ (D) With competing sugar and 10 mM Ca++

Fig. 1 : BSM binding by lectinized liposomes and plain liposomes prior to and after the challenge of the competing sugar, alpha-methyl mannoside

Experiments performed in the presence of α-methyl mannoside are presented in bar diagram (B and D). In the case of plain liposomes (control) the results remained unvaried for liposome-mucin interaction either in the presence or in the absence of the specific sugar (for Con-A). In contrast, the interactions between lectinized system and mucin decreased significantly on addition of competitive sugar. The results clearly reveal that lectinized liposomes possess the sugar specificity that corresponds to the native lectin.

Although there is no substitute for the *in vivo* assessment of targeting efficiency, nevertheless it is desirable to have an in vitro protocol for assaying the effectiveness of targeting of liposomes; bearing site directing surface immobilized lectin. The efficiency of targeting of lectinized liposomes to *S. mutans* suspension culture has been measured in terms of % G.I. Lectinized liposomes followed by plain liposomes were found superior in maintaining a higher value of % G.I. over a prolonged period of time.

The quantitation of liposomal (containing antimicrobial) system-bacterial interaction was assessed in terms of percentage bacterial growth inhibition (%GI). Percent Growth Inhibition was calculated as the ratio of optimal density (at 550 mm) of a given test mixture against that of tubes containing *S.mutans* alone. The % GI was calculated using the formula as given below:

$$\% \text{ GI} = \frac{[\text{OD of test organism - OD of test mixture}]}{[\text{OD of test organism at a given time}]} \times 100$$

The increase in optical density caused by addition of liposomes (final lipid concentration in culture media was 532 μm) was not significantly different, at any time, from that of tubes containing medium alone. The tubes containing liposomes and culture media were included in order to ascertain whether lipid peroxidation products of any other residual component, if present, contributed to the bactericidal action exhibited by the liposomal mixture.

A series of experiments was carried out to assess microbial growth profile of the various bacteria-vesicle systems. All the results of liposomal bacterial interactions are presented graphically (Fig. 2). Bacterial growth was significantly inhibited by all the selected plain and lectinized systems to the levels of significance (Rank sum test). Further, the difference in growth inhibition when compared amongst the formulation was statically significant ($P<0.05$). The results of the bacterial growth by the developed systems were comparable with the effect of free antimicrobial. These results demonstrate that the lectinized liposomes caused a significantly higher % G.I. in the bacteria growth at an equivalent MIC value of encapsulated drug (MIC_{50}) compared to that of plain liposomal formulations. In other words lectinized liposomes exhibited superior % antibacterial activity compared to that of plain liposomes or free drug as estimated from triplicates of representative experiments. The maximum average % G.I. values recorded for plain drug (55.1±1.5% GI), plain vesicles (97.1±1.5% GI), and lectinized vesicles (100 % GI) could be compared (Fig. 2).

Control tubes containing bacteria and liposomal system filled with buffer to check any antimicrobial activity of the constitutive lipids or immobilized lectin. The growth inhibition provided by the control tubes were 17.5±0.9% for control 1 and 41.1±1.1% G.I. for control 2, respectively. These observations suggest intrinsic anti-bacterial characteristics of these modules but these could be due to their interactions with and peptizaton of the bacterial surface and not to the anti-microbial properties of these constructs.

Lectin (immobilized on the surface of liposomes) may simply arrest glyco-calyx covering (glycoprotein and glycosphingolipids) by its multivalency characteristics and may cause peptization and sequestration of bio-films. These bio-film fusogenicity characteristics could be ascribed to the significant growth inhibition offered by control formulations.

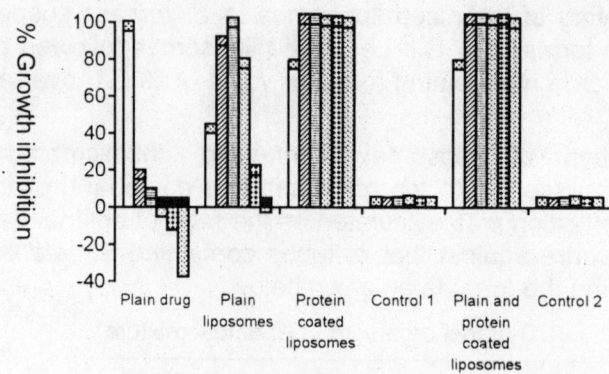

□ 30 Min ☒ 60 Min ▦ 90 Min ▦ 120 Min ▦ 240 Min ▦ 360 Min

Fig. 2 : % growth inhibition achieved by lectinized and plain liposomes at 0.5 MIC (~18 µg/ml) as compared against plain drug

The interaction of the plain vesicles could be ascribed to the structural similarity of the liposomes with bio-membrane, leading to fusion and eventually the translocation of contents, whereas the role of lectin (receptor) mediated bacterial adhesion could lead to the synergistic bio-events. The lectin-appended system was proven to be the most effective in bringing the maximum growth inhibition upto 100% and maintaining it for nearly 360 minutes. Statistical analysis of data revealed that there were significant difference in % G.I. of plain and coated modules at 5% level of significance (PC< 0.05).

The effects shown by placebo formulations could be ascribed to the intrinsic properties of constituting lipids and lectin. Liposomal fusion with the bacterial film may retard functionality of the bacterial surface and may simply arrest the growth, a bacteriostatic type of effect.

Plain liposomal formulation has been found to provide a higher % GI compared of plain drug. This could be attributed to intrinsic protection of antimicrobial encapsulated in the liposomes from β-lactamases and exogenous enzymes. Change in the bacterial cell envelope permeability facilitating the fusion/diffusion of the drug across the bacterial envelope, followed by translocation of the contents, could also be cited as another possibility [17,18]. The constitutive lipids (DSPC) with a high Tc^0 upon interaction and fusion with the cell membrane may become less rigidized and leaky. This fluidization of the bilayer may provide burst release in the vicinity of the target cell lines. Vesicles constructed from high transition temperature lipids were found to provide better in vitro targetability from both coated and uncoated liposomes as compared against vesicles constructed only from plain PC. Another point to be considered in enhanced anti-bacterial study is the use of stearoylamine based coated liposomes as cationic liposomes have shown to enhance affinity towards bacterial bio-film [19].

Coated liposomal formulation produced more or less similar levels of % G.I. with respect to plain module, but a comparatively better %GI value was recorded, which could be due to one or more of the proposed mechanisms. The multi or poly valency characteristics of the lectin, i.e., binding to a target site through multiple interactions can be proposed to partially explain the enhanced activity of coated module [20]. Further carbohydrate adherin receptors (mainly lectins) on the bacterial surface could be exploited to route the antimicrobial into the interior of cell targets. It has been proposed that lectinized liposomal systems with affinity to the lectin receptors of oral and skin associated bacteria are instrumental in pursuing better result [21]. Specificity of lectins to bind selectively to bacterial "glyco-calyx" (composed of surface glycoproteins and glycolipids) can possibly be proposed for its selective interaction with bacterial cell lines (lectin mediated bio-signaling). These findings are based on the fact that lectin and the complementary carbohydrates are located on the surfaces of opposing cells, which may of the same type or different cells [22]. Cells of bacterial bio-film may interact with lectin immobilized vesicles via bridge formed by soluble glycoconjugates that bind to the immobilized lectins. Alternatively, the immobilized lectin may combine with carbohydrate of insoluble component of the extracellular matrix that promotes vesicular-cell adhesion. Con-A has specificity for glucose and mannose residues [23], which constitute part of surface polymer of bacterial glyco-calyx. In the light of these considerations, it can be suggested that the developed system(s) may offer potential in alleviating drug bacterial resistance problems, and could be used clinically for periodontal pocket bacterial diseases as well as to bring about resultant healing of infected site(s).

ACKNOWLEDGEMENTS

We are thankful to UGC and CSIR, New Delhi for financial assistance to two authors (PD & VS) respectively.

REFERENCES

1. Potera, C. (1996). **Science** 273, 1795-1797.

2. Banker, C.N., Stocker, S.A., Culver, D.H. and Thornbberry, C., (1991). **J. Clin. Microbiol. 29,** 533-538.

3. Agrawal, B.B.L. and Goldstein, I.J. (1967). **Biochim. Biophys. Acta**. 33, 376-379.

4. Adamson, A.W. (1967). Physical chemistry of surface, II ed., Ch. 9, Interscience, New York, 223.

5. Zaraparkar, S.S., Dhanvate, A.A., Doshi, V.J. , Salunke, V.B. and Sawant, S.V. (1994). **Ind. Drug.** 31, 468-470.

6. Barlett, G.R. (1959). **J. Biol. Chem.** 234, 466-468.

7. Bottcher, C.J.F., van Gent, C.M. and Pries, C. (1961). **Anal. Chem. Acta.** 24, 203-204.

8. Honda, S. and Suzuki, S. (1984). **Anal. Biochem.** 142, 167-174.

9. Kottgen, E., Hell, B., Muller, C. and Tauber, R. (1988). **Biol. Chem. Hoppe-Seyler** 369, 1157-1166.

10. Wang, C.S. and Smith, R.L. (1975). **Anal. Biochem.** 63, 414-417.

11. Nacucchio, M.C., Bellora, M.J.G., Sordelli, D.O. and D'aquino, N. (1988). **J. Microencap.** 5, 303-309.

12. Goldstein, I.J. and Poretz, R.D., (1986). In: The lectins, Functions and Applications in Biology and Medicine, (Edt. by I.E. Liener et al.), Academic Press, New York, 103-115.

13. Rademacher, T.W., Parekh, R.B. and Dwek, R.A. (1988). **Annu. Rev. Biochem.** 57, 785-838.

14. Hutchinson, F.J. and Jones, M.N. (1988). **FEBS Lett.** 234, 493-496.

15. Bogdanov, A.A., Gordeeva, L.V., Torchilin, V.P. and Margolis L.B. (1989). **Exp. Cell Res.** 181, 362-374.

16. Farajollahi, M.M., Cook, D.B., Self, C.H. (1998). **Anal. Biochem.** 261, 118-121.

17. Brayn, L.E. (1979). In: Clinical manifestations of infection and current therapy, (Edt. by R.G. Doggest), Academic Press, New York, 219-244.

18. Nacucchio, M.C., Bellora, M.J.G., Sordelli, D.O. and D'aquino, N. (1985). **Antimicrob. Agents Chemother.** 27, 137-142.

19. Sanderson, N.M. and Jones, M.N. (1996). **J. Drug Target.** 4, 181-189.

20. Matrosovich, M.N. (1989). **FEBS Lett.** 252, 1-4.

21. Jones, M.N., Kaszuba, M. and Lyle, I.G. (1992). Treatment composition. British patent application No. 9208339.3, filed April 15th

22. Sharon, N. and Lis, H. (1989). **Science** 246, 227-234.

23. Palomino, E. (1994). **Adv. Drug Deliv. Rev.** 13, 311-323.

LIGAND DIRECTED MACROPHAGE TARGETING OF AMPHOTERICIN B LOADED LIPOSOMES:
Development and Characterisation

S.P. VYAS*, Y.K. KATARE, V. MISHRA and V. SIHORKAR

Department of Pharmaceutical Sciences,
Dr. H.S. Gour Vishwavidyalaya, Sagar, M.P., INDIA

- Introduction
- Materials and Methods
- Results and Discussions

- Conclusion
- References

INTRODUCTION

Macrophages are phagocytic cells present either in circulating plasma (wandering macrophages) or in endothelial lining and the reticular spaces of the connective tissues of the mammals (fixed or tissue macrophages). They have a pivotal role in the defensive responses and serve to protect the host against a wide variety of invading microorganisms and developing neoplasms through triggering of humoral as well as intracellular oxidative and hydrolytic activities.

In a number of microbial and metabolic diseases these protective responses are overwhelmed, pre-engaged or arrested and as a result these protective cells become the focal point in a large number of parasitic diseases. For diseases of microbial etiology, the intracellular localization of the pathogens necessitates the administration of relatively high doses of the cytotoxic drugs for the effective killing of the pathogens, thereby causing the side effects, which are often unacceptably severe. The rationale approach to the problem requires that drugs should be targeted to the macrophages in such a way that the interaction of the free drug with non-target tissues could be minimized.

Targeted drug delivery to the macrophages has also been appreciated as a strategy for achieving other diverse objectives like treatment of lysosomal storage diseases [1], targeting of immunomodulators to achieve macrophage activation [2] cell or cell product depletion [3] and blockade of the macrophages [4]. Many approaches for targeting the drugs to the macrophages have been developed, which are largely represented by liposomes [5,6]. Although liposomes show natural affinity towards the macrophages and passively targeted to them; yet inclusion of the macrophage receptor(s) specific ligands may significantly enhance the rates and extent of liposomal uptake by the macrophages.

Mannose/fucose receptors, expressed abundantly in liver, spleen and alveolar macrophages have been most widely utilised for targeting bioactives to the macrophages. The receptor facilitates endocytosis of glycoproteins terminated with mannose, fucose and glucosamine. Mannose residues have been appended to the liposomes in the form of mannosylated albumin [7]; palmitoylated derivatives of polysaccharides like pullulan, amylopectin and mannan [8]; mannobiose arachidonic esters [9]; mannose terminated glycolipids of natural and synthetic origin [10]; mannopyranoside [11] and mannose terminated glycoproteins [12,13] for macrophage targeting.

Amphotericin B is a drug of choice in systemic fungal infections. The drug is also used in the treatment and management of leishmaniasis. Amphotericin B manifests serious adverse complications related to dose dependent acute and chronic toxicity. Maximum tolerated dose of amphotericin B is considerably low in mice; LD_{50} is 1.2 mg/kg and doses higher than 1.6 mg/kg cause acute toxic reactions followed by cardio-respiratory arrest [14]. Treatment of disseminated fungal infections by liposomal Amphotericin B results in a lower toxicity and significantly increased survival times. It has been proposed that increased concentrations of drug in macrophages through passive uptake may improve its therapeutic index. Toxicological comparisons of free and liposomally formulated amphotericin B in mice has revealed that maximum tolerated dose has been significantly increased. The LD_{50} has been found to increase from 1.2 mg/kg to more than 12 mg/kg in the case of mice [14]. Although liposomal formulations of amphotericin B could considerably reduce the toxicity of the drug and subsequently make it possible to enhance the therapeutic index, however, doses required to obtain improved survival times are still very high.

Amphotericin B bearing liposomes investigated so far have been small unilamellar or multilamellar vesicles [15]. Most of the work was aimed at reducing the toxicity of the drug by entrapping it in liposomes. It was expected that ligand mediated active targeting to the macrophages would significantly increase the rate and extent of drug uptake quantitatively. This may reduce the required doses of liposomal Amphotericin B in diseases like hepato-splenic fungal infections and leishmaniasis.

The present work was programmed for designing an actively targeted system of Amphotericin B based on liposomes. The macrophages being the target were assessed for selective accessibility through receptor-mediated endocytosis using O-palmitoylated mannan (OPM) and p-aminophenyl-mannopyranoside (PAM) as specific ligand modules. Comparative *in vivo* distributions and targeting profiles of O-palmitoylated mannan and P-aminophenyl-mannopyranoside anchored liposomes against plain liposomes were studied.

MATERIALS AND METHODS

Materials

Amphotericin B was obtained as a gift sample from M/S Ambalal Sarabhai Enterprises, Vadodara, India. Soya PC, cholesterol (Chol), phosphatidyl-ethanolamine (PE), P-aminophenol mannopyranoside (PAM), stearylamine, mannan and conconavalin A were purchased from Sigma (USA). Palmitoyl chloride (Fluka, Switzerland), glutaraldehyde (Loba-Chemie, India), absolute alcohol (Bengal

Chemicals, India) were purchased and used as supplied. All other chemicals were of Anal R grade until otherwise stated.

Preparation and optimisation of MLVs containing Amphotericin B

Multilamellar vesicles (MLVs) containing amphotericin B were prepared by the method described by Lopez-Berestein and co-workers [12]. Soya PC and Cholesterol were dissolved in the minimum amount of chloroform and a methanolic solution (60 µg/ml) of Amp B was added to it. Soya PC to Cholesterol ratio (8:2 m mol ratio) was kept constant while amp B content was varied at different mole percent ratio levels, i.e. (20, 16, 12, 8, 4, 2 and 1% moles of the total lipids) in different preparations for determining optimum Amp B content. The organic solvent mixture was removed using a rotary flash evaporator under reduced pressure. The dried film was hydrated with 0.9% NaCl solution at 40±1°C for 60 minutes and subsequently at room temperature for 6 hours. The dispersion was centrifuged at 60000 rpm for 4 hours and the pellet was resuspended in 0.9% NaCl solution.

Resulting formulations were evaluated for lamellarity, shape and size of the vesicles formed. The formulations which were free from undesired and unspecified liposomal structures were evaluated for the entrapment efficiency by the method described by New [16]. The liposomal formulations were centrifuged through Sephadex G-50 minicolumn at 2000 rpm for 3 minutes for the separation of unentrapped drug. The liposomal fraction was added with minimum amount of triton X-100 (0.5% w/v), drug content was determined spectrophotometrically at 404 nm and percent drug entrapment was calculated. MLVs with optimum Amp B to lipid ratio were optimized for optimum Soya PC to Cholesterol ratio in terms of % drug entrapment and toxicity towards erythrocytes. The MLVs with different Soya PC to Cholesterol ratios (90:10, 80:20, 70:30, 60:40, 50:50 mMol ratios) were prepared. Amp B content however was kept constant at its optimum concentration level. The liposomes were prepared and evaluated for % entrapment and toxicity to mammalian cells in terms of % hemolysis. Percent hemolysis was determined by the method described by Mehta et al., [17]. Liposomal dispersions containing equivalent amount of Amp B (50 µg/ml) were incubated with 1.0 ml mammalian blood at 37±1°C for 45 minutes, centrifuged at 60000 rpm for 4 hr and hemoglobin released in the supernatant was measured spectrophotometrically at 550 nm [17]. For control, blood was similarly incubated with 0.9% NaCl solution. Blood was incubated with same volume of distilled water (100% hemolysis). From the hemoglobin released in supernatant, percent hemolysis in each case was computed and assessed. Percent hemolysis and % entrapment were plotted against Soya PC to cholesterol ratio, from which optimum Soya PC to Chol ratio was determined.

MLVs coated with O-palmitoyl mannan (OPM)

O-palmitoylated mannan was synthesised from the yeast mannan by the process reported elsewhere in the literature [18]. O-Palmitoyl mannan (OPM), in brief, was prepared by reacting mannan (1.0 g) in dry DMF at 60°C with palmitoyl chloride (0.1 g) in DMF in the presence of dry pyridine (1.0 ml). The mixture was stirred at 60°C for 6 hours and slowly poured into absolute ethanol (100 ml) under vigorous stirring. The precipitate of OPM, thus obtained was collected and washed with 50 ml of absolute ethanol and 25.0 ml of dry diethyl ether, and dried in vacuo at $50\pm1°C$ for 1 hour. O-palmitoyl mannan (OPM) was characterised by IR spectroscopy to identify carbonyl groups, and thus, to ascertain that mannan is covalently bound to palmitoyl anchor. Characteristic peaks were recorded at 2650 cm^{-1}, 1480 cm^{-1}, 1690 cm^{-1}, 1210-1190 cm^{-1}, and 3400 cm^{-1}.

Coating was affected by incubating 1.0 ml liposomal suspension with the dispersion of optimised amount of OPM (0.5 : 1 w/w OPM : PC) in 0.9% NaCl solution. The dispersion was stirred gently at room temperature for 4 hours. Excessive, unbound polysachharide was removed by spinning the resulting suspension through a sephadex G-50 mini-column at 2000 rpm for 5 minutes. For optimisation of OPM:PC ratio and incubation time required for the effective coating, positively charged MLVs were prepared by incorporating stearylamine as one of the phospholipids at 0.5 mole % level of the total lipidic contents. These MLVs were incubated with varying amounts of OPM, i.e. w/w ratios based on PC weight (0.01:1, 0.05:1, 0.1:1, 0.15:1, 0.20:1, 0.25:1 and 0.5:1 w/w ratio) for 4 hours. After removing excessive, unbound polysaccharide specific electrical conductance of these liposomes was determined [19]. Conductivity was measured at an applied voltage of 10 mV using Systronics Conductivity Bridge 305 (India) and the measurements were made in micromhos. Specific electrical conductance was plotted against the OPM:PC ratio and optimum OPM:PC ratio was determined from the plot as one, at or beyond which no further changes in the conductance recorded. Similarly, to obtain optimum incubation time, formulations were incubated at optimum OPM concentration for different time intervals (0.5, 1.0, 1.5, 2.0, 2.5, 3.0 and 4.0 hours), and specific electrical conductance of these vesicles was recorded after separating the excessive, unbound polysaccharide. From the plot of Specific electric conductance against incubation time, optimum incubation time was determined to be one, at or beyond which no significant changes in the conductance were recorded.

Preparation of mannopyranoside (PAM) linked MLVs containing Amp B

MLVs containing optimum amount of amphotericin B (from the earlier experiment) and different molar ratios of PC, PE and Cholesterol were prepared by the method discussed. MLVs obtained were evaluated for the shape, size, percent drug entrapment and toxicity to mammalian cells in terms of percent hemolysis. From these parameters optimum proportions of the phospholipids were determined and selected.

P-aminophenyl mannopyranoside was linked to PE containing MLVs by the method described by Ghosh et al., [19]. A 1.0 ml liposomal dispersion (containing $\cong$ 30 mg lipids/ml) in 0.9% w/v aqueous NaCl solution was mixed with 20.0 mg P-aminophenyl mannopyranoside contained in 2.0 ml of aqueous NaCl solution. Glutaraldehyde was then slowly added to the suspension to a concentration level 3 mM and the mixture was incubated for 5 minutes at 20°C. Uncoupled glycosides and glutaraldehyde were removed by dynamic dialysis technique against 0.9 % NaCl solution.

Characterisation of mannose terminating ligand coated liposomes

Developed formulations were characterized prior to and after surface ligand anchoring. Lamellarity of the vesicles and shape of the vesicle was determined by the microscopic method (Leitz-Biomed, Germany). Transmission electron microscopy (Geol, Japan) was performed on carbon coated sample using 1.0 % phosphotungstic acid as the negative stain (Photomicrographs 1-3). Size distribution of the MLVs was determined by microscopic method using phase contrast compound microscope (Leitz-Biomed, Germany). Average diameter of the vesicles was determined in each case, with the help of calibrated ocular micrometer. Percent of amphotericin B entrapped in the MLVs was determined by the method described by New, [16]. Drug content of the MLVs was determined by the method given by Lopez-Berestein et al. [14], following the disruption of liposomal pellets by adding triton X 100 (0.5% w/v). The presence of mannose residues on the surface of liposomes was detected by agglutination of the vesicles with concanavalin A. In the case of mannopyranoside linked liposomes, the percent of total PE that gets modified with the mannopyranoside linkage was determined by titrating amino groups of liposomal PE with trinitrobenzene sulphonic acid in the presence of 0.5% triton X-100.

Stability in serum

The stability of liposomes in the serum was determined by observing vesicle disruption and intact vesicles count and drug leaching following incubation of MLVs with serum at 37 ±1°C. 1.0 ml suspension of the MLVs was incubated with 2.0 ml serum at 4 ± 1°C and 37± 1°C for 2 hours and the MLVs counts per cubic mm of the dispersion were recorded by the microscopic method using haemocytometer and nauebaer chamber (Japan). % Vesicles remaining in dispersion as intact was calculated. The drug content of the MLVs was determined by the method given by Lopez-Berestein et al., [14]. 1.0 ml of each formulation was incubated with 2.0 ml serum at 37±1°C for 1, 2, 4, 6 and 24 hours. After specified time intervals, suspensions were centrifuged at 60000 rpm for 4 hours and supernatant was filtered through 0.45 μm membrane filter. The filtrate was analyzed for drug content by reverse phase HPLC method as described elsewhere [20].

Determination of *In vivo* target specificity

Albino rats of either sex weighing about 150 to 200 g each were divided in 7 groups of 6 rats each. Food and water were allowed *ab libitum* during the study period. Free amp B (0.8 mg per Kg body weight), ligand appended formulations and their respective non-ligand anchored counterparts containing equivalent doses of amp B (0.8 mg per Kg body weight) were administered intravenously to different groups.

In order to observe the effect of hydrolyzed mannan on the uptake of ligand appended liposomes, two groups were administered with 10mg hydrolyzed mannan i.v. prior to the administration of OPM coated and P-aminophenyl mannopyranoside anchored formulations. Three albino rats from each group were sequentially sacrificed at 15 min, 30 min, 1, 2, 4 and 24 h after administration of the formulations. Blood was collected by cardiac puncture method. Different organs (liver, spleen, lungs, kidney) were excised, isolated, washed with distilled water and were blot dried using tissue papers [21]. Drug content in the blood and organs was determined by

HPLC method [20]. Drug localization index for each organ at different time intervals was calculated by the formula given by Gupta and Hung, [22].

$$\text{Drug localization index} = \frac{\text{Drug concentration in target tissue at time 't' after administration of test delivery system}}{\text{Drug concentration in target tissue at time 't' after administration of free drug}}$$

RESULTS AND DISCUSSIONS

At higher concentrations (8-20 mole % of the total lipids) of Amp B ribbons and unspecified structures were observed. However, some liposomes of sizes lower than 1.6 μm were also observed. As the concentration of Amp B was gradually lowered, relative numbers of ribbons and unspecified structures decreased down while number of liposomes being formed increased (Table 1).

With an increase in concentration of Amp B, the average size of liposomes was found to decrease. This may be attributed to the lower magnitude of rigidity of the bilayers on the incorporation of the amp B molecules that relieve the stress involved in the formation of small vesicles. It is also speculated that the association of amp B molecule with cholesterol may result in leaky membrane formations leading to lower entrapped volume and hence lower size of the vesicles. This hypothesis however, needs confirmation from experimental studies. When molar concentration of Amp B was used at 2% of the total lipids, liposomal formulation was observed to be free of other undesired structures and average vesicle size measured was 2.37±0.76 μm.

Table 1. Types of structures formed with different molar ratios of Amp B to lipids

Amp B content*	Types of Structures formed	Entrapment efficiency (n=3)
20	Comma shaped ribbons & other unspecified structures	Not Determined
16	Unspecified structures, ribbons and some liposomal population.	Not Determined
12	Distorted liposomes, ribbons & some intact liposomes	Not Determined
8	Mostly liposomes, some ribbons & distortedliposomes	Not Determined
4	Only liposomes of size range lower than 1.6μm to 4.8μm with average size 1.86μm	68.9 ± 1.23%
2	Only liposomes of size range lower than 1.6μm to 6.4 with average size 2.37 μm	79.2 ±1.56%
1	Liposomes of size range 1.6um to 4.8um with average size 3.86 μm	84.1 ± 1.33%

* % molar ratio of Amp B to total lipids

In another variation, with an increase in cholesterol concentration in liposomes at constant concentration of Amp B, a distinctive reduction in toxicity to the erythrocytes and % entrapment of Amp B was observed. On increasing the mM ratio of Chol:PC from 10:90 to 40:60 the % hemolysis was found to decrease from 11.2±1.09% to 1.0±0.19% (Fig. 1). The mechanism operative behind this toxicity reduction of Amp B upon liposomal entrapment is still undefined. However, it seems to be attributed to the more stable and compact configuration of bilayers as such; and of Amp B intercalation in the bilayers. Probably increased interaction of Amp B molecules with cellular cholesterol restricts their lateral interaction with cholesterol present in the erythrocyte membranes. An increase in the concentration of cholesterol resulted in to relatively low % entrapment of amp B (Fig. 1). It may probably be due to sterically favorable and hence, preferential accommodation of the cholesterol molecules in the bilayer assemblages. Optimum PC:Chol ratio however, was found to be 7:3 mM which could entrap maximum amount of drug (79.2±1.29) while manifest toxicity towards erythrocytes to an apparently acceptable lower limits (% hemolysis = 1.1±0.18).

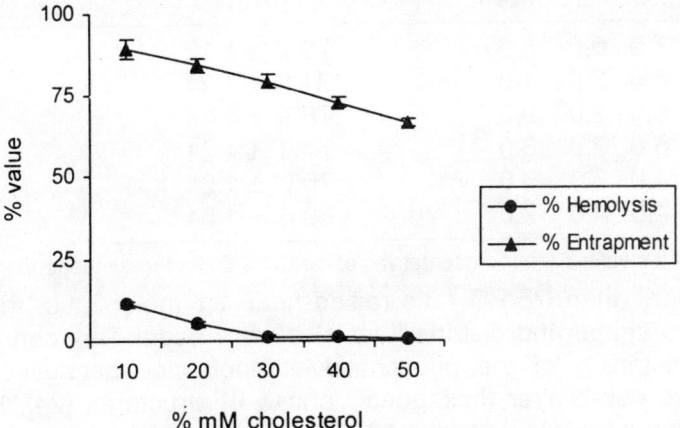

Fig. 1 : Optimisation of cholesterol content in MLVs containing amphotericin B in terms of % hemolysis and % entrapment.

Comparison of the infra red spectra of O-palmitoylated mannan with mannan revealed the presence of extra peaks due to C-C band deformation (2850 cm^{-1}) and C-H deformations (1480 cm^{-1}) arising from alkyl group in the product. Peak due to C=O stretching vibrations which was expected at 1735 cm^{-1} [23] appeared with a shift at 1695 cm^{-1}. It may be a consequence of intra-molecular hydrogen bonds between carbonyl and hydroxyl groups which suppress the stretching force constant of C=O bond. The presence of hydrogen bonding was confirmed by the lower frequency stretching vibrations of the O-H band (at about 3388 cm^{-1}) and also by its higher intensity and larger band width. C-O stretching vibrations appeared as a characteristic band in the range 1210-1190 cm^{-1}. All these peaks in the infra red spectra provided convincing evidences of the formation of an ester bond between mannan and O-palmitoyl anchor.

The OPM:PC ratio and incubation time were optimized by measuring the changes in electrical conductance of stearylamine containing liposomal suspension with varying concentrations of OPM as well as with variation in incubation time. Electrical conductance remained nearly constant on addition of OPM after an optimized value. This indicates no further charge based interaction of the components of the bilayer and is suggestive of the completion of coating. The optimum OPM:PC ratio was found to be 0.15:1, while optimum incubation time (the time that corresponds to completion of OPM coating under the experimental condition) was found to be 1.5 hours. At the optimum OPM concentration level, the optimum incubation time was recorded to be one after which electrical conductance remained fairly constant at 2388 ±12.7 µMhos.

PE containing liposomes were also optimized for total PE content. It was found that addition of PE with an equivalent reduction of PC exhibited no significant effect on the toxicity of Amp B to the erythrocytes as well as on percent entrapment in so far the concentration of cholesterol was kept constant (Table 2).

Table 2. Optimization of PC:PE:Chol ratio

Millimolar Ratios PC : PE : Chol	Percent Entrapment* (n=3)	Percent Hemolysis* (n=3)
7.0 : 0.0 : 3.0	79.2 ± 1.12	1.5 ± 0.021
6.0 : 3.0 : 1.0	81.8 ± 1.24	13.1 ± 0.85
6.0 : 2.0 : 2.0	78.9 ± 1.18	6.9 ± 0.54
5.0 : 2.0 : 3.0	74.2 ± 1.21	1.6 ± 0.036
4.0 : 3.0 : 3.0	70.0 ± 1.24	1.8 ± 0.054
4.0 : 4.0 : 2.0	69.8 ± 1.54	7.3 ± 0.63

* All the values are representatives of mean ±S.D. for three independent determinations

However, when PE:PC ratio raised near 1:1 molar ratio, the vesicles were off spherical in shape and distorted vesicles were seen. This can be attributed to the reported instability of the phosphatidylethanolamine because of its rapid phase transition to non-bilayer (hexagonal phase II) structures [24]. However, when the PE:PC ratio was decreased relatively stable vesicles were obtained, owing to increased stabilizing contribution of PC and Chol and hence less membrane defects. Optimum PC:PE:Chol ratio was found to be 5:2:3 mM. Liposomes formed at this composition were absolutely spherical within a size range 1.66 µm to 4.98 µm. 87±2.5% of liposomal population was lower than 3.50 µm in size (Fig. 3). The average size of the vesicles was 1.78±0.35 µm, which increased marginally on anchoring P-aminophenol mannopyranoside residues via glutaraldehyde spacer arm (Table 3).

Table 3. Formulation codes, composition and characterisation of various ligand anchored and plain formulations

Codes	Composition	Nature of ligand	Encapsulation*	Avg. size*
PC3	PC:Chol (7:3mMol ratio)	----	79.6±1.8	2.35±0.25
OPMPC3	PC:Chol (7:3mMol ratio)	O-palmitoyl mannan	78.6±2.1	3.04±0.18
CE3	PC:PE:Chol (5:2:3 mMol ratio)	---	74.2±1.7	1.78±0.35
MAPCE3	PC:PE:Chol (5:2:3 mMol ratio)	P-aminophenyl-mannopyranoside	73.9±1.9	2.10±0.06

*All the values are representatives of mean ±S.D. for three independent determinations

Microscopic observation revealed the spherical shape of the liposomes. The presence of coating on the liposomal surface could be appreciated from the transmission electron microscopy, which indicates surface intervening and anchoring of mannose terminating ligands (Photomicrographs 1-3). The coating on the surface of liposomes was also confirmed qualitatively by the agglutination of liposomes by concanavalin A [25]. Size of non coated PC:Chol liposomes was found to be within the range 1.84 μm to 5.6 μm, with more than 70% population of liposomes being below 3.3 μm (Fig. 3). Average size of plain liposomes was 2.35±0.25 μm. The ligand coating of OPM resulted in an increase in the size of liposomes. The percent of liposomes below 3.3 μm size in coated formulation was 60±1.7 with an average size of coated liposomes to be 3.04±0.18 μm. The % of Amp B entrapped in the uncoated liposomal formulation was found to be 79.6±1.8% and noted to remain fairly unaffected by the coating or ligand anchoring process (Table 3).

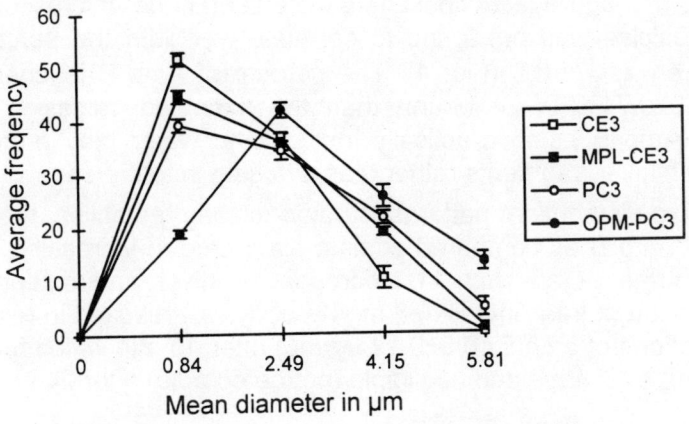

Fig. 3 : Size distribution of MLVs in different formulations

The percent entrapment of Amp B in the non-mannopyranoside anchored formulation was found to be 74.2±1.7 %. It was observed that drug content of the ligand anchored liposomes was comparable to the plain (non-ligand anchored) liposomes (Table 3). The findings suggest that surface ligand anchoring and the process used did not affect the entrapment efficiency of liposomal system as preformed vesicles were used in the process. The presence of p-aminophenyl mannopyranoside on liposomal surface was qualitatively confirmed with the help of concanavalin A induced vesicle agglutination [25]. The titration of liposomal PE groups with trinitrobenzene sulphonic acid revealed that about 15-18% of the total amino groups was modified via covalent coupling of p-aminopohenyl mannopyranoside (data not shown). This finding suggests that only surfacial PE was involved in the covalent linking whilst the PE present in the inner lamellae remained unaffected.

The stability of liposomes (both plain and surface modified) was found to be adversely affected on incubation with freshly pooled rat serum. However, the liposomal preparations intended for targeting to macrophages are reported to be cleared from the circulation within a very short span of time [19]. Therefore the observed instability is of a little relevance.

Stability in serum was reflected in terms of the % vesicles remaining intact per cu mm after the incubation for two hour. After two hour of incubation at 37±1°C all the preparations displayed a significant loss, i.e., 15-20% vesicles disrupted. The percent residual vesicles found to be the lowest in the case of phosphatidyl-ethanolamine based liposomes (20.5±1.5% vesicles disrupted). O-palmitoylated mannan coated vesicles displayed better stability (15.0±0.9 % vesicles disrupted) as compared to their uncoated counterparts (17.4±2.1% vesicles disrupted). Similarly, linking of P-aminophenyl glycosides also offered stabilization effect (18.7±1.7% vesicles disrupted) as compared to their respective non-ligand appended formulation (20.5±1.5% vesicles disrupted). The loss of vesicles can be attributed to disruption and aggregation of the vesicles. The disrupted vesicles appearing as unspecified structures and aggregated liposomes were seen under microscopic observation. The loss of vesicles was not found to correlate well with the percent drug leached in serum even at 37±1°C (Fig. 4). The percent of Amp B leached in the serum was lower (7.9±0.71% in 24 hours) than the expected values. This is presumably because Amp B being practically insoluble in water may prefer to remain in the disrupted bilayer fragments rather than diffusing in to the serum.

The bio-distribution patterns studied clearly establish the superiority of the liposomal amp B as compared against plain drug in increasing the accumulation of amp B in the organs rich in macrophages (liver and spleen). The intravenous administration of free Amp B (0.8 mg/Kg body wt.) resulted in relatively lower plasma concentrations of amp B (0.9±0.12 µg/mL) after 15 min which further declined to 0.2 ±0.1 µg/mL after 4 hrs and negligible (not detectable) after 24 hrs (Fig. 4).

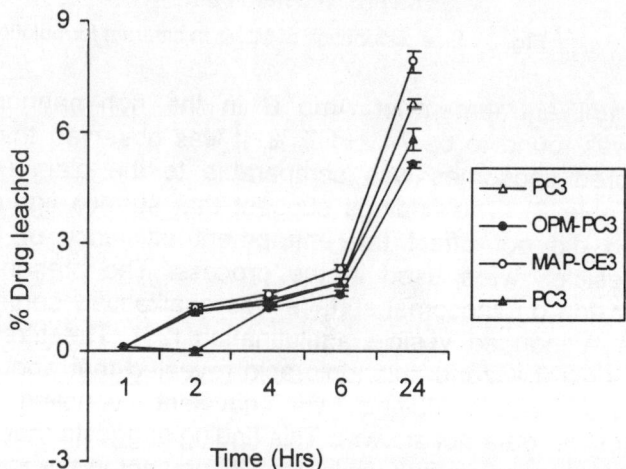

Fig. 4 : Blood concentrations of amp B following the intravenous administration of free amp B, PC3, CE3, OPMPC3 and MAPCE3

The fraction of administered dose recovered from macrophage rich organs like liver, spleen and lungs were also lower than that obtained in the case of liposomal formulations. This suggested that the lower plasma concentrations probably resulted from the rapid tissue distribution of the drug to the tissues other than macrophages.

Plasma concentrations of amp B estimated as free and liposomal encapsulated amp B after the administrations of plain liposomes were significantly higher, i.e., 4.6±0.7 µg/mL and 4.9 ±1.1 µg/ml after 15 min respectively in the case of formulations PC-3 and CE-3 (Fig. 4).

The higher blood concentrations of amp B upon liposomal encapsulation are in agreement with the observations made by earlier workers [21]. However, the relative fraction of administered dose recovered from blood was lower than that reported by the same workers. The probable reason for this effect may be accounted for the vesicle type as MLVs, which were used in the study, were of considerably larger in size than the SUVs used by van Etten et al. [21]. The large sized liposomes exhibit greater rates and extent of passive uptake by phagocytes upon intravenous administrations [26]. Ligand anchored liposomes (OPMPC3 and MAPCE3) exhibited blood concentrations higher (3.1±0.9 and 2.9±1.1 µg/ml, respectively after 15 min) than that of free drug, but it was noticeably lower than that obtained after the administration of their plain counterparts (Fig. 4).

This decrease in blood concentration was accompanied by corresponding increase in the accumulation of drug in macrophage rich organs like liver, spleen and lung. The subsequent lower blood concentrations may be attributed to the enhanced hepato-splenic and lung clearance of ligand anchored liposomes and entrapped amp B. It is interesting to note that free drug concentrations in the blood following the administration of the liposomal formulation were far lower than that obtained after the administration of the free drug. Most of the drug present in the blood was associated with liposomes; which is considerably less toxic to the mammalian cells.

Estimation of Amp B accumulated in various organ reveals that liposomal Amp B significantly alters its bio-distribution pattern (Fig. 5). Although free Amp B itself accumulates to a significant extent in liver, spleen, lung and kidney, yet the rate, extent and duration of accumulation are significantly higher after the administration of liposomally entrapped Amp B. When compared amongst the respective groups, the difference was statistically different (P< 0.05). The maximum accumulation of Amp B after the administration of the free drug (in terms of % dose administered) in different organs was found to be 35.6 ±2.15% (in liver), 7.1 ±1.1% (in spleen), 3.8 ±0.91% (in lungs) and 6.8±0.95% (in kidney). All the organs except kidney exhibited maximum accumulation after the first hour of intravenous administration of free drug. The intravenous administration of the both the plain liposomal formulations exhibited augmented rates and higher extent of uptake by liver, spleen and lungs whereas a concomitant decreases in drug accumulation in kidney. In the case of non-OPM coated formulation the maximum uptake was found to be 56.1±4.63, 13.9±1.2, 6.8 ±0.86and 2.3±0.64% respectively in the liver, spleen, lungs and kidney.

Coating of liposomes with OPM further enhanced the accumulation of amp B selectively in liver (from 56.1±3.86% to 66.1±4.7%), spleen (from 13.9 ±1.4% to 17.1±1.5%) and lungs from (6.8±0.94% to 10.9±1.23%). Similar results were obtained following the administration of p-aminophenyl mannopyranoside (PAM) linked formulation, where uptake by liver, spleen and lungs was significantly higher when compared against respective plain (non-ligand anchored) formulations. The higher accumulations in liver, spleen and lungs were 70.80±2.5%, 19.6±1.7% and

6.1±0.9% respectively. The faster rates and higher extent of uptake of liposomes by liver, spleen and lungs on anchoring mannose terminated ligands to them has been reported by various workers [13,27,28]. Studies utilizing radiolabelled encapsulated materials have revealed that macrophages present in these organs are mainly responsible for increased uptake [27,28].

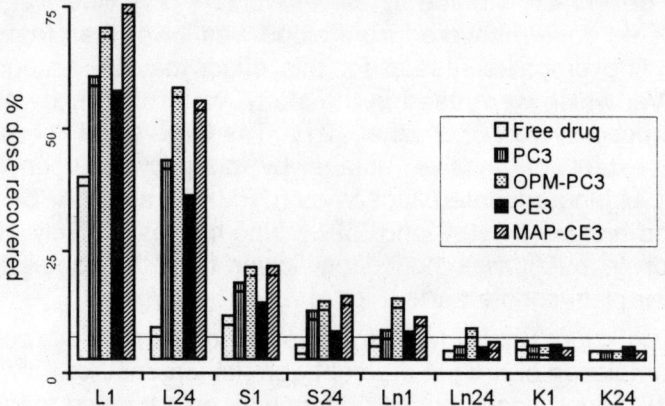

Fig. 5 : Percent dose recovered from liver (L1 and L24), spleen (S1 and S24), lungs (Ln1 and Ln24) and kidney (K1 and K24) respectively after 1 and 24 h of intravenous administration of different formulations

Comparison of the bio-distribution patterns after the administration of OPM coated and PAM linked liposomes suggest that both the formulations exhibit a higher accumulation in liver and spleen as compared against plain liposomes containing an equivalent dose of Amp B. Significant (P<0.05 in a rank sum test) statistical difference in the resulting bio-distribution patterns rules out the probability of inter/intra-subject variations suggesting the role of ligand-receptor interaction mediated phenomenon.

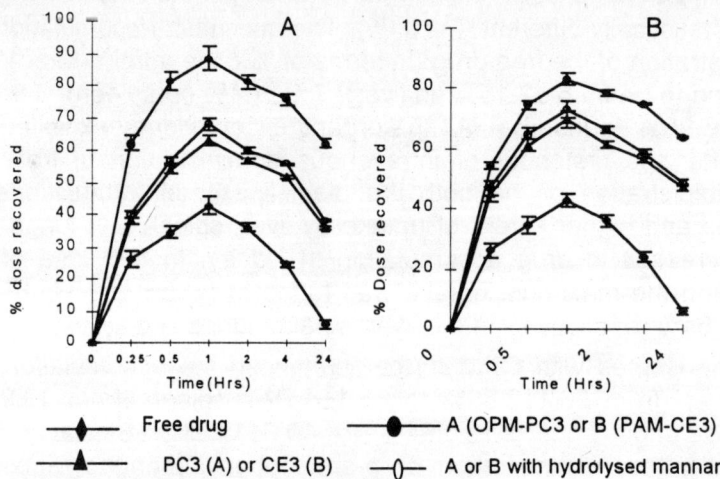

Fig. 6: The effect of liposomal encapsulation and subsequent ligand anchoring on the hepato-splenic uptake of amp B. Liposomal encapsulation enhanced the accumulation which was further enhanced on anchoring ligands, mannopyranoside (A) or coating OPM (B) on to the liposomal surface.

However, the relative hepato-splenic accumulation of the Amp B entrapped in the PAM linked liposomes was higher. The results of bio-distribution studies also suggest that OPM coated liposomes are more effective than mannopyranoside linked liposomes in targeting bioactives to the lungs as the accumulation of OPM coated formulation was quantitatively higher (10.9±0.7) than that of PAM linked formulation (6.9±0.3) in lungs. The augmented lung uptake of the liposomes coated with derivatives of polysaccharides like amylopectin and mannan has already been reported [29,30]. The same effect has also been reported with oil droplets in O/W emulsion coated with polysaccharides using a hydrophobic anchor [25].

Studies involving fluorescent probe encapsulated OPM coated liposomes have shown that alveolar macrophages and phagocytes are mainly involved in the uptake of such liposomes [8]. The increased lung uptake is not completely inhibited by the preinjection of hydrolysed mannan; which suggests that some other mechanisms besides mannose/fucose receptor mediated endocytosis are also involved in mediating an enhanced lung uptake. We speculate that probably uptake via anionic scavenger receptor mediated endocytosis is in part responsible for the observed higher uptake. This hypothesis, however, need confirmation through the competitive inhibition studies. The hepato-splenic quantitative uptake of OPM coated and PAM linked liposomes were significantly low when 10 mg hydrolyzed mannan was administered intravenously prior to injecting the formulations (Fig.7). This qualitatively suggests the possible involvement of mannose receptors expressed onto the membrane of macrophages. The later may be involved in the selective and higher uptake of the ligand appended liposomes.

The analysis of the data obtained from the drug localization index calculations revealed that in the case of liver and spleen, drug localization indices calculated after different time intervals following the administration of various ligand appended formulations were distinctively higher than those corresponding to non-ligand appended formulations. It is realized that the drug localization index in various organs remained significantly higher over 24 h and even after in the case of both ligand appended formulations. These findings help conclude that considerably higher concentrations of the drug could be maintained in the organs over the protracted period of time.

On comparing the drug localization indices of ligand appended formulations it is seen that drug localization indices in liver and spleen are higher in the case of PAM linked formulation than in the case of OPM coated formulation. In the case of lungs however, OPM coated liposome was found to exhibit a better drug localization index. The results are in accordance to the bio-distribution studies obtained as discussed earlier. The observed values suggest that the ligand anchored liposomes are not only effective in rapid attainment of high drug concentrations in macrophage rich organs but also maintain the same over the prolonged period of time, when compared against the free drug. This establishes the significance of the targeting potential of the developed systems.

CONCLUSION

The developed systems (mannose terminating ligand-anchored liposomes) can be proposed for the treatment of hepato-splenic candidiasis and leishmaniasis specifically. Furthermore, in systemic fungal infections the systems can be used for rapid loading of RES organs by the encapsulated drug for the complete eradication of the intracellular pathogens from these organs. It is also concluded that targeting profile of OPM coated liposomes can further be explored for targeting amp B to lung tissues in pulmonary fungal infections and other bioactives' in the treatment of infectious diseases of respiratory tract. Bio-response modifiers can also be incorporated in such systems for achieving effective macrophage activation that can serve as powerful synergistic effect to the therapy of opportunistic infections.

ACKNOWLEDGEMENTS

One of the authors (YKK) is thankful to UGC, New Delhi, for providing financial assistance (JRF). The facilities provided by the Head, Department of Pharmaceutical Sciences is duly acknowledged.

REFERENCES

1. Gordon, S. and Rabinowitz, S. (1989). **Adv. Drug Deliv. Rev.** 4, 27-47.

2. Fidler, I.J. (1988). **Adv. Drug Deliv. Rev.** 2, 69-106.

3. Rooijen, N.V. and Sanders, A. (1994). **J. Immunol. Method.** 174, 83-93.

4. O'Mullane, J.E., Artursson, P. and Tomlinsson, E. (1987). In: Biological approaches to the controlled delivery of drugs (Juliano, R.L. Ed.), Annals. NY Acad. Sci. 507, 120-140.

5. Alving, C.R. (1982). In: Targeting of Drugs (Gregoriadis, G., Senior, J. and Trouet, A. Eds.), Plenum press, New York, 285-312.

6. Bakker-Wouderberg, I.A., Storm, G. and Woodle, M.C. (1994). **J. Drug Target.** 2(5), 363-371.

7. Garcon, N., Gregoriadis, G. and Taylor, M. (1988). **Immunology** 64, 743-748.

8. Sunamoto, J., Gato, M., Iida, T., Hara, K., Saito, A. and Tomonega, A. (1985). In: Receptor mediated targeting of drugs, (Gregoriadis, G., Senior, J. and Trouet, A. Eds), Plenum Press, NewYork, 359-371.

9. Yachi, K., Kikuchi, K., Yamauchi, H., Hirota, S. and Tomikawa, M. (1995). **J. Microencap.** 12 (4), 377-388.

10. Baratt, G.a and Schuber, F. (1992). In: Liposome Technology (Gregoriadis, G. Ed.), CRC Press, Boca Raton, FL, 199-218.

11. Bachhawat, B. K., Das, P.K. and Ghosh, P.K. (1984). In: Liposome Technology (Gregoriadis, G. Ed.), CRC Press, Boca Raton, FL, 117-138.

12. Ponpipon, M.M., Shen, T.Y., Baldeshwieler, J.D. and Wu, P.S. (1984). In: Liposome Technology (Gregoriadis, G. Ed.), CRC press, Boca Raton, 3, 95-125.

13. Szoka, F. C., Jr. and Mayhew, E. (1983). **Biochim. Biophys. Res. Commun.** 110, 140-147.

14. Lopez-Berehtein, G., Mehta, R., Hopffer, R., Mills, K., Kasi, L., Mehta, K., Fainstein, V., Luna, M., Harsh, E.N. and Juliano, R. (1983). **J. Infect. Dis.** 147 (5), 939-945.

15. Hiemenz, J.W.and Walsh, T.J. (1996). **Clin. Infect. Dis.** 22, (S-2) S133-S144.

16. New, R.R.C. (1990). In: Liposomes: A practical approach, Oxford University Press, Oxford, 125-126.

17. Mehta, R., Lopez-Berehtein, G., Hopffer, R., Mills, K. adn Juliano, R.L. (1984). **Biochim. Biophys. Acta.** 770, 230-234.

18. Hammerling, U. and Westphal, O. (1967). **Eur. J. Biochem.** 1, 46-50.

19. Jaitely, V. and Vyas, S.P. (1999). **J. Drug Target.** 6, 315-322.

20. Van Etten, E.W.M., Van den Heuvel-de Groot, C. and Bakker-Wouderberg, I.A.J.M. (1993). **J. Antimicrob. Chemother.** 32, 723-729.

21. Van Etten Els, W.M., OtteLambillion, M., Van Vianen, W., TenKate, M.T. and Bakker-Wouderberg, I.A.J.M. (1995). **J. Antimicrob. Chemother.** 35, 509-515.

22. Gupta, P.K. and Huang, C.T. (1989). **J. Microenap.** 6, 427-462.

23. Pavia, D.L., Lampman, G.L. and Kriz, G.S. (1979). In: Introduction to spectroscopy: A guide for students of organic chemistry. (Hoit, Rinehart and Weinstein, Eds.) Saunder's College, Philadelphia, 13-15.

24. Rodeny, J.Y.H., Rouse, B. T. and Huang, L. (1986). **Biochim. Biophys. Acta.** 138(2), 931-937.

25. Iwamoto, K., Kato, T., Mosahiro, K., Koyama, N., Watanabe, S., Miyake, Y. and Sunamoto, G. (1991). **J. Pharm. Sci.** 80 (3), 219-214.

26. Juliano, R.L. and Layton, D. (1980). In: Drug delivery systems: Characteristics and biomedical applications (Juliano, R.L. Ed.), Oxford University Press, New York, 189-236.

27. Ghosh, P. and Bacchawat, B. K. (1980). **Biochim. Biophysic. Acta.** 632, 560-565.

28. Das, P.K., Murray, G.J., Zairzow, G.C., Brady, R.O. and Barranger, J.A. (1985). **Biochem. Med.** 33, 124-131.

29. Takada, M., Yuzuriha, T., Katayama, K. Iwamoto, K. and Sunamoto, J., (1984). **Biochim. Biophys. Act.** 802, 237-244.

30. Deol, P. and Khuller, G.K. (1997) **Biochim. Biophys. Acta.** 1334, 161-172.

23

POLYSACCHARIDE COATED LIPOSOMES FOR ORAL IMMUNIZATION

N. VENKATESAN AND S.P. VYAS*

Department of Pharmaceutical Sciences,
Dr. Harisingh Gour Vishwavidyalaya,
Sagar (M.P.) 470 003. INDIA

- Introduction
- Materials and Methods
- Characterization

- Results and Discussion
- References

INTRODUCTION

Immunization is the most efficient and cost-effective means for the prevention of various diseases. The mucosal surface of the human body is a major site of entry for pathogens. However, no significant means of immunization have been brought about to prevent this. Historically, immunization has relied on the induction of humoral immunity by parenteral administration of vaccines. Moreover, antibodies induced in this manner, does not always reach the mucosal surfaces which is the predominant site for most of the infectious pathogens.

Among the antibodies induced in this manner, it is not always necessarily reach the mucosal surfaces which is the predominant site for most infectious pathogens. Among the antibodies produced in the body, antibodies produced by humoral immune responses at the mucosal surfaces are of importance in fighting against pathogens at the mucosal surface. One such antibody is the secretory IgA (sIgA). Secretory IgA is the predominant antibody isotype present at the mucosal sites which prevents the attachment of bacteria and viruses to mucosa and thereby prevents any possible damage to the host.

Mucosal immunity provides the first line of immunological defense. However, to induce antibodies at the mucosal surfaces, administration of antigen directly to the mucosal site is required. Oral immunization offers the safest and most convenient way to induce mucosal immunity [1]. Orally administered antigens are taken up through the specialized epithelial cells called M cells, overlaying Peyer's patches which are the major component of the gut associated mucosal immune system. The picked up antigens are transported in to the regional lymphoid tissues, processed and stimulate antigen specific B lymphocytes in the germinal centres of follicles located beneath domes.

Oral administration of vaccines generally requires large doses of antigen due to insufficient stimulation of gut associated lymphoid tissue (GALT). In addition oral administration of antigens must overcome several challenges. To, overcome these disadvantages, encapsulation of antigens and delivering it in a safer way in order to stimulate mucosal immunity has been proposed over the years.

Among other delivery systems for oral immunization, liposomes have a number of potential advantages [2,3]. Other delivery systems studied include, microspheres [4], alginate microparticles [5], polymerized liposomes [6], hydrogels [7], niosomes [8], Novasomes® [9], etc.

The susceptibility of conventional liposomes to bile salt caused dissolution and enzymatic degradation in the g.i. tract, however, remains to be as the main barrier for their beneficial utilization in oral delivery [2]. Therefore, to exploit the full potential of liposomes as immunological carriers for oral delivery, we have developed and evaluated stable liposomal adjuvant utilizing a novel technique reported by Sunamoto et al. [10].

The aim of the work was to synthesize and characterize a modified polysaccharide, O-palmitoyl pullulan (OPP) and to use it for coating of unilamellar vesicles containing the model antigen, bovine serum albumin (BSA). The so prepared liposomes were characterized for their size, shape, stability and their antibody stimulating efficiency following oral administration.

MATERIALS AND METHODS

Materials

Egg phosphatidylcholine (PC), cholesterol, phosphatidylethanolamine (PE), bovine serum albumin (BSA), pullulan were obtained from Sigma. Palmitoyl chloride from Fluka Chemika. All other chemicals and reagents were obtained from Merck, India and used as supplied.

Synthesis and characterization of O-palmitoylpullulan

O-palmitoylpullulan was prepared by a method described earlier by Sunamoto et al. [11]. Briefly, 1 g of pullulan was dissolved in 11 ml of dry dimethylformamide at 60°C. To the resulting solution, 1 ml of dry pyridine and 0.1 g of palmitoyl chloride dissolved in 0.24 ml of dry dimethylformamide were added. The mixture was stirred at 60°C for 2 h followed by 1 h at room temperature. This mixture was then slowly poured into 70 ml of absolute ethanol under stirring. The so formed precipitate was collected and washed with 80 ml of absolute ethanol and 60 ml of dry diethyl ether. The white solid material obtained was dried in vacuum at 50°C for 2 h.

The synthesized polymer was characterized by IR and ^{1}H-NMR. The IR spectrum of OPP (1%) was taken by incorporating it into a compressed KBr pellet. Similarly, a ^{1}H-NMR spectrum was obtained in deuterated dimethylsulfoxide solution (DMSO-d_6) using tetramethylsilane (TMS) as internal standard. Additionally, a ^{1}H-NMR spectrum of pullulan was also obtained.

Preparation of liposomes

Liposomes were prepared by reverse phase evaporation technique as reported by Sazoka et al. [12] with slight modifications. Briefly, PC, cholesterol and PE were taken in different mole fractions (Table 1) and dissolved in 5 ml of diethylether to which 2ml of aqueous phase, i.e. phosphate buffer saline (PBS) (pH 7.4) containing 2 mg of BSA was added. The mixture was sonicated (Soniweld) for 10 minutes (with an interval of 2 minutes after 5 minutes). A thick emulsion was formed which was then kept over a vortex mixer in order to remove any residual ether. To this emulsion, 3 ml of warm PBS (pH 7.4) was added in order to hydrate the vesicles.

CHARACTERIZATION

Encapsulation efficiency

The prepared liposomes were taken and the free (unentrapped) antigen was separated by sephadex G-25 minicolumn using centrifugation technique [13]. The method was repeated thrice with a fresh syringe packed with gel each time. The fraction was finally collected which was free from unentrapped antigen.

The isolated liposomes were centrifuged at 60,000 rpm for 4 h. The pellets were challenged with triton X-100 (0.2%) to disrupt the vesicles and the liberated antigen was estimated by Bradford method [14]. The percent fraction of antigen entrapped was calculated and recorded (Table 1).

Table 1. Various formulation code and encapsulation efficiency and size of liposomes

Formulation code	Molar lipid ratio (PC:CH:PE)	% encapsulation efficiency	Size (µm)
P1	9:1:0	37.5 ± 0.9	4.3 - 5.4
P2	7:2:1	40.3 ± 1.8	2.5 - 3.3
P3	5:4:1	35.6 ± 1.2	5.9 - 8.5

Coating of liposomes

OPP was dissolved in 2ml of PBS (pH 7.4). Liposomes were coated with OPP by adding 2ml of solution to 4ml of liposome dispersion under constant stirring. Stirring was continued for 1h in order to ensure complete coating of the liposome [15].

Measurement of zeta potential

The movement of a charged surface with respect to an adjacent liquid phase is the basic principle underlying this technique. Malvern zetasizer was used in the present study to calculate the zeta potential (ζ). The results are as recorded in table 2.

Table 2. Formulation code with varying polysaccharide to lipid ratio and their zeta potential values

Formulation code	OPP:Lipid (w/w)	Size (µm)	Zeta potential (mV)
PC1	0:10	2.5±0.63	88.5±6.0
PC2	1:9	2.80±0.59	65.5±4.0
PC3	2:8	3.25±0.74	40.2±5.0
PC4	3:7	3.8±0.68	18.0±3.0
PC5	4:6	4.1±0.54	4.5±1.0

Measurement of Size

Mean particle size of liposomes was measured by photocorrelation spectroscopy with an Autosizer II C apparatus (Malvern Instruments, UK).

Stability in simulated gastric fluid (pH 1.5)

The present study involves the delivery of OPP-coated liposomes via oral route. Henceforth, it was necessary to study stability of the vesicle in simulated gastric fluid (SGF). One ml of coated and uncoated liposomal suspension was taken in two separate dialysis tubing (Sigma, USA) and was placed in a beaker containing 250 ml of SGF. The beaker was placed over a magnetic stirrer and stirred continuously for 3 h. The mean vesicle size and number of vesicles per cu mm before placing in the SGF and 3 h after placing in SGF was determined. The results are as recorded in table 3.

Table 3. Mean vesicle size and number of vesicles before and after incubation in SGF for 3 h

Formulation code	Mean vesicle size (μm)		No. of vesicles per cu mm (No. x 10^3)	
	Before incubation	After incubation	Before incubation	After Incubation
PC5	4.1 ± 0.54	4.8 ± 0.38	47	46
P2	2.5 ± 0.63	5.3 ± 0.47	50	42

Immunization protocols

Ten groups of albino rats (Wistar strain) weighing 120-150 g were used with three rats in each group. On day 1, groups of rats were administered orally with preparations containing BSA equivalent to 100μg. A similar group of mice was injected intraperitoneally. Secondary immunization was done on day 15 with formulations containing BSA equivalent to 100 μg. Blood was collected from the orbital plexus on day 15 and 21 and the production of anti-BSA IgG and IgA antibody in the serum was quantified.

Measurement of IgG and IgA by ELISA

Specific anti-IgG and IgA antibody levels in the serum were determined by ELISA [16]. Each well of microplate (Dynatech) was coated with 50μl of a BSA (100μg/ml) solution in 50mM carbonate buffer (pH 9.6) at 4°C overnight. After being washed three times with 10mM phosphate-buffered saline containing 0.05% Tween 20 (PBS-Tween), the wells were coated with 100 μl of 3% skim milk in PBS-Tween for 1 h at room temperature to block non-specific adsorption of the antibodies. After washing with PBS-Tween diluted serum (50μl/well) was added. Following incubation at 25°C for 2 h and washing, horseradish peroxidase-conjugate antibodies having specificity for rat IgG or IgA (Sigma) diluted with PBS-Tween (500ng/ml) were added (50μl/well).

The plates were incubated at 25°C for 2 h then washed and 50μl of 0.015% H_2O_2 containing 2,2'-azino-bis(3-ethylbenzthiazoline-6-sulfonic acid) (15 μg/ml) dissolved in 0.1M citrate buffer (pH4.0) were added to each well. The wells were incubated at 37°C for 20 min., absorbance at 405nm was measured with a microplate reader (Molecular device).

RESULTS AND DISCUSSION

Characterization of OPP

Pullulan a naturally occurring polysaccharide produced by the yeast like fungus *Pullalaria pullulans* is known to protect plasma membranes against physicochemical stimuli such as osmotic pressure and ionic strength. However, when adsorbed on to the liposomal surface it is easily removed on dilution. Therefore, it was necessary to chemically modify pullulan by conjugating it to a hydrophobic group which allows the polysaccharide to intereligitate with the liposomal membrane [17]. The, pullulan used in present study was chemically modified by esterification with palmitoylchloride. The resultant product was characterized by IR and ^{1}H-NMR spectrum. The results are as in table 4.

Table 4. IR spectral data of OPP

Observed values (cm^{-1})	Expected values (cm^{-1})	Functional group	Interpretation
1685	1750-1735	C=O	Carbonyl band stretching
3460	3600-3200	Free-OH	Stretching vibration of O-H bond
2940	2960-2850	CH_2CH_3	C-H stretching
1100	1150-1040	C-O	C-O stretching

Characterization of OPP by IR spectroscopy helped identification of carbonyl groups. Pavia et al. [18] reported that a characteristic stretching vibration is observed at about 1735 cm^{-1} due to carbonyl (C=O) bond. However, here in the synthesized OPP the stretching vibration was observed at 1685 cm^{-1}. This shift in frequency may be attributed to the intermolecular hydrogen bonding between the carbonyl and hydroxyl group. The presence of hydrogen bonds was confirmed from the OH stretching vibration at 3460 cm^{-1}. This represents a polymeric band. However, there Is a shift in band from 3600-3200 cm^{-1} to 3460 cm^{-1}, which may be attributed to the intramolecular single bridge hydrogen bonds and the intermolecular bridge between hydrogen bonds. A characteristic C-H stretching vibration was observed at 2940 cm^{-1} and a C-O stretching at 1100 cm^{-1}. From these observations it can be concluded that there exists an ester bond between pullulan and palmitoyl residues suggesting palmitoylation of pullulan.

The OPP formation was further confirmed by ^{1}H-NMR resonance spectroscopy (Table 5). The protons corresponding to the terminal methyl group of the palmitoyl chain was observed at 0.850 ppm, that of the 12-methylene groups was observed at 1.20 ppm while those at 1.234 and 2.38 ppm were indicating the presence of β and α methylene groups respectively. These observations were in accordance with those found by Moreira et al. [19]. Two peaks at the down field at 4.996 and 4.647 ppm were observed which indicated C_1 position of α1,4 and α1,6 glycosidic bonds respectively. It was possible to identify a range of protons from 2.546-3.568 ppm corresponding to the glucose residue units at positions C_2-C_6. This observation was in accordance with Akiyoshi et al. [20] where they reported a range of 2.60-4.20ppm. From these observed data, the formation of OPP was further confirmed.

Table 5. Proton NMR resonance spectral data of OPP

Observed values (ppm)	Expected values (ppm)	Functional group	Interpretation
0.858	0.9	$-CH_3$	Terminal methyl group
1.20	1.17	$-(CH_2)_{12}$	Methylene group
1.234	1.4	$-CH_2\beta$	β-methylene group
2.38	2.3	$-CH_2\alpha$	α-methylene group
4.647	4.54	$-H$	at C_1 position of $\alpha 1,6$ glycosidic bond
4.996	5.04	$-H$	at C_1 position of $\beta 1,6$ glycosidic bond
2.546-3.568	2.60-4.20	$-H$	at C_2-C_6 positions glucose residues

Characterization of liposomes

It is apparent from table 1 that the variation in phospholipid ratio used in the preparation of liposomes demonstrated a significant difference in their size and encapsulation efficiency of liposomes. Encapsulation efficiency in the case of P1 was found to be 37.5±0.9% while for P2 and P3 it was 40.3±1.8% and 35.6±1.2% respectively. The low percent encapsulation in the case of formulation P1 may be due to the formation of a leaky vesicle, as the cholesterol content in this formulation was relatively less. Similarly, a lower encapsulation value was obtained with formulation P3. Here, the cholesterol content was higher enough probably beyond its optimum concentration ratio resulting into packing with decreased fluidity. Similarly, the vesicle size in case of P1 and P3 showed great deal of variation with high dispersibility index an indicative of heterogenecity in liposome population. The wide range of vesicle size in case of P3 (5.4-8.5 µm) may be due to the reduction in area which might have raised due to condensation of the membrane. In case of P1 the vesicle size were found ranging between 4.3-5.4µm. This may be due to the formation of leaky, less rigid leading to fusion of vesicles contributing larger vesicles. From the three formulations prepared as mentioned in Table 1, formulation P2 was chosen for further coating of the liposomes with OPP, where cholesterol ratio was considered to be at optimum level (PC:CH:PE , 7:2:1).

Coating of liposomes

Based on encapsulation efficiency (40.3%) and size (2.5-3.35 µm), formulation P2 was selected for further studies. Liposomes were coated using OPP. The coating process of liposomes with OPP was optimized by varying different polysaccharide:lipid ratio (Table 2). The coating of liposomes was indirectly measured using Malvern zetasizer. The observations as noted from table 2 indicate that on increasing the polysaccharide ratio (w/w) from 1 to 4, there was a decrease in zeta potential by 88.5±2.5, 65.5±1.5, 40.0±2.5, 18.0±3.0 and 4.5±1.5 µm for formulations PC1 to PC5 respectively. From these results it can be concluded that the initial, high zeta potential values are ascribed to the charge on the surface of the liposomes imparted by phosphatidylethanolamine. On addition of the negatively charged OPP, the charge on the liposomes is being neutralized due to the charge induced coating of the negatively charged OPP on the positively charged liposomes. The resultant fall in zeta potential was found to be very significant in the case of formulation PC4. On further increasing the OPP concentration, the zeta potential approached near zero value. This is an indication of the almost complete intrinsic charge of quenching on coating of the liposomes with OPP. Hence, the formulation PC5 with polysaccharide:lipid ratio (w/w) of 4:6 was selected as an ideal one and used in further studies. The coated vesicles did not show any significant increase in vesicle size (Table 2).

Stability in SGF

The mean vesicle size of uncoated liposomes (P2) was 2.5±0.63 μm and that of coated liposomes (PC5) was 4.1±0.54 μm before incubation in SGF. The number of vesicles per cu mm were 50 x 10³ in case of P2 and 47 x 10³ in case of PC5. The mean vesicle size increased dramatically from 2.5 μm to 5.3 μm in case of formulation P2 which was further confirmed by the fall in number of vesicles per cu mm. However, the mean vesicle size as well as the number of vesicles per cu mm did not show any significant change in case of formulation PC5 following their incubation in SGF for a period of 3 h. This clearly indicated that the polymer-coated vesicles are stable in SGF.

Systemic IgG and IgA responses

Rats which were inoculated with BSA in liposomes coated with OPP by oral administration exhibited an increased serum IgG and IgA titers against BSA in other forms (Fig.1 and 2). The antibody titre values recorded as optical density, following oral administration of liposomes coated with OPP was found to be 0.134 and that after intraperitoneal administration, it was 0.139. This shows that there was no significant effect dictated by the route of administration on secretion of IgA. However, there was a significant change in IgG levels due to the route of administration, was observed.

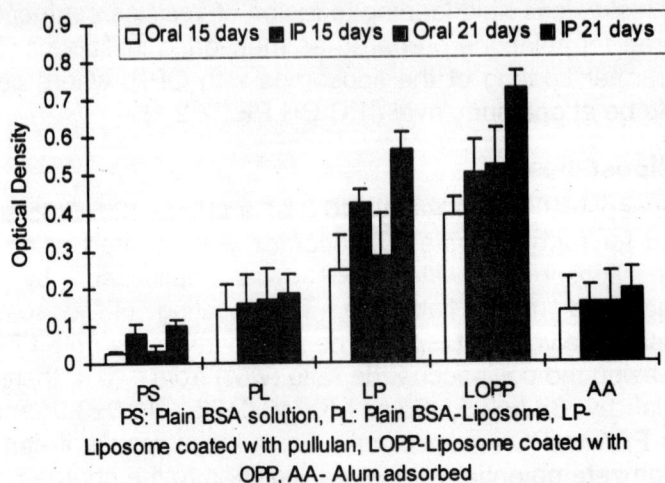

PS: Plain BSA solution, PL: Plain BSA-Liposome, LP-
Liposome coated with pullulan, LOPP-Liposome coated with
OPP, AA- Alum adsorbed

Fig. 1: Serum IgG level in rats following oral and IP administration of various formulations

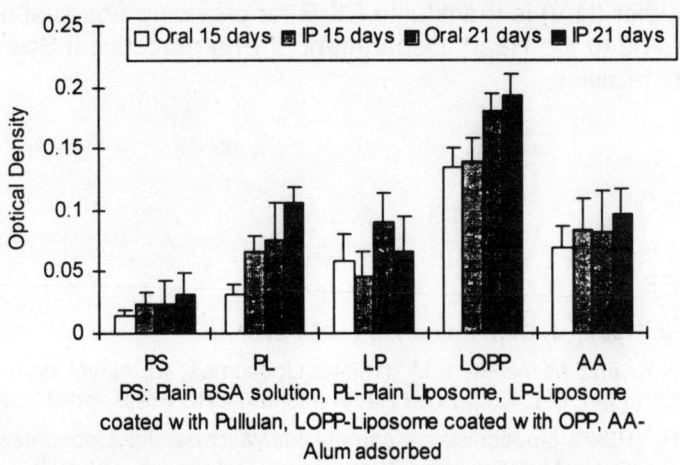

Fig.2 : Serum IgA level in rats following oral and IP administration of various formulations

Serum IgG level on day 15, in case of orally administered OPP coated liposomes were found to have an O.D. of 0.394 while that administered via intraperitoneal route showed a O.D of 0.500. Antibody levels on administration of liposomes coated with pullulan alone, did elicit an immune response better than plain liposomes. This may be attributed to the pullulan, that itself possesses some antigenicity [19].

The pullulan borne antigenicity may lead to an increase in serum IgG levels. However, the serum IgA level recorded was lower as compared to its palmitoyl derivative coated liposomes. The increased IgA level obtained following oral administration of OPP coated liposomes as compared to plain liposomes or pullulan coated liposomes signifies that the OPP coated liposomes are stable even after passing through the stomach and might be taken up by the Peyer's patches.

In our study, we observed that there was a significant level of IgA secretion following primary immunization whilst earlier, reports using biodegradable microspheres for oral immunization showed a significant IgA secretion only after secondary immunization [21]. Even though biodegradable microspheres have been studied exhaustively for oral immunization, the method involved in preparation of these microspheres may lead to lose in the antigenicity. To overcome this, alginate microspheres are being studied [5,22]. However, the control of microsphere size below 10µm, which tend them capable of passing through Peyer's patches is of importance. Liposomes in present study used were in the size range of 2.5-3.35 µm and as a result might have been responsible for their uptake by the Peyer's patches. In addition, liposomes are protected from acids, proteolytic enzymes, lipases and bile salts by OPP coating (net).

Several groups [2,23,24] have studied liposomes as an immunoadjuvant for mucosal immunization. However, their stability was a cause of concern, which we have tried to alleviate by coating them with OPP. Moreover, further studies are being carried out to elucidate whether the coated liposomal systems are capable of stimulating antibody clones over a prolonged period of time.

ACKNOWLEDGEMENTS

One of the author (N.V) is thankful to CSIR for providing financial assistance to carry out this work and to the Head, Department of Pharmaceutical Sciences for providing the necessary facilities.

REFERENCES

1. Mestecky, J. (1987). **J. Clin. Immunol.** 7, 265-276.

2. Childers, N.K. and Michalek, S.M. (1994). Liposomes, In: Novel delivery systems for oral vaccines (O'Hagen, D.T. Ed.), Boca Raton, Florida, CRC Press, pp. 175-205.

3. Alving, C.R. (1987). Liposomes as carriers for vaccines, In: Liposomes: from biophysics to therapeutics (Ostro, M.J. Ed.), New York, Marcel Dekker, pp. 195-218.

4. Moloveanu, Z., Novak, M., Huan, W.Q., Gilley, R.M., Staas, J.K., Schafer, D., Compans, R.W. and Mestecky, J. (1993). **J. Infect. Dis.** 167, 84-90.

5. Bowersock, T.L., HogenEsch, H., Suckow, M., Porter, R.E., Jackson, R., Park, H. and Park, K. (1996). **J. Control. Rel.** 39, 209-220.

6. Chen, H., Torchilin, V. and Langer, R. (1996). **J. Control. Rel.** 42, 263-272.

7. Bowersock, T.L., Shalaby, W.S.W., Levy, M., Blevins, W.E., White, M.R. Borie, D.L. and Park, K. (1994). **J. Control. Rel.** 31, 245-254.

8. Brewer, J.M. and Alexander, J. (1992). **Immunology** 75, 570-575.

9. Gupta, R.K., Varanelli, C.L., Griffin, P., Wallach, D.F.H. and Siber, G.R. (1996). **Vaccine** 14, 219-225.

10. Sunamoto, J., Iwamoto, K., Takada, M., Yuzuriha, T. and Katayama, K. (1984). Improved drug delivery to target specific organs using liposomes as coated with polysaccharides. In: Polymers in Medicine: Biomedical and Pharmaceutical Applications (Chiellini, E. and Giustic, P. Eds.). Plenum press, New York, pp. 157-168.

11. Sunamoto, J., Sato, T., Taguchi, T. and Hamazaki, H. (1992). **Macromolecules** 25, 5665-5670.

12. Sazoka, F.C., Papahadjopoulos, D. (1978). **Proc. Natl. Acad. Sci USA** 75, 4194-4198.

13. Fry, D.W., White, J.C., Goldman, I.D. (1978). **Anal. Biochem.** 90, 809-815.

14. Bradford, M.M. (1976). **Analyt. Biochem.** 72, 248.

15. Sunamoto, J., Sato, T., Hirota, M., Fukishima, K., Hiratani, K. and Hara, K., A. (1987). **Biochim. Biophys. Acta.** 898, 323-330.

16. Michalek, S.M., Morisaki, I., Harmon, C.C., Hamada, S. and McGhee, J.R. (1989) **Infect. Immun.** 39, 645-654.

17. Sato, T. and Sunamoto, J. (1992). **Prog. Lipid Res.** 31, 345-372.

18. Pavia, D.L., Lampman, G.M. and Kriz, G.S. (1979). Infrared absorption process, In: Introduction to spectroscopy: a guide for students of organic chemistry (Holt, Rinehart, Winston Eds.), Saunder College, Philadelphia, pp13-15.

19. Moreira, J.N., Almeida, L.M., Geraldes, C.F., Madeira, V.M.C. and Costa, M.L. (1997) **Int. J. Pharm.** 147, 153-164.

20. Akiyoshi, K., Deguchi, S., Moriguchi, N., Yamaguchi, S. and Sunamoto, J. (1990). **Macromolecules** 26, 3062-3068.

21. Challacombe, S.J., Rahman, D., Jeffery, H., Davis, S.S. and O'Hagan, D.T. (1992). **Immunology** 76, 164-168.

22. Cho, N.H., Seong, S.Y., Chun, K.H., Kim, Y.H., Kwon, I.C., Ahn, B.Y. and Jeong, S.Y. (1998). **J. Control. Rel**. 53, 215-224.

23. Michalek, S.M., Childers, N.K. and Dertzbaugh, M.T. (1995). Vaccination strategies for mucosal pathogens In: Virulence mechanisms of bacterial pathogens (Roth, J.A., Bolin, C.A., Brogden, K.A., Minion, F.C. and Wannemuehler, M.J. Eds.). 2ed. ASM publications, Washington DC, pp. 269-302.

24. Kersten, G.F.A. and Crommelin, D.J.A. (1995). **Biochim.Biophys.Acta**, 1241, 117-138.

SUBJECT INDEX

SUBJECT INDEX